Stroke Nursing
Certification Review

Kathy J. Morrison, MSN, RN, CNRN, SCRN, FAHA, is a certified neuroscience nurse, a certified stroke nurse, a Fellow of the American Heart Association, and a recipient of the prestigious Pennsylvania State Nightingale Award for Clinical Nursing Excellence. She played a pivotal role in Penn State Hershey Medical Center's attainment of The Joint Commission Comprehensive Stroke Center certification and has mentored many stroke program coordinators through the process of attaining Primary and Comprehensive Stroke Center certification. Ms. Morrison is the author of *Fast Facts for Stroke Care Nursing* as well as the *Stroke Certification Study Guide for Nurses*, a chapter contributor for the American Association of Neuroscience Nurses Core Curriculum and Online CNRN Review Course, and a contributing author for the American Heart Association's Stroke Education online series. In 2010, she established the Stroke Coordinators of Pennsylvania (SCoPA)—a group of stroke coordinators whose collaborative work has resulted in significant improvements in stroke care and outcomes in community hospitals across central Pennsylvania. Ms. Morrison is a board member of the Susquehanna Valley Chapter of the American Association of Neuroscience Nurses and is a board member of the Stroke Survivors Foundation.

Stroke Nursing Certification Review

Kathy J. Morrison, MSN, RN, CNRN, SCRN, FAHA

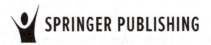
SPRINGER PUBLISHING

Springer Publishing Company, LLC
11 West 42nd Street, New York, NY 10036
www.springerpub.com
connect.springerpub.com/

Acquisitions Editor: Jaclyn Koshofer
Compositor: DiacriTech

ISBN: 978-0-8261-8405-4
ebook ISBN: 978-0-8261-8406-1
DOI: 10.1891/9780826184061

22 23 24 25 26 / 5 4 3 2 1

The author and the publisher of this Work have made every effort to use sources believed to be reliable to provide information that is accurate and compatible with the standards generally accepted at the time of publication. Because medical science is continually advancing, our knowledge base continues to expand. Therefore, as new information becomes available, changes in procedures become necessary. We recommend that the reader always consult current research and specific institutional policies before performing any clinical procedure or delivering any medication. The author and publisher shall not be liable for any special, consequential, or exemplary damages resulting, in whole or in part, from the readers' use of, or reliance on, the information contained in this book. The publisher has no responsibility for the persistence or accuracy of URLs for external or third-party Internet websites referred to in this publication and does not guarantee that any content on such websites is, or will remain, accurate or appropriate.

Library of Congress Cataloging-in-Publication Data
LCCN: 2022902844

Contact sales@springerpub.com to receive discount rates on bulk purchases.

Publisher's Note: **New and used products purchased from third-party sellers are not guaranteed for quality, authenticity, or access to any included digital components.**

Printed in the United States of America.
Printed by Hatteras, Inc.

SCRN® is a registered service mark of American Board of Neuroscience Nursing (ABNN). ABNN does not sponsor or endorse this resource, nor does it have a proprietary relationship with Springer Publishing.

Contents

Contributors

Ritu C. Light, PharmD, is a graduate of the Wilkes University Nesbitt School of Pharmacy in Wilkes-Barre, Pennsylvania, and completed a Pharmacy Practice Residency (PGY1) at WellSpan York Hospital in York, Pennsylvania. She has experience in the hospital, administrative, and ambulatory pharmacy settings. She has been at the Penn State Health Milton S. Hershey Medical Center in Hershey, Pennsylvania, since 2014 as a transitional care pharmacist for the stroke program. In this role, she works with the pharmacy department's bedside discharge medications program, completes transitional care activities for the stroke population, and staffs at the institution's Anticoagulation Clinic. Ritu shares her expertise in educating the community and her interdisciplinary colleagues.

Cesar Velasco, BSN, RN, ASC-BC, is a former emergency department nurse who has adapted the critical care experience within his current role as a stroke program coordinator for Penn State Health. Earning his Advanced Stroke Program Coordinator certification has enhanced Cesar's ability to engage with various stakeholders with the focus of delivering safe and quality stroke care. His commitment to improving clinical practice has motivated Cesar to inspire nurses at the bedside to help champion stroke program goals. He is an advocate for change and creating opportunity for nurses to be influential in this change when it pertains to the implementation of best practice in stroke care. He is a member of the American Association of Neuroscience Nurses and the Association of Neurovascular Clinicians.

Preface

Stroke care nursing is multifaceted and requires a specialized body of knowledge and a specific skill set to meet the complex care needs of patients. Over the past 15 to 20 years, nurses who found themselves working with this distinct population (and many did not consciously seek out the challenge) also found the need for collaboration and support from their peers across the country. As research evidence led to practice standards and stroke center certification, nurses recognized that a specialty was being born.

This review and study guide is a combination of my first two books, *Fast Facts for Stroke Care Nursing* and *Stroke Certification Study Guide for Nurses*. The feedback I received from those books has been overwhelmingly positive. I've heard from nurses who discovered a passion for stroke care and others who developed increased confidence in their stroke care competence, nurses who utilized the book to help their organization prepare for and attain stroke center certification, nurses who expressed gratitude for a pocket-sized reference that was quick and easy to use, and nurses who described these books as key to their success with the American Board of Neuroscience Nursing's Stroke Certified Registered Nurse (SCRN®) exam. It just made sense to combine these two into one comprehensive resource.

Each chapter is designed with stroke care information including clinical pearls, followed by knowledge check questions and a case study specific to that chapter. The questions will be valuable not only for those preparing for the exam but also for nurses helping their colleagues to prepare for stroke center certification visits and for internal stroke education hours at their organization. The book's format includes the SCRN exam categories, as well as distinct chapters on medication, diagnostic tests, and neurological assessment. There is a practice test with 170 questions, and along with the case study questions and knowledge check questions, there are a total of over 400 questions in this comprehensive resource. The number of questions in each category matches the percentage of the test dedicated to that category. The medications chapter, provided by my colleague, a stroke clinical pharmacist, Ritu C. Light, will provide an overview and clinical tips on the most common medications prescribed for stroke patients. Case studies are a valuable tool used in nursing education, so in addition to those included in each specific chapter, my colleague and one of the best stroke coordinators I know, Cesar Velasco, has provided a collection of 10 case studies that span the continuum of stroke care to further stimulate your critical thinking. I've retained the neuroscience terms appendix for quick reference of the most used—and sometimes confounding—neuroscience terms.

Few of us could have imagined the phenomenal evolution of stroke care and the leadership role that nurses play in all aspects of research, publication, oversight, and delivery of stroke care. I am grateful to the many nurses who have utilized my books and to those who took the time to provide feedback; it has been invaluable in guiding me to this new comprehensive review and study guide.

If you have any comments or suggestions for this book, or want to contact me, please do so at kmorrison98@gmail.com.

Kathy J. Morrison

Pass Guarantee

If you use this resource to prepare for your exam and you do not pass, you may return it for a refund of your full purchase price. To receive a refund, you must return your product along with a copy of your original receipt and exam score report. Product must be returned and received within 180 days of the original purchase date. Excludes tax, shipping, and handling. One offer per person and address. Refunds will be issued within 8 weeks from acceptance and approval. This offer is valid for U.S. residents only. Void where prohibited. To begin the process, please contact customer service at CS@springerpub.com.

Foundations of Stroke Care

Although healthcare professionals have been caring for stroke patients for hundreds of years, the past 20 years have been marked by dramatic changes in the way care is delivered. While rehabilitation is an important aspect of stroke recovery, stroke is no longer just rehabilitation focused but is recognized as true emergency. Along with the multitude of research studies, evidence-based practice is the cornerstone of stroke nursing. Although the specialty of neuroscience nursing has been well established for over 40 years, it has shown remarkable growth with the surge of interest in cerebrovascular nursing. Accompanying advancements in neuroelectrophysiology and neuro-oncology, cerebrovascular nursing has contributed to the phenomenon of neuroscience nursing as nursing's new frontier.

BRIEF HISTORY OF STROKE CARE

Stroke care nursing is not new. The first time the term *stroke* was noted in English literature in reference to a health condition was in 1689 by William Cole. Hippocrates is credited with coining the word *apoplexy* in 400 BCE to represent episodes of convulsions and paralysis, typically on the opposite side of the body from the injury. He also described episodes of impaired speech, similar to what is known today as *aphasia*. The ancient Greeks believed that someone suffering a stroke had been struck down suddenly, without consciousness or motion, retaining pulse and respiration (Engelhardt, 2017).

Stroke care first appeared in nursing texts in 1890, but only with brief discussions (Nilsen, 2010). The treatment then was supportive care and rehabilitation, but only if the patient survived the stroke and avoided the multitude of secondary injuries that could occur.

The World Health Organization (WHO) defined *stroke* in 1970 as "rapidly developing clinical signs of focal or global disturbance of cerebral function, lasting more than 24 hours or leading to death, with no apparent cause other than that of vascular origin" (Sacco et al., 2013, p. 2065). This definition is still used today; but with advances in knowledge about the nature, timing, recognition, and imaging of stroke, an update to this definition is needed (Sacco et al., 2013).

▶ ADVENT OF EMERGENCY TREATMENTS

The year 1996 could be considered the watershed moment for acute stroke care. It is the year the U.S. Food and Drug Administration (FDA) approved intravenous (IV) alteplase as the first medication for the treatment of acute ischemic stroke. The research outcome found that patients who received IV alteplase would have 30% better functional outcomes at 3 months than those who did not receive it. The FDA's approval of IV alteplase has become known as the turning point for acute stroke care. Stroke is now an emergency, a "brain attack." In 2004, the first mechanical clot removal device received FDA approval for recanalization, or restoring circulation to a blocked cerebral artery. In 2015, mechanical thrombus removal became the standard of care after five landmark studies demonstrated overwhelmingly the benefit of this treatment for large-vessel occlusions (LVO).

▶ INTRODUCTION OF THE BRAIN ATTACK COALITION

The Brain Attack Coalition (BAC) was established in 1991 by a group of neurosurgeons who conceptualized improving stroke care through standardization and evidence-based guidelines. They were inspired by the improved patient outcomes seen after institution of trauma guidelines. The BAC has grown to include membership from 16 professional organizations. This group of highly educated professionals, passionate about stroke care, reviewed over 600 research articles related to stroke care and, in 2000, published "Recommendations for the Establishment of Primary Stroke Centers" in the *Journal of the American Medical Association* (Alberts et al., 2000). These recommendations, coming just 4 years after FDA approval of IV alteplase, contributed to the buzz that was developing in the more progressive healthcare organizations around the country; that is, stroke patients should receive care that had been proven through research to improve outcomes. This meant that hospital organizations had the opportunity and responsibility to support evidence-based practice for stroke care. The BAC continues to be a driving force for stroke care across all levels of hospital organizations. In 2005, their "Recommendations for Comprehensive Stroke Centers" (Alberts et al., 2005) was published in the journal *Stroke*, and in 2013, their "Formation and Function of Acute Stroke–Ready Hospitals Within a Stroke System of Care" was also published in the journal *Stroke* (Alberts et al., 2013).

BAC MEMBER ORGANIZATIONS

- American Academy of Neurological Surgeons
- American Academy of Neurology
- American Association of Neuroscience Nurses
- American College of Emergency Physicians
- American Society of Neuroradiology
- American Stroke Association
- Centers for Disease Control and Prevention
- Congress of Neurological Surgeons
- National Association of EMS Physicians
- National Association of State EMS Officials
- National Institute of Neurological Disorders and Stroke
- National Stroke Association
- Neurocritical Care Society
- Society of NeuroInterventional Surgery
- Stroke Belt Consortium
- Veterans Administration (Brain Attack Coalition, 2013)

STROKE CERTIFICATION OVERSIGHT

Between 2000 and 2004, numerous hospitals reviewed the BAC's Primary Stroke Center (PSC) recommendations and determined for themselves whether all the criteria were met. Many then advertised themselves as PSCs, but who could attest to whether that level of care was actually provided? In 2003, in a study published in the journal *Neurology*, 77% of nearly 1,000 respondents indicated that they met the criteria for PSC, but only 7% actually met all the criteria (Kidwell et al., 2003). It was time for an oversight body for stroke care, similar to the Trauma Systems Foundation. The Joint Commission (TJC) was the first organization to provide PSC certification based on the BAC recommendations, with others following.

▶ ORGANIZATIONS THAT PROVIDE STROKE CERTIFICATION

THE JOINT COMMISSION

- Founded in 1951 with the mission of improving healthcare
- Oldest and largest accrediting and standards-setting organization in healthcare
- First organization to establish a program for PSC certification in 2003 through its Disease-Specific Care Division; also has Acute Stroke–Ready Hospital (ASRH), Thrombectomy-Capable Stroke Center (TSC), and Comprehensive Stroke Center (CSC) certification programs (www.jointcommission.org/about_us/history.aspx)
- Certification is valid for 2 years

● CLINICAL PEARL

Many nurses have the misconception that TJC is responsible for coming up with the standards for PSCs, probably because they were the first to offer certification, coupled with their reputation as an authority on hospital accreditation. However, it was the BAC that established these standards.

HEALTHCARE FACILITIES ACCREDITATION PROGRAM (HFAP)

- Created in 1945 for the purpose of review of osteopathic hospitals (www.hfap.org/)
- Broadened its scope to all hospitals in 1965
- Since 2008 has provided PSC certification; also provides Stroke Ready Hospital (SRH), TSC, and CSC certifications
- Certification is valid for 3 years

DET NORSKE VERITAS

- Founded in Norway; Det Norske Veritas (DNV) established an American presence in 1897 with an initial focus on risk management consulting for the maritime industry (www.dnv.us/assurance/healthcare/stroke-certs.html)
- Healthcare division approved by Centers for Medicare & Medicaid Services (CMS) in 2007 as an accrediting organization
- Certification is valid for 3 years; provides Acute Stroke Ready (ASR), PSC, Primary Stroke Center + thrombectomy (PSC+), and CSC certifications

CENTER FOR IMPROVEMENT IN HEALTHCARE QUALITY (CIHQ)

- Founded in 1999 in McKinney, Texas
- The Disease-Specific certification, of which stroke is a part, was founded in 2019
- Certification is valid for 3 years; provides ASRH and PSC certifications

CLINICAL PEARL

Several states provide stroke center certification either by adopting TJC, HFAP, or DNV criteria, or through their own distinct processes and criteria. In 2004, Florida, New Jersey, Massachusetts, and New York became the first states to enact legislation or to develop regulations for state-level PSC designation.

UNRAVELING THE STROKE MEASURES

The original 10 stroke performance measures were developed in November 2004, by the BAC, in collaboration with the American Heart Association/American Stroke Association (AHA/ASA). The purpose was to support PSC certification. These 10 measures were based on research evidence of processes that resulted in improved outcomes for stroke patients. Organizations pursuing PSC certification and recertification had to demonstrate compliance with—or performance improvement strategies toward—all 10 of the measures.

From 2008 to 2015, eight of the 10 stroke performance measures were endorsed by the National Quality Forum (NQF) as Core Measures and were aligned with the CMS's measures. The two that were not endorsed were dysphagia screening and tobacco-cessation counseling. Dysphagia screening was not endorsed because of the lack of a valid, reliable, standardized screening tool or process supported by research (NQF, 2009), although it is recognized as an important aspect of prevention of aspiration pneumonia. Smoking cessation was not endorsed as it was deemed to have already been met by organizational initiatives and through documentation of teaching or counseling provided.

The Stroke Core Measures were retired as Core Measures on December 31, 2015, by the CMS, but continue to be required for performance measure reporting for stroke center certification, and thus are performance measures. It is not uncommon for healthcare professionals to continue to refer to them as Core Measures, although technically incorrect.

With the growth of additional stroke center certification levels, there have come along additional stroke measures. Tables 1.1, 1.2, 1.3, and 1.4 provide an overview of the current measures for which compliance is required for stroke center certification.

Table 1.1 Stroke Measures

STK-1	VTE Prophylaxis
STK-2	Discharged on Antithrombotic Therapy
STK-3	Anticoagulation Therapy for Atrial Fibrillation/Flutter
STK-4	Thrombolytic Therapy
STK-5	Antithrombotic Therapy by End of Hospital Day 2
STK-6	Discharged on Statin Medication
STK-8	Stroke Education
STK-10	Assessed for Rehabilitation

STK, stroke measures; VTE, venous thromboembolism.

Table 1.2 Stroke Outpatient Measures

STK-OP-1	Door to Transfer to Another Hospital
STK-OP-1a	Overall Rate
STK-OP-1b	Hemorrhagic Stroke

(continued)

Table 1.2 Stroke Outpatient Measures (*continued*)

STK-OP-1d	Ischemic Stroke; No IV Alteplase Prior to Transfer, LVO and MER Eligible
STK-OP-1e	Ischemic Stroke; No IV Alteplase Prior to Transfer, LVO and NOT MER Eligible
STK-OP-1f	Ischemic Stroke; No IV Alteplase Prior to Transfer, No LVO
STK-OP-1g	Ischemic Stroke; IV Alteplase Prior to Transfer, LVO and MER Eligible
STK-OP-1h	Ischemic Stroke; IV Alteplase Prior to Transfer, LVO and NOT MER Eligible
STK-OP-1i	Ischemic Stroke; IV Alteplase Prior to Transfer, No LVO

IV, intravenous; LVO, large-vessel occlusion; MER, mechanical endovascular reperfusion; OP, outpatient; STK, stroke measures.

Table 1.3 Outpatient Stroke Measures

OP-23	Head CT or MRI Scan Results for Acute Ischemic Stroke or Hemorrhagic Stroke Patients Who Received Head CT or MRI Scan Interpretation Within 45 Minutes of ED Arrival

OP, outpatient.

Table 1.4 Comprehensive Stroke Measures

CSTK-01	NIHSS Performed for Ischemic Stroke Patients
CSTK-03	Severity Measurement Performed for SAH and ICH Patients
CSTK-04	Procoagulant Reversal Agent Initiation for ICH Patients
CSTK-05	Hemorrhagic Transformation
CSTK-06	Nimodipine Treatment Administered
CSTK-08	TICI Posttreatment Reperfusion Grade
CSTK-09	Arrival Time to Skin Puncture
CSTK-10	Modified Rankin Score (mRS at 90 Days: Favorable Outcome)
CSTK-11	Rate of Rapid Effective Reperfusion From Hospital Arrival
CSTK-12	Rate of Rapid Effective Reperfusion From Skin Puncture

CSTK, comprehensive stroke measures; ICH, intracerebral hemorrhage; mRS, modified Rankin Scale; NIHSS, National Institutes of Health Stroke Scale; SAH, subarachnoid hemorrhage; TICI, Thrombolysis In Cerebral Infarction.

NURSING CERTIFICATIONS

Certifications in nursing signify the attainment of a higher level of knowledge and competence in a specialty area. Unlike licensure requirements, certifications are optional, although the popularity—and number—of nursing certifications continues to grow. As far back as 1997, Barbara Stevens Barnum wrote, "We are in the throes of a love affair with certification in this country, and virtually every RN has a string of (possibly) inexplicable certification initials following their signature" (Barnum, 1997). Certification requirements ensure that continuing education and clinical experience are maintained, a practice proven to raise the level of nursing professional practice. Some of the most popular stroke-related nursing certifications are the following:

CNRN—Certified Neuroscience Registered Nurse, established in 1978 by the American Board of Neuroscience Nursing (ABNN); aann.org

SCRN—Stroke Certified Registered Nurse, established in 2012 by the ABNN; aann.org

NVRN—Neurovascular Registered Nurse, established in 2007 by the Association of Neurovascular Clinicians (ANVC); anvc.org

ANVP—Advanced Neurovascular Practitioner, established in 2007 by the ANVC; anvc.org

ASC-BC—Advanced Stroke Coordinator–Board Certified, established in 2019 by the ANVC and is the first stroke coordinator certification; anvc.org

CRRN—Certified Rehabilitation Registered Nurse, established in 1984 by the Association of Rehabilitation Nurses; rehabnurse.org

NET SMART is a unique program that offers postgraduate neurovascular fellowship training for RNs and advanced practice clinicians. NET SMART, which stands for Neurovascular Education and Training in Stroke Management and Acute Reperfusion Therapy, was established by Anne Alexandrov in 2007; learnstroke.com

CLINICAL PEARL

The 1990s were designated as the Decade of the Brain by President George W. Bush in collaboration with the Library of Congress, the National Institute of Neurological Disorders and Stroke, and the National Institute of Mental Health. Numerous programs were developed to bring increased awareness about brain research to the members of Congress and the general public. Acute stroke care got rolling in the 1990s, with the foundation of the BAC, the American Stroke Association, and the National Stroke Association, coupled with approval of IV tissue plasminogen activator (tPA). Even more has been accomplished since 2000; perhaps, the 21st century should be designated as the Century of Stroke Innovation (Figure 1.1).

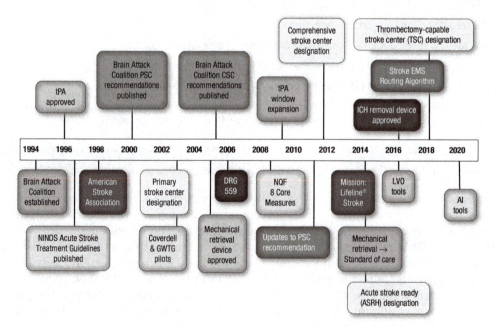

Figure 1.1 Acute stroke milestones.

ASRH, acute stroke–ready hospital; CSC, comprehensive stroke center; DRG, diagnosis-related group; EMS, emergency medical services; GWTG, Get With The Guidelines; ICH, intracerebral hemorrhage; LVO, large-vessel occlusion; NINDS, National Institute of Neurological Disorders and Stroke; NQF, National Quality Forum; PSC, primary stroke center; TSC, thrombectomy-capable stroke center; tPA, tissue plasminogen activator; AI, artificial intelligence.

REFERENCES

Alberts, M., Hademenos, G., Latchaw, R., Jagoda, A., Marler, J., Mayberg, M., Starke, R. D., Todd, H. W., Viste, K. M., Girgus, M., Shephard, T., Emr, M., Shwayder, P., & Walker, M. (2000). Recommendations for the establishment of primary stroke centers. *Journal of the American Medical Association, 283*(23), 3102–3109. https://doi.org/10.1001/jama.283.23.3102

Alberts, M. J., Latchaw, R. E., Selman, W. R., Shephard, T., Hadley, M. N., Brass, L. M., Koroshetz, W., Marler, J. R., Booss, J., Zorowitz, R. D., Croft, J. B., Magnis, E., Mulligan, D., Jagoda, A., O'Connor, R., Cawley, C. M., Connors, J. J., Rose-DeRenzy, J. A., Emr, M., Warren, M., Walker, M. D., & the Brain Attack Coalition. (2005). Recommendations for comprehensive stroke centers: A consensus statement from the Brain Attack Coalition. *Stroke, 36*(7), 1597–1616. https://doi.org/10.1161/01.STR.0000170622.07210.b4

Alberts, M. J., Wechsler, L. R., Jensen, M. E. L., Latchaw, R. E., Crocco, T. J., George, M. G., Baranski, J., Bass, R. R., Ruff, R. L., Huang, J., Mancini, B., Gregory, T., Gress, D., Emr, M., Warren, M., & Walker, M. D. (2013). Formation and function of acute stroke–ready hospitals within a stroke system of care: Recommendations from the Brain Attack Coalition. *Stroke, 44*(12), 3382–3393. https://doi.org/10.1161/STROKEAHA.113.002285

Barnum, B. (1997). Licensure, certification, and accreditation. *Online Journal of Issues in Nursing, 2*(3). http://ojin.nursingworld.org/MainMenuCategories/ANAMarketplace/ANAPeriodicals/OJIN/TableofContents/Vol21997/No3Aug97/LicensureCertificationandAccreditation.html

Brain Attack Coalition. (2013). *Member organizations.* https://www.brainattackcoalition.org/organizations.html

Engelhardt, E. (2017). Apoplexy, cerebrovascular disease, and stroke: Historical evolution of terms and definitions. *Dementia & Neuropsychologia, 11*(4), 449–453. https://doi.org/10.1590/1980-57642016dn11-040016

Kidwell, C. S., Shephard, T., Tonn, S., Lawyer, B., Murdock, M., Koroshetz, W., Alberts, M., Hademenos, G. J., & Saver, J. L. (2003). Establishment of primary stroke centers: A survey of physician attitudes and hospital resources. *Neurology, 60*(9), 1452–1456. https://doi.org/10.1212/01.wnl.0000063314.67393.58

National Quality Forum. (2009). *National voluntary consensus standards for stroke prevention and management across the continuum of care: A consensus report.* Author. https://www.qualityforum.org/Publications/2010/02/National_Voluntary_Consensus_Standards_for_Stroke_Prevention_and_Management_Across_the_Continuum_of_Care.aspx

Nilsen, M. L. (2010). A historical account of stroke and the evolution of nursing care for stroke patients. *Journal of Neuroscience Nursing, 42*(1), 19–27. https://doi.org/10.1097/jnn.0b013e3181c1fdad

Sacco, R. L., Kasner, S. E., Broderick, J. P., Caplan, L. R., Connors, J. J., Culebras, A., Elkind, M. S. V., George, M. G., Hamdan, A. D., Higashida, R. T., Hoh, B. L., Janis, L. S., Kase, C. S., Kleindorfer, D. O., Lee, J., Moseley, M. E., Peterson, E. D., Turan, T. N., Valderrama, A. L., & Vinters, H. V. (2013). An updated definition of stroke for the 21st century: A statement for healthcare professionals from the American Heart Association/American Stroke Association. *Stroke, 44*(7), 2064–2089. https://doi.org/10.1161/STR.0b013e318296aeca

About the SCRN® Exam

CERTIFICATION EXAM OVERVIEW

The American Board of Neuroscience Nursing (ABNN) is a not-for-profit corporation with the purpose of creating and overseeing programs for certification of professional nurses within neuroscience nursing (www.abnncertification.org).

The American Association of Neuroscience Nurses (AANN) was founded in 1968 with the purpose of advancing the science and practice of neuroscience nursing. It accomplishes this through provision of continuing professional education, information sharing, research support, standard setting, and advocacy of not only neuroscience nursing but also advocacy of patients and their families (www.aann.org).

These two organizations work closely together for the mutual goal of advancement of stroke nursing certification via the SCRN® (Stroke Certified Registered Nurse) exam. The SCRN certification exam is only available through the ABNN and the AANN. The SCRN certification is valid for 5 years.

▶ SCRN ELIGIBILITY CRITERIA

1. A current, unrestricted RN license in the United States, Canada, or a U.S. territory that utilizes the U.S. State Board Test Pool Exam or National Council for Licensure Exam. Audits to validate current licensure will be conducted. Candidates from other countries must meet comparable license requirements and must be able to read and understand English, as the test is administered in English.
2. Professional nurses working in stroke care at the bedside (direct practice) or researcher, educator, administrator, or consultant (indirect practice)—with a minimum of 1 year full-time (2,080 hours) stroke care experience as an RN within the past 3 years—are eligible.
3. Completion of the online certification application and submission with fee must be received by ABNN prior to the application deadline.

   Questions about eligibility can be addressed by emailing info@abnncertification.org.

▶ EXAM FORMAT

- The SCRN exam is a computer-based test (CBT) in a multiple-choice format. Each question has four answer options with only one of the answers being correct. There are 170 questions (20 of which are possible future questions and do not count toward your score), with 3 hours allowed for completion.
- The exam will be automatically terminated after 3 hours. A digital clock is included for tracking time; this feature may be turned off during the exam if desired.

- The questions are presented one at a time, with the question number appearing in the lower right area of the screen. You may change your answer as many times as you want until the allotted time is exhausted. To advance to the next question, click on the forward arrow (>) in the lower right area of the screen.
- Questions can be bookmarked for later review by clicking on the blank square to the right of the Time button. To advance to the next unanswered or bookmarked question, click on the double arrow (>>) icon.

▶ EXAM CATEGORIES

The ABNN has based the exam categories and percentage of the total score dedicated to each category on extensive research of stroke and stroke care nursing. The content is divided as follows:
- Anatomy and physiology: 21%
- Hyperacute care: 24%
- Acute care: 31%
- Postacute care: 12%
- Preventive care: 12%

▶ NOTIFICATION OF EXAM RESULTS

- Exam results will be provided to the test taker upon completion of the exam, and certificates will be mailed to those who achieved the passing score.
- Those who fail the exam may reapply and retake it. The eligibility criteria must be met each time, along with a new application and fee.

▶ EXAM ADMINISTRATION

- Examination services are provided by Applied Measurement Professionals (AMP), a PSI business, in contract with ABNN.
  - The exam is offered three times each year in February, May, and September. Registration at a testing site will be possible after you receive confirmation of the completed online exam application from ABNN. For a list of test sites, see https://schedule.psiexams.com/
- Two forms of identification (ID) are required on the day of the exam, and both must be valid and include your current name and signature. One of them must be from this list:
  - Driver's license with photograph
  - State ID card with photograph
  - Passport
  - Military ID card with photograph

Examples of acceptable forms for the second ID include social security card with signature, employment or student ID card with signature, or credit card with signature.

▶ SCHEDULING AN EXAM APPOINTMENT

- Online: https://schedule.psiexams.com/ and select "Test takers."
- By phone: call toll-free 833-333-4755. Be prepared to confirm a date and location for testing and to provide your name and candidate ID number (from AMP's email scheduling notice).

▶ RESCHEDULING, POSTPONING, OR CANCELING AN EXAM APPOINTMENT

- You may reschedule your exam appointment **one time** at no charge as long as the new date is within your eligibility window. To do so, call AMP at 833-333-4755 at least two business days prior to your scheduled appointment date.
- If your exam has not yet been scheduled, you may postpone your exam window to the next exam window **one time**; contact AMP: 833-333-4755.
- If you have completed the application process but have not yet scheduled your exam date and wish to cancel your application, contact ABNN at info@abnncertification.org. Refunds (minus a $100 administrative fee) will only be made for requests received a minimum of 7 days prior to the scheduled exam window.

This information, along with more details, is available at www.abnncertification.org or www.aann.org.

▶ COMMON QUESTIONS ABOUT THE SCRN EXAM

1. Do I have to be a member of AANN to take the SCRN exam?
   Answer: No, nonmembers can take the test. Members receive a discounted exam fee.
2. Is there a penalty for guessing on the SCRN exam?
   Answer: No, there is no penalty for guessing, so do not leave unanswered questions.
3. Can I skip a question and return to it later?
   Answer: Yes, questions can be left unanswered and returned to later during the exam time period.
4. How soon can I retake the exam if I fail it?
   Answer: The ABNN does not specify a waiting period to retake the exam, only that it cannot be in the same eligibility window and that the exam cannot be taken more than three times in 12 months.
5. What if I do not think any of the answer choices for a question are correct?
   Answer: You will need to make your best guess from the choices provided. Be assured that the test questions have been reviewed by multiple content experts at AANN. It is possible to post an online comment by clicking on the button displaying an exclamation point to the left of the time button. The comments will be reviewed, but an individual response will not be provided.
6. What is a passing score for this exam?
   Answer: The passing score is determined by a procedure that involves the judgment of national neuroscience nursing experts and professional psychometricians from AMP, the company that administers the exam, so there is no specific passing score. A scaled score is utilized to ensure a consistent scale of measurement, regardless of which exam

a candidate was given. In other words, the raw score of a more difficult version of the exam would not equate with the raw score of a less difficult version. So, the raw scores are converted to scaled scores for determination of pass or fail.

7. What if there is a snowstorm, hurricane, tornado, tsunami, earthquake, or massive highway closure on the day of my exam and I cannot get to the testing site?

    Answer: The testing administrator, AMP, will determine if circumstances warrant cancellation or rescheduling. Scheduled candidates will be notified regarding rescheduling if this occurs. You can also visit their website at https://schedule.psiexams.com/ for information.

8. Which certification should I pursue, the SCRN or the Certified Neuroscience Registered Nurse (CNRN), or both?

    Answer: This is a personal choice based on professional experience, goals, and employment setting. Neuroscience nurses working in a setting that includes a variety of neuroscience populations, including stroke, might be interested in pursuing both certifications. Stroke is covered on the CNRN exam, but obviously not in the detail that it is covered in the SCRN exam. It might help to understand the distinctions between the two certification exams (see Table 2.1).

Table 2.1 Comparison of SCRN and CNRN Exams

	SCRN	CNRN
Year of origination	2013	1978
Number certified	Over 6,500	Over 4,400
Experience required	1-year full-time stroke care nursing in past 3 years	1-year full-time neuroscience nursing in past 3 years
Duration of certification	5 years	5 years
Cost of certification	Same for both—AANN members $300, nonmembers $400	
Categories covered	Adult stroke–specific	Pediatric and adult neuroscience spectrum
Number of questions	170 (150 count toward score)	220 (200 count toward score)
Testing time	3 hours	4 hours

AANN, American Association of Neuroscience Nurses; CNRN, Certified Neuroscience Registered Nurse; SCRN, Stroke Certified Registered Nurse.

MAXIMIZING YOUR SCORE

Consider attending a review course if there is one available. Also, consider a group of colleagues who might be interested in studying together for the SCRN certification exam. Each member could outline a different topic to present to the group.

Familiarize yourself with the generic names of common stroke medications (refer to the list provided in this study guide). The test will only refer to the generic names, so be prepared.

A few weeks before your exam date, design a notes sheet that you will memorize right before the exam. Common items might be the cranial nerves or generic/trade names of important drugs.

▶ THE NIGHT BEFORE THE EXAM

Ensure that you have your two forms of ID and the test date confirmation information to take along with you. Verify that you know the route to the testing center and plan for extra time to get there. Get adequate sleep—avoiding heavy meals and alcohol 3 to 4 hours prior to bedtime is helpful.

▶ THE DAY OF THE EXAM

Arrange for a wake-up time that allows you to get ready and eat without rushing. Avoid a heavy breakfast and try to include a combination of protein and complex carbohydrates for sustained energy. When you start the exam, utilize any time left from the tutorial session and jot down the notes you have memorized. This often helps you to relax as you know you have those things jotted down now. The first several questions are often some of the hardest. Keep this in mind and remember to use the feature that allows you to mark a question so you can skip it and come back to it later after you've gotten into your rhythm with more questions. If the choices of a particular question do not make sense to you, try reading them in reverse order—the last one first. Sometimes there is more information provided than is needed. Try not to read into the questions or answer choices—take them at face value. If there is a large paragraph, consider reading the last sentence first to get an idea of what they're asking, then read the paragraph. Do not leave any questions unanswered. Remember, there is no penalty for guessing, so you have a 25% chance of being right, which is better than a 0% if you leave it blank.

If you find yourself feeling panicked or overwhelmed, consider a quick break. There is no pause in the time window for breaks, so keep it to less than 5 minutes. But a change of scenery, a quick drink, a bathroom stop, and maybe even splashing water on your face may be helpful. Also remember the simple technique of slow, deep breaths.

When you have finished, take the time to congratulate yourself and your colleagues for having the discipline and focus to prepare for and take this important certification exam.

● REFERENCE

American Board of Neuroscience Nursing. (2022). *Stroke Certified Registered Nurse (SCRN®) 2022 candidate handbook*. Author. https://abnncertification.org/uploads/SCRN/ABNN_2022_SCRN_Handbook_Final.pdf

Anatomy, Physiology, and Etiology of Strokes

Knowledge of the anatomy and physiology of the brain is critical for neuroscience nurses. With advances in acute interventions, more patients are surviving large-vessel strokes, driving the need for nurses to be prepared to care for increasingly complex neurovascular patients. The changes that occur during the hours and days after the initial insult are often subtle and require stroke-knowledgeable neuroscience nurses to recognize them and take appropriate action.

BRAIN STRUCTURE AND FUNCTION

The brain is made up of multiple lobes and is divided into two halves, called *hemispheres*, which are separated by the medial longitudinal fissure (Figure 3.1). The hemispheres are connected physically by the corpus callosum, which also facilitates communication between the hemispheres (Figure 3.2).

The outer portion of the hemispheres is the cerebral cortex, also known as the *gray matter*. It contains numerous sulci and gyri, which are the terms for the grooves and folds that increase the surface area of the cortex. Beneath the cortex is the white matter, which contains tracts of axons.

CLINICAL PEARL

The terms **gray matter** and **white matter** originated from research using slices of tissue dyed to differentiate structures for microscopic examination. The cells that make up the cortex stained easily; the myelin-covered tracts of subcortical structures did not.

The surfaces of the brain and spinal cord are covered by the meninges, a series of three protective membranes. Starting with the outermost layer to the innermost layer, they are as follows:

- Dura mater: Composed of thick, fibrous connective tissue that closely lines the inside of the skull.
  - There are two notable dural folds, the falx and the tentorium; the falx separates the right and left hemispheres of the brain, and the tentorium separates the cerebrum from the cerebellum.
- Arachnoid mater: A delicate fibrous membrane attached to the dura mater.
  - Named for the delicate, spiderweb-like filaments that extend to the pia mater.
- Pia mater: A thin membrane that covers the surface of the brain.
  - Fits the brain like a latex glove fits the hand, following the surface detail of the sulci and gyri (Figure 3.3).

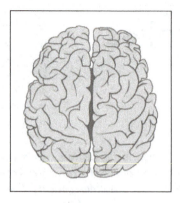

Figure 3.1 Brain showing two hemispheres.

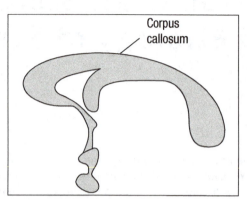

Figure 3.2 Corpus callosum.

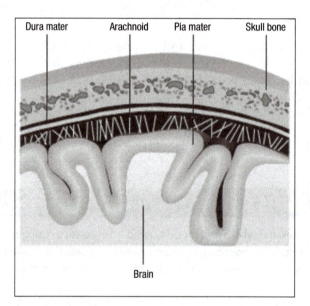

Figure 3.3 Meninges layers.

CLINICAL PEARL

The subarachnoid space is where most major cerebral blood vessels lie. Aneurysms commonly form on these vessels and, when they rupture, result in subarachnoid hemorrhage (SAH).

▶ FRONTAL LOBE

- Anterior/superior portion of the hemispheres.
- Functions are reasoning, emotions, judgment, and voluntary movement.
- Broca's area, located in the frontal lobe, is responsible for language production.

- The most anterior portion is called the *prefrontal lobe* or *prefrontal cortex* and specifically functions in planning and initiation, personality expression, and moderation of social behaviors.
- The posterior portion of the frontal lobe contains the motor neurons and is called the *primary motor cortex* or *motor strip*; it is also called the *precentral gyrus* because it lies in front of the central sulcus, which separates the frontal lobe from the parietal lobe (Figure 3.4).

CLINICAL PEARL

When the frontal lobe is damaged, patients are sometimes said to be acting "frontal," meaning that they are exhibiting inappropriate behavior. This is due to the frontal lobe not functioning correctly regarding judgment and reasoning.

▶ PARIETAL LOBE

- Sits directly behind the frontal lobe.
- The anterior portion of the parietal lobe is called the *primary sensory cortex* or *sensory strip*; it is also called the *postcentral gyrus*; this area functions to process sensory input.
- Right parietal lobe: Responsible for interpretation of the position of the body in accordance to the other objects in its surroundings.
- Left parietal lobe: Function includes the ability to understand numbers and manipulation of objects.
- Parieto-occipital sulcus: Separates the parietal lobe from the occipital lobe (Figure 3.4).

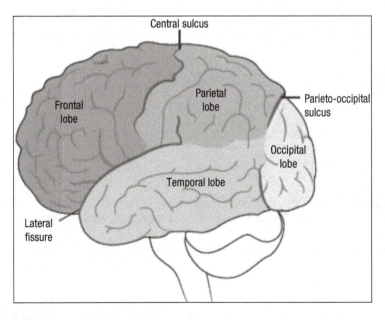

Figure 3.4 Side view of the brain: frontal, parietal, and occipital lobes; central sulcus; and parieto-occipital sulcus.

CLINICAL PEARL

The homunculus is a diagram that depicts which parts of the body are controlled by the motor and sensory strips. The top of the motor/sensory strip controls the lower portion of the body (legs and feet), whereas the bottom of the motor/sensory strip controls the upper portion of the body (face and arms; Figure 3.5).

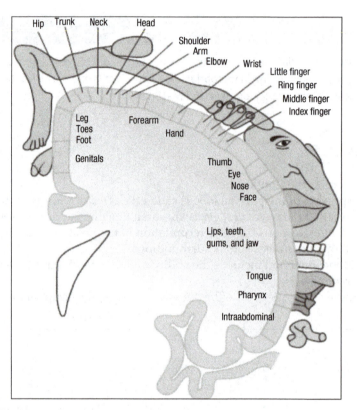

Figure 3.5 Homunculus.

▶ OCCIPITAL LOBE

- The most posterior portion of the cerebral cortex and the smallest of the lobes.
- Functions are visual spatial processing, color recognition, and motion perception (see Figure 3.4).

▶ TEMPORAL LOBE

- Positioned below the parietal lobe and separated from the other lobes by the lateral sulcus or Sylvian fissure.
- Functions are hearing, memory, facial and object recognition, and receptive speech.
- Wernicke's area is located in the area of the temporal lobe called the *primary auditory cortex* and is responsible for hearing and speech processing (see Figure 3.4).

CLINICAL PEARL

A simple way to remember where each speech area is located and its specific function is to look at the first vowels in each area:

Broca's area
*Located in: Fr*o*ntal lobe*
*Controls: M*o*tor speech*
Wernicke's area
*Located in: T*e*mporal lobe*
*Controls: R*e*ceptive speech*

DIENCEPHALON: THALAMUS, HYPOTHALAMUS, AND PITUITARY GLAND

These portions of the brain are located between the hemispheres and are considered gray matter like the cortical structures (Figure 3.6).

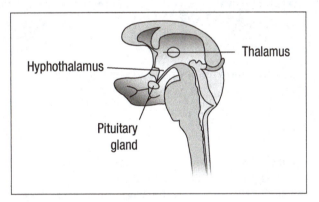

Figure 3.6 Thalamus, hypothalamus, and pituitary gland.

▶ THALAMUS

- Serves as a relay station between the cerebral cortex and the brainstem structures.
- Relays auditory, somatosensory, visual, and gustatory signals.
- Influences arousal and consciousness.

▶ HYPOTHALAMUS

- Its name describes its position, that is, below the thalamus.
- Functions in its connection between the cortex and the pituitary gland.
- Controls the release of eight major hormones by the pituitary gland.
- Controls body temperature, blood pressure (BP), hunger and thirst, sexual behavior, and circadian rhythms.

▶ PITUITARY GLAND

- Located below the hypothalamus, connected by the pituitary stalk.
- Referred to as the *master gland* because it directs other organs and endocrine glands, such as the adrenal glands, to suppress or induce hormone production.
- Anterior portion releases hormones that influence BP, metabolism, gluconeogenesis, lactation, ovulation, growth, and immune response.
- Posterior portion releases hormones that influence labor, birth, lactation, and BP.

BASAL GANGLIA

- Subcortical structure, located near the thalamus.
- Composed of gray matter and contains the caudate nucleus and the lenticular nucleus, the latter consisting of the putamen and the globus pallidus.
- Serves as the connection between the primary motor cortex and the brainstem, and thus controls voluntary movement and coordination of movement.

BRAINSTEM STRUCTURES: MIDBRAIN, PONS, AND MEDULLA OBLONGATA

The brainstem structures are made up of gray and white matter.

▶ MIDBRAIN

- Uppermost portion of the brainstem, superior to the pons (Figure 3.7).
- Motor and sensory tracts pass through the midbrain.
- The red nuclei, the substantia nigra, and the origin of cranial nerves III and IV are located here.
- Functions along with other structures in vision, hearing, motor control, sleep and wake cycles, arousal (alertness), and temperature regulation.

▶ PONS

- Located below the midbrain (Figure 3.7).
- Contains motor and sensory tracts.
- Serves as a communication and coordination center between the cerebrum and the cerebellum.
- Cranial nerves V, VI, VII, and VIII originate here.

- Controls sleep, respiratory drive, swallowing, hearing, balance, bladder control, taste, eye movement, facial expression, and sensation.
- The reticular formation, which controls consciousness, is located here.

CLINICAL PEARL

A pontine stroke can result in the syndrome referred to as locked-in syndrome, characterized by quadriplegia and the inability to do anything except blink the eyes. Cognition is usually preserved, and these patients communicate via eye blinks.

▶ MEDULLA OBLONGATA

- Lowest portion of the brainstem, connecting to the spinal cord at the foramen magnum (Figure 3.7).
- Controls respiratory and heart rates and digestive processes as well as vomiting, coughing, sneezing, swallowing, and balance.
- Cranial nerves IX, X, and XII originate here.

CEREBELLUM

- Also referred to as the *little brain*.
- Located below the cortex and behind the brainstem (Figure 3.7).
- Communicates with the pons and spinal cord to coordinate motor movement and maintain balance.
- Contributes to cognitive function, particularly language, in ways that are not yet well understood.

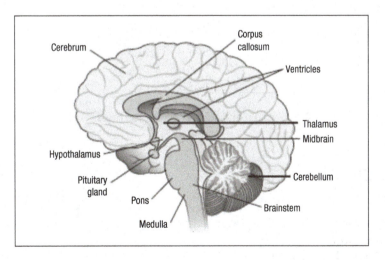

Figure 3.7 Midbrain, pons, and medulla.

BRAIN VASCULATURE

The entire blood supply of the brain depends on two sets of branches from the aorta—the common carotid arteries and the subclavian arteries. The internal carotid arteries (ICA) are branches of the common carotid arteries, and the vertebral arteries arise from the subclavian arteries (Figure 3.8). The ICA branch to form two major cerebral arteries: the anterior cerebral arteries (ACA) and middle cerebral arteries (MCA). The right and left vertebral arteries come together at the level of the pons to form the midline basilar artery (Figure 3.9).

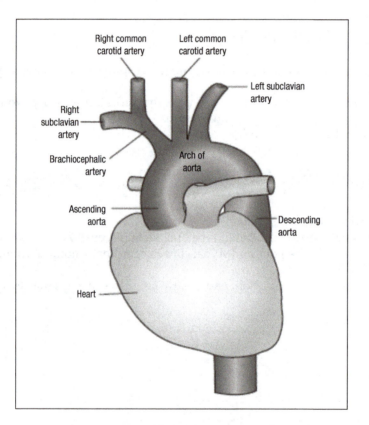

Figure 3.8 Aortic arch and subclavian and carotids.

▶ THE CIRCLE OF WILLIS

- ICA
- ACA
- Anterior communicating artery
- Posterior cerebral arteries (PCA)
- Posterior communicating arteries
- Not considered to be part of the circle of Willis (Figure 3.9) are the MCA, vertebral arteries, and the basilar artery

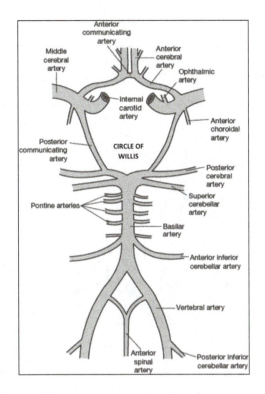

Figure 3.9 Circle of Willis and other anterior and posterior vessels.

CLINICAL PEARL

As much as 50% to 75% of the population has an incomplete circle of Willis, reminding us that collateral circulation is a very important concept in cerebrovascular anatomy. There have been 22 variations of the circle of Willis documented.

▶ ANTERIOR CIRCULATION

Supplies the anterior portion of the cerebrum—the frontal lobe, temporal lobes, and majority of parietal lobes (Figures 3.10 and 3.11).

Table 3.1 Anterior Circulation Arterial Anatomy

ICA	Connect aorta and anterior brain vessels
MCA	Supply blood to most of frontal and parietal lobes, the lateral portion of temporal lobes, the internal capsule, and the basal ganglia
ACA	Supply blood to the medial portion of the frontal lobe, the medial and superior portions of the parietal lobes, and portions of the corpus callosum, basal ganglia, and internal capsule
Anterior communicating artery	Connects the left and right ACA

ACA, anterior cerebral arteries; ICA, internal carotid arteries; MCA, middle cerebral arteries.

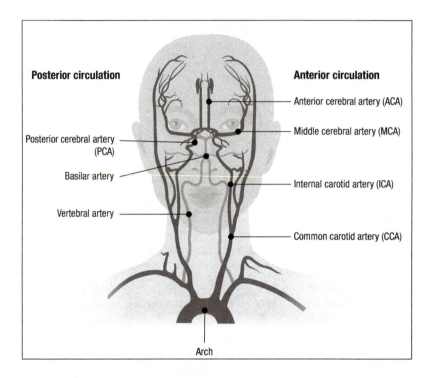

Figure 3.10 Neurovascular anatomy.

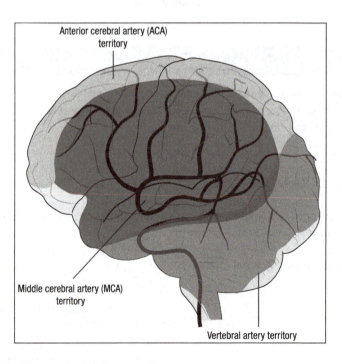

Figure 3.11 Large vessel territories.

▶ POSTERIOR CIRCULATION

Supplies the posterior portion of the cerebrum—the posterior parietal lobes, occipital lobe, cerebellum, and brainstem.

Table 3.2 Posterior Circulation Arterial Anatomy

Vertebral arteries	Connect the subclavian arteries (which arise from the aorta) and the posterior brain
Basilar artery	Supplies blood to the cerebellum via the PICA, the AICA, and the superior cerebellar arteries; it also supplies blood to the pons
PCA	Supply blood to the occipital lobe, inferior portion of the temporal lobe, and the thalamus
Posterior communicating arteries	Connect the anterior and posterior portions of the circle of Willis

AICA, anterior inferior cerebellar artery; PCA, posterior cerebral artery; PICA, posterior inferior cerebellar artery.

▶ PENETRATING ARTERIES

- Penetrating arteries are smaller branches of the large cerebral arteries that extend throughout the brain tissue and provide blood flow to all areas of the brain.
- Overlap of these vessels accounts for "collateral" flow.
- For instance, if a distal portion of the middle cerebral vessel is occluded, the area it normally supplies can be perfused by a distal branch of nearby vessels. But if a proximal portion of the MCA is occluded, there will be a large area of infarction that may not be able to be supplied by smaller, nearby vessels (Alexander, 2013).

● CEREBRAL VENOUS CIRCULATION

- Cerebral venous circulation serves as the brain's drainage system.
- Dural venous sinuses (also called *dural sinuses, cerebral sinuses*, or *cranial sinuses*) are venous channels found between layers of dura mater in the brain.
- The venous sinuses collect the blood from the brain and empty it into the internal jugular veins (Figure 3.12).

● STROKE TYPES

Figure 3.13 shows the associated likelihood of different stroke subtypes.

▶ ISCHEMIC STROKE

Eighty-eight percent of all strokes are ischemic strokes that occur due to lack of blood to part of the brain caused by narrowing or occlusion of vessels or by systemic hypotension. High BP is the most common risk factor because it damages the intima of blood vessels and

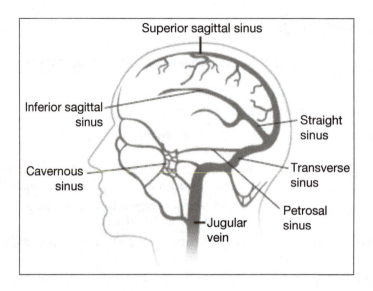

Figure 3.12 Venous system, jugular veins.

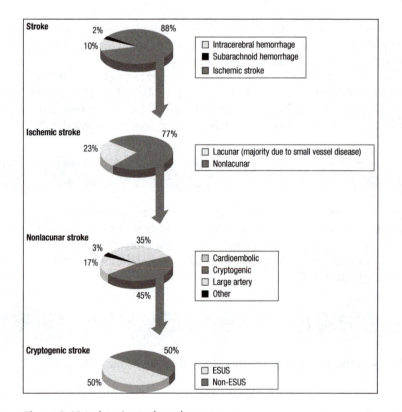

Figure 3.13 Ischemic stroke subtypes.

Source: Reprinted with permission. *Stroke*.2021;52:e364-3467. ©2021 American Heart Association, Inc.

ESUS, embolic stroke of undetermined source.

causes hypertrophic cardiomyopathy, which leads to atrial fibrillation. Other risk factors are cigarette smoking, uncontrolled diabetes, high cholesterol, physical inactivity and obesity, and certain blood disorders. Systemic hypoperfusion is a little-understood cause of stroke; it occurs when the systemic BP is too low and too little blood reaches the brain.

PHYSIOLOGY OF CEREBRAL ISCHEMIA

- Normal cerebral blood flow is 45 to 60 mL/100 g/min. When it drops below 18 mL/100 g/min, brain tissue infarction can occur if cerebral blood flow is unresolved for up to 4 hours. This process is known as the *ischemic cascade*.
- The ischemic cascade is a series of biochemical reactions that are initiated within minutes of brain ischemia.
  - Carbon dioxide retention and adenosine triphosphate (ATP) breakdown occur, activating sodium/hydrogen exchange transporters.
  - Disruption of normal cellular exchange results in cell death.
  - Cell death releases toxic chemicals that damage the blood–brain barrier.
  - Large molecules, such as albumin, pass through the damaged barrier, pulling water with them by the process of osmosis.
  - The result is tissue swelling and edema—the ischemic penumbra.

ISCHEMIC PENUMBRA

- The area surrounding the infarcted tissue.
- The area is still viable, often supported by collateral circulation, but is at risk of proceeding to infarction, like the core of the stroke (original area of infarcted tissue).
- If the area proceeds to infarct, it is referred to as *extending the stroke*, because the core has now been enlarged.
- The tissue is swollen, resulting in diminished function, increased intracerebral pressure (ICP), and somnolence.
- Resolution of edema generally occurs within 72 hours, as demonstrated by improvement of some deficits and by patients being more awake and alert (Figure 3.14).

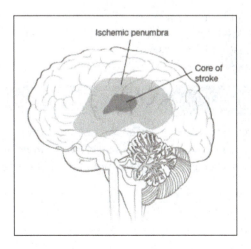

Figure 3.14 Ischemic penumbra.

▶ THROMBOTIC STROKE

- Thrombotic stroke is caused by a stationary blood clot (thrombus) or stenosis in an artery going to the brain.
- Blood clots usually form in arteries damaged by plaque.
- Plaque accumulation occurs over time, resulting in narrowing (stenosis) of the vessel lumen.

▶ EMBOLIC STROKE

- Embolic stroke is caused by a traveling clot (embolus) that is formed elsewhere (usually from the heart or neck arteries).

CLINICAL PEARL

Understanding the physiology of the penumbra will help the neuroscience nurse to educate the patient's family and allay some of their anxiety during the first few days. For example, a patient with a right MCA infarct is admitted with left arm weakness. On day 2, the patient is hard to arouse, and the left leg is not working properly due to the penumbra swelling into the motor strip area controlling the leg. The nurse can explain this, along with the reassurance of close monitoring and careful medical management, indicating that in another day or two the swelling will subside, the patient will be more awake, and the leg will work again.

▶ LACUNAR STROKE

- Seventy-seven percent of ischemic strokes are lacunar strokes.
- A lacunar stroke is caused by occlusion of smaller, penetrating arteries, blocking blood flow to small portions of the brain.
- Also referred to as *pure motor* or *pure sensory* stroke because the territory of infarct is so small as to only affect motor or sensory fibers, usually not both. The surrounding brain tissue often quickly takes over the function of the infarcted territory; thus, the symptoms may only last a few hours.

CLINICAL PEARL

In the past, lacunar strokes were often mistaken for transient ischemic attacks (TIAs) because the symptoms only lasted a few hours, with no imaged infarct. Improved imaging has made it possible to see tiny infarcts, even in the case of symptom resolution. See Chapter 4 for more information on TIAs.

WATERSHED STROKE

- A watershed stroke occurs at the junction of distal fields of two nonanastomosing (nonconnecting) arterial systems.
- A watershed stroke is more common in the presence of vascular disease.
- There are two types:
  - Cortical watershed (CWS): This type occurs between the territories of the ACA, MCA, and PCA.
  - Internal watershed (IWS): This stroke occurs in the white matter along and slightly above the lateral ventricle, between the deep and the superficial arterial systems of the MCA, or between the superficial systems of the MCA and ACA.
- A watershed stroke is caused by systemic hypoperfusion or microemboli from carotid artery disease.

CLINICAL PEARL

An example of a watershed stroke is the patient who awakens after surgery with new neuro deficit, but no evidence of embolic source. Patients with vascular disease and/or history of hypertension are less tolerant of anesthesia and resultant lower BP that doesn't perfuse their distal vascular beds. Astute anesthesia providers will be aware of their history and manage BP accordingly during surgery.

SILENT STROKES

- Ischemic: Imaging or pathophysiological evidence of infarction without a history of acute neurological dysfunction attributable to the lesion.
- Hemorrhagic: Focal collection of chronic blood products within the brain parenchyma, subarachnoid space, or ventricular system on neuroimaging or neurophysiological exam that is not caused by trauma and without a history of acute neurological dysfunction attributable to the lesion (Sacco et al., 2013).

CRYPTOGENIC STROKES

- Cryptogenic strokes refer to strokes confirmed by imaging with no source found despite a thorough diagnostic workup.
- Further subdivided into embolic stroke of undetermined source (ESUS) or non-ESUS; in other words, if imaging confirms that the stroke is not lacunar, and no source is found, then it is ESUS.

⬤ LARGE-VESSEL SYNDROMES

- Large-vessel syndromes occur when the blood supply is suddenly restricted or occluded in one of the large cerebral arteries, resulting in a "syndrome" or specific set of symptoms that are often dramatic.
  - Large-vessel occlusions can be gradual, which allows collateral circulation to expand to assume the responsibility of supplying the affected region with blood, and stroke does not necessarily occur.
- Symptoms are dependent on the area of the specific artery that is affected: Proximal occlusions will result in a broader set of symptoms, whereas distal occlusions will result in smaller territories of ischemia, thus a smaller set of symptoms.

▶ ANTERIOR CEREBRAL ARTERY SYNDROME

- Signs and symptoms of ACA syndrome are contralateral hemiparesis of lower limbs (see Figure 3.5 to visualize the lower limb portion of the homunculus and Figure 3.11 for vascular supply to that area), urinary incontinence, and apraxia.

▶ MIDDLE CEREBRAL ARTERY SYNDROME

- Signs and symptoms of MCA syndrome are contralateral hemiparesis and hemisensory loss in the face and arms (see Figure 3.5 to visualize the face and arm portion of the homunculus and Figure 3.11 for the vascular supply to that area).
- If the dominant side is affected, speech impairments occur, particularly aphasia, because Broca's and Wernicke's areas are part of the MCA territory.
- If the occlusion is proximal at the origin of the MCA, the result is a devastating, large-territory stroke, with 80% mortality.

▶ VERTEBRAL ARTERY SYNDROMES

- Signs and symptoms of vertebral artery syndromes vary considerably depending on the area affected.
- The most common syndromes are the following:
  - Wallenberg's syndrome: Symptoms are nausea, vomiting, vertigo, nystagmus, tachycardia, dysarthria, dysphagia, imbalance, and crossed signs.
  - Cerebellar infarction: Causes incoordination, ataxia, and dysarthria.
  - Locked-in syndrome: Caused by infarction of upper central pons; results in quadriplegia with preserved consciousness.
  - PCA occlusion: Causes hemianopia and macular sparing.

CLINICAL PEARL

The MCA territory is the most common site for embolic ischemic stroke. Because it supplies the face and arm territory of the motor/sensory strip, as well as the speech center territories, it makes sense that the face, arm, speech, time (FAST) mnemonic is so popular—these are the most common signs of stroke.

HEMORRHAGIC STROKE

Twenty percent of strokes are hemorrhagic strokes, which happen when a blood vessel ruptures in or near the brain, disrupting blood flow to a part of the brain. The two main types of hemorrhagic strokes are SAH and intracerebral hemorrhage (ICH), as illustrated in Figure 3.15.

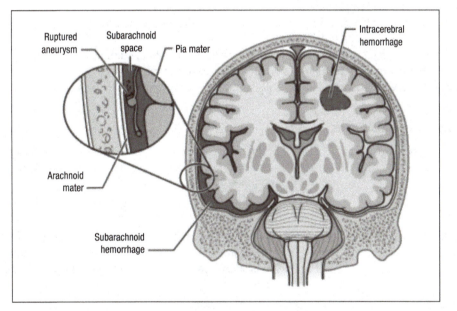

Figure 3.15 Intracerebral and subarachnoid hemorrhages.

CLINICAL PEARL

Due to the pressure of the blood spurting from an aneurysm (SAH) or from a broken vessel into the brain tissue (ICH), the most common symptom of hemorrhagic stroke is "the worst headache of my life."

▶ SUBARACHNOID HEMORRHAGE

- Ruptured cerebral aneurysms are the cause of 85% of SAHs. This causes blood to collect in the subarachnoid space. It is prevented from getting into the brain tissue (parenchyma) by the pia mater.
- Most common sites for aneurysms are the anterior communicating artery (29%), followed by the posterior communicating artery (19.6%), the basilar artery (14.7%), and the MCA (11.8%).
- Large amounts of subarachnoid blood can block circulation of cerebrospinal fluid (CSF), resulting in hydrocephalus; this usually occurs later during recovery and may appear as progressive dementia.
- Cerebral vasospasm occurs due to cerebral arteries in the subarachnoid space being surrounded by blood, which is irritating to the muscular arterial walls, resulting in spasms.
- Seizures occur in 7% of patients and may signal rebleeding.
- Rebleeding occurs in 17% of patients, typically within first 24 hours.
- Secondary ischemic stroke occurs in 30% of these patients, a condition referred to as *delayed cerebral ischemia (DCI)*.
- Cerebral edema also develops due to an SAH's effects on the blood–brain barrier, contributing to increased ICP.
- Release of catecholamines results in cardiac abnormalities, such as arrhythmias, tachycardia, and hypertension, as well as increased troponin levels.
- Mortality rate at 30 days is 40%.

Table 3.3 Aneurysmal Types

Saccular, also known as "berry" due to its shape	Occurs at arterial bifurcations and branches of the large arteries at the base of the brain—the circle of Willis Comprises 80%–90% of cerebral aneurysms
Fusiform	An outpouching of artery that is expanded in all directions Has no stem and seldom ruptures
Infective, also known as mycotic aneurysm	Infectious emboli mainly originate in left-sided bacterial endocarditis Can produce aSAH or ICH depending in which vessel the emboli lodge

aSAH, aneurysmal subarachnoid hemorrhage; ICH, intracerebral hemorrhage.

● CLINICAL PEARL

Aneurysms are weakened "ballooned" segments of arterial walls. Over time, and in the presence of hypertension, the aneurysm walls become stretched to the point of breaking. Other causes of aneurysms are sepsis, anticoagulation, and trauma. Referred to as aSAH, the "a" designates that the SAH is caused by an aneurysm.

▶ INTRACEREBRAL HEMORRHAGE

ICH is also known as *intraparenchymal hemorrhage (IPH)*. It occurs about twice as often as SAH.

- Caused by rupture of a penetrating artery, which releases blood directly into the brain tissue; in essence, this is a hematoma in the brain.
- The result is an inflammatory response with accompanying edema very similar to the ischemic penumbra; however, its duration is longer than that of the ischemic penumbra.
- The resulting increase in ICP contributes to a reduction in venous outflow, secondary ischemia (which initiates the ischemic cascade), and breakdown of the blood–brain barrier.
- Fifty percent of ICHs occur in the basal ganglia (rupture of lenticulostriate branches of the MCA), whereas 33% occur in the cerebral hemispheres (rupture of penetrating cortical branches of the anterior, middle, and PCA).
- Hypertension is the single most important risk factor due to its dilatation of the cerebral vessels, separating the normally tight endothelial junctions of the blood–brain barrier, thus lowering the threshold for ICH.
- Other risk factors are anticoagulation, cigarette smoking, alcohol consumption (more than two drinks daily), cocaine or amphetamine use, malignant neoplasms, and arteriovenous malformations (AVMs).
- Mortality rate at 30 days is 34% to 50%; the mortality rate is much higher for those who are comatose on arrival.

● CLINICAL PEARL

Up to 73% of spontaneous ICHs expand over the first 24 hours (Davis et al., 2006); so, close neurological monitoring for deterioration is essential.

A nurse attends an autopsy of a patient who had an ischemic stroke and heart attack simultaneously on Tuesday and died on Wednesday. They were 48 years old with a past medical history of diabetes and hypertension and were noncompliant with their medications for both. Their stroke symptoms started Tuesday morning, manifested as a numbness and weakness of the left arm. On admission, their blood sugar was 401 mg/dL, and their blood pressure (BP) was 210/105 bpm.

1. Considering their presenting symptoms, in which area of the brain is infarcted tissue expected?

    A. Left hemisphere
    B. Brainstem
    C. Occipital lobe
    D. Right hemisphere

2. As the pathologist starts to examine the brain further, they note that some tissue appears gray, and some appears white. Which color is the cortex?

    A. White
    B. Gray
    C. Mottled gray/white
    D. None of the above

3. The motor and sensory strips sit adjacent to each other but in different lobes. Please indicate which combination is correct for motor/sensory strip locations.

    A. Frontal/parietal
    B. Parietal/occipital
    C. Frontal temporal
    D. Parietal/temporal

4. The pathologist points out the infarcted tissue and notes that there is significant swelling of the brain tissue surrounding the core stroke. This is known as what?

    A. Encephalomalacia
    B. Hemorrhagic transformation
    C. Penumbra
    D. Exophthalmos

5. The pathologist also notes that the circle of Willis is incomplete, which is common in up to 75% of the population. They comment that this patient must have had adequate _____ to compensate for this.

    A. Lipoprotein balance
    B. Collateral circulation
    C. Hippocampal tone
    D. Venous sinus drainage

1. D) Right hemisphere
The motor and sensory fibers cross at the level of the brainstem; so, right-side infarct produces left-sided symptoms. Therefore, the numbness and weakness of the left arm indicates that the infarcted tissue would appear in the right hemisphere. Since fibers cross, left-sided infarct would not result in left-sided symptoms; brainstem infarcts result in a mixed presentation; and occipital lobe infarcts do not produce motor symptoms.

2. B) Gray
The cortex is made up of gray matter. These cells stain easily in the lab and appear gray, while the myelin-covered subcortical tissue does not and appears white. There is no area of the brain that appears mottled gray/white.

3. A) Frontal/parietal
The motor strip sits at back of the frontal lobe, while the sensory strip sits at the front of the parietal lobe; they are adjacent to each other. The temporal lobe is located below the frontal and parietal lobe, and the occipital lobe is located at the back of the brain. Both the temporal and occipital lobes do not contain the motor and sensory strips.

4. C) Penumbra
The penumbra is the swollen area of salvageable tissue surrounding the core of the stroke. Encephalomalacia is known as the softening or loss of brain tissue that follows a cerebral infarction. Hemorrhagic transformation would be seen as blood, not swelling; exophthalmos is the medical term that describes bulging eyes. It is unrelated to the anatomy of the brain.

5. B) Collateral circulation
Good collateral circulation provides blood supply to areas of the brain that might not receive it via the usual pathway, for example, an artery in circle of Willis that wasn't developed. An adequate lipoprotein balance, hippocampal tone, or venous sinus drainage will not compensate for an incomplete circle of Willis.

6. The pathologist begins to quiz the nurse, peeling away one of the membranes covering the brain. They are very impressed that the nurse instantly identifies the membrane as the pia mater because

A. It is the outermost layer
B. It is a delicate, spider-like membrane
C. It fits the brain like a latex glove fits your hand
D. It is thick and fibrous and very tough

(See answers next page.)

6. C) It fits the brain like a latex glove fits your hand
The pia mater is the innermost layer, clinging to the brain surface, following the contours of the sulci and gyri. The outermost layer is the dura mater, which is thick, fibrous, and tough; the delicate spider-like membrane is the arachnoid mater.

1. Aneurysmal rupture most commonly results in which type of stroke?

   A. Subdural hemorrhage
   B. Watershed hemorrhage
   C. Subarachnoid hemorrhage
   D. Intracerebral hemorrhage

2. The cerebrum is separated from the cerebellum by which dural fold?

   A. Corpus callosum
   B. Tentorium
   C. Falx
   D. Foramen magnum

3. Which of the following would be affected by a parietal lobe stroke?

   A. Wernicke's area
   B. Motor strip
   C. Sensory strip
   D. Globus pallidus

4. The postcentral gyrus is located in the

   A. Parietal lobe
   B. Occipital lobe
   C. Pons
   D. Cerebellum

5. The homunculus is represented by which of the following?

   A. Diagram that depicts what body parts are controlled by the motor/sensory strips
   B. Another name for the large third ventricle
   C. Diagram that represents the ischemic cascade
   D. Portion of cerebellum responsible for being awake and aware

6. Which of the following is a common nickname for the thalamus?

   A. Optic chiasm
   B. Reticular activating system
   C. Relay station
   D. Horner's knob

1. C) Subarachnoid hemorrhage

Large arteries are located in the subarachnoid space, and most aneurysms are associated with large arteries. Subdural hemorrhage is usually the result of trauma. Watershed hemorrhage would be called petechial hemorrhage and is result of small vessel rupture. Intracerebral hemorrhage rarely is the result of aneurysm rupture; predominantly, it is the result of simple arterial rupture.

2. B) Tentorium

The tentorium is also called the tentorium cerebelli and means "tent of the cerebellum," so picture it as a tent over the cerebellum, separating it from the cerebrum. The corpus callosum is a band of fibers that connects the two hemispheres. The falx is a dural fold that separates the two hemispheres, and the foramen magnum is the opening in the skull through which the spinal cord passes.

3. C) Sensory strip

Although the sensory strip lies right next to the motor strip, it is located at the front of the parietal lobe; the motor strip is located at the back of the frontal lobe. Wernicke's area is located in the temporal lobe near the junction of the temporal and parietal lobes. The globus pallidus is in the basal ganglia, a subcortical structure.

4. A) Parietal lobe

The postcentral gyrus is where the sensory strip lies, in the parietal lobe. The postcentral gyrus is not located in the occipital lobe, pons, nor cerebellum.

5. A) Diagram that depicts what body parts are controlled by the motor/sensory strips

The homunculus comes from the 16th century alchemist's description of a "little man." This term has been used to describe the location of the motor and sensory control of the body. The homunculus is not another name for the large third ventricle, is not the diagram the represents the ischemic cascade, and does not refer to the portion of the cerebellum responsible for being awake and aware.

6. C) Relay station

The thalamus relays auditory, somatosensory, visual, and gustatory signals between the cortex and the brainstem structures and is often given the nickname "relay station." The optic chiasm is where the optic nerves cross; the reticular activating system is a network of nerve pathways in the brainstem that mediate level of consciousness; there is no structure called Horner's knob.

7. Collectively, the thalamus, hypothalamus, and pineal gland are known as the

   A. Cerebral trifecta
   B. Diencephalon
   C. Penumbra
   D. Caudate nucleus

8. Someone who cannot understand what is said to them has had an infarct of the

   A. Frontal lobe
   B. Occipital lobe
   C. Temporal lobe
   D. Brainstem

9. Damage to this brainstem structure that connects to the spinal cord results in cardiac arrhythmias and respiratory dysfunction.

   A. Medulla oblongata
   B. Pons
   C. Hypothalamus
   D. Cerebellum

10. Mr. Spade presents to the ED with staggering gait and slurred speech. He swears he hasn't been drinking, and his alcohol level is normal. Where is the most likely location of an infarct on the CT scan?

    A. Midbrain
    B. Right parietal lobe
    C. Occipital lobe
    D. Cerebellum

11. Which statement would not be accurate for a provider to say to someone about the cause of their ischemic stroke?

    A. "We discovered that your circle of Willis is incomplete"
    B. "We found a carotid dissection on your left side"
    C. "You have atrial fibrillation on your electrocardiogram"
    D. "You have clot in your middle cerebral artery (MCA)"

12. A patient ended up with just a small core of stroke despite having had a large penumbra. They would be described as having good

    A. Communicating circulation
    B. Intracellular circulation
    C. Collateral circulation
    D. Borderline circulation

7. B) Diencephalon
The thalamus, hypothalamus, and pineal gland are collectively referred to as the diencephalon, which relays sensory information among brain regions and controls many autonomic functions of the peripheral nervous system. There is no structure known as the cerebral trifecta; the penumbra is the swollen tissue surrounding the stroke core; and the caudate nucleus is involved in learning and planning of motor activities.

8. C) Temporal lobe
The temporal lobe is where Wernicke's area is located. It is responsible for receptive speech. Someone with damage to this area might have trouble understanding spoken or written language. Damage to the frontal lobe would result in difficulty producing speech or writing words; damage to the occipital lobe would result in visual deficits; and damage to the brainstem would result in a variety of mixed motor/sensory signs as well as locked-in syndrome if the pons were affected.

9. A) Medulla oblongata
The medulla oblongata is sometimes called the extension of the spinal cord within the skull. It controls heart rate and respiration. Without its proper function, humans cannot survive. Damage to the pons would result in locked-in syndrome; the hypothalamus and cerebellum are not brainstem structures.

10. D) Cerebellum
The cerebellum is responsible for coordination and balance. When damaged, it can produce symptoms that have been mistaken for inebriation. Damage to the midbrain would result in a mixed set of symptoms not including gait or slurred speech. Damage to the parietal lobe would result in left-sided numbness or extinction. Damage to the occipital lobe would result in visual deficits.

11. A) "We discovered that your circle of Willis is incomplete"
The majority of the adult population has an incomplete circle of Willis, with no correlation to increased stroke risk; therefore, it is incorrect for a provider to note it as a cause of an ischemic stroke. Possible causes of ischemic stroke include carotid dissection, atrial fibrillation, and MCA clot.

12. C) Collateral circulation
Collateral circulation refers to the "detoured" circulation via small vessels that circumvent a blocked larger vessel. It provides circulation to the penumbra on the outer edges. Communicating circulation, intracellular circulation, and borderline circulation would not affect the size of the stroke core.

13. Of the choices below, which would not be a true statement regarding the cause of your patient's ischemic stroke?

    A. Embolus at the bifurcation of the left and right basilar arteries
    B. Thrombus in the right vertebral artery
    C. Embolus in the right cerebellar artery
    D. Thrombus in the left posterior cerebral artery

14. Your patient is acting "frontal." What is the patient doing?

    A. Having trouble hearing
    B. Exhibiting left arm numbness
    C. Behaving inappropriately
    D. Seeing double

15. Which of the following is *not* a lacunar syndrome?

    A. Disconjugate gaze syndrome
    B. Pure motor syndrome
    C. Pure sensory syndrome
    D. Dysarthria–clumsy hand syndrome

16. Another term for intracerebral hemorrhage is

    A. Subdural hemorrhage
    B. Subarachnoid hemorrhage
    C. Intraparenchymal hemorrhage
    D. Intraventricular hemorrhage

17. A patient who must communicate through eye blinks has had a stroke in which area of the brain?

    A. Central occipital lobe
    B. Pons
    C. Thalamus
    D. Right cerebellum

18. A patient awakens from surgery with deficits. The CT shows a stroke in the territory between two adjacent cerebral arteries called a/an

    A. Sublacunar infarct
    B. Watershed infarct
    C. Subsurgical infarct
    D. Associated infarct

13. A) Embolus at the bifurcation of the left and right basilar arteries

There is only one basilar artery, so there is no bifurcation of the left and right basilar arteries. Emboli and thrombi of any of these cerebral vessels are causes of ischemic stroke.

14. C) Behaving inappropriately

The frontal lobe is responsible for many things, including motor function, problem solving, spontaneity, memory, language, initiation, judgment, impulse control, and social and sexual behavior. Damage to the frontal lobe can result in inappropriate behavior that is often sexual in nature. Trouble hearing would be the result of temporal lobe damage; arm numbness would be the result of parietal lobe damage; and seeing double is likely the result of cerebellar damage.

15. A) Disconjugate gaze syndrome

Lacunar syndromes are small infarcts of territories supplied by a penetrating artery branch of one of the major cerebral arteries. The area involved is small with finite impact on function. Pure motor syndromes produce only motor symptoms; pure sensory syndromes produce only sensory symptoms; and dysarthria–clumsy hand syndromes produce dysarthria and mild hand weakness. There is no formal term as disconjugate gaze syndrome

16. C) Intraparenchymal hemorrhage

Intracerebral hemorrhage and intraparenchymal hemorrhage both refer to blood within the brain, also known as parenchymal tissue. Subdural hemorrhage is under the dura mater, between the dura mater and arachnoid mater, so not within the brain tissue; subarachnoid hemorrhage is under (sub) the arachnoid mater, between the arachnoid mater and the pia mater; and intraventricular hemorrhage is blood in the ventricles, which may have come from either a subarachnoid hemorrhage or an intracerebral hemorrhage.

17. B) Pons

The pons is located between the midbrain and medulla and serves as a communication and coordination center between the cerebrum and the cerebellum. Damage results in inability to move anything but the eyes, a condition referred to as locked-in syndrome. Damage to the central occipital lobe, thalamus, or right cerebellum would likely not result in locked-in syndrome.

18. B) Watershed infarct

Watershed infarct refers to stroke in the space between two adjacent cerebral arteries that is supplied by tiny penetrating vessels that are the first to collapse in the setting of hypoperfusion. This space is called the watershed territory. Lacunar infarcts refer to small territory infarcts; there is no such thing as sublacunar infarct, nor are there subsurgical or associated infarcts.

19. Which of the following best describes the cerebral cortex?

   A. Folds of gray matter playing an important role in consciousness
   B. Folds of white matter playing an important role in consciousness
   C. Tracts of white matter playing an important role in autonomic function
   D. Tracts of gray matter playing an important role in motor function

20. The band of white matter fibers that facilitates communication between the left and right hemispheres is known as

   A. Foramen magnum
   B. Corpus callosum
   C. Basal ganglia
   D. Midbrain

19. A) Folds of gray matter playing an important role in consciousness
The cerebral cortex is composed of gray matter. Gray matter tracts do not exists; there are only white matter tracts.

20. B) Corpus callosum
The corpus callosum is a band of white matter fibers that connects the left and right cerebral hemispheres. The foramen magnum is the name for the hole in the skull base that the spinal cord passes through. The basal ganglia and midbrain are subcortical structures responsible for motor control and other functions unrelated to the communication of brain hemispheres.

REFERENCES

Alexander, S. (Ed.). (2013). *Evidence-based nursing care for stroke and neurovascular conditions*. Wiley-Blackwell.

Davis, S. M., Broderick, J., Hennerici, M., Brun, N. C., Diringer, M. N., Mayer, S. A., Begtrup, K., & Steiner, T. (2006). Hematoma growth is a determinant of mortality and poor outcome after intracerebral hemorrhage. *Neurology*, *66*(8), 1175–1181. https://doi.org/10.1212/01.wnl.0000208408.98482.99

Kleindorfer, D. O., Towfighi, A., Chaturvedi, S., Cockroft, K. M., Gutierrez, J., Lombardi-Hill, D., Kamel, H., Kernan, W. N., Kittner, S. J., Leira, E. C., Lennon, O., Meschia, J. F., Nguyen, T. N., Pollak, P. M., Santangeli, P., Sharrief, A. Z., Smith Jr, S. C., Turan, T. N., & Williams, L. S. (2021). 2021 guideline for the prevention of stroke in patients with stroke and transient ischemic attack: A guideline from the American Heart Association/American Stroke Association. *Stroke*, *52*(7), e364–e467. https://doi.org/10.1161/STR.0000000000000375

Sacco, R. L., Kasner, S. E., Broderick, J. P., Caplan, L. R., Connors, J. J., Culebras, A., Elkind, M. S. V., George, M. G., Hamdan, A. D., Higashida, R. T., Hoh, B. L., Janis, L. S., Kase, C. S., Kleindorfer, D. O., Lee, J. M., Moseley, M. E., Peterson, E. D., Turan, T. N., & Hellips Vinters, H. V. (2013). An updated definition of stroke for the 21st century: A statement for healthcare professionals from the American Heart Association/American Stroke Association. *Stroke*, *44*(7), 2064–2089. https://doi.org/10.1161/STR.0b013e318296aeca

Associated Stroke Disorders

The disorders discussed in this chapter are not viewed as types of stroke, but often lead to stroke. Transient ischemic attack (TIA), in particular, can be a difficult condition to diagnose with confidence but is strongly associated with stroke.

TRANSIENT ISCHEMIC ATTACK

- TIA causes focal neurological deficits similar to stroke symptoms, but the deficits completely resolve with no MRI and/or CT findings of acute cerebral infarction (Easton et al., 2009).
- Historically, TIA was defined by time-based parameters (i.e., symptom resolution within 24 hours).
- With improved CT and MRI technology, TIA is now defined by tissue-based parameters (i.e., absence of infarction on brain imaging, along with complete resolution of symptoms).
- The incidence of TIA leading to stroke has dropped dramatically over the past 10 years as the result of more aggressive treatment of TIA.
- Another term for TIA is *ministroke*; some practitioners use the term *ministroke* when referring to tiny, lacunar strokes, which can lead to considerable confusion.

CLINICAL PEARL

TIA is to stroke what angina pectoris is to myocardial infarction (MI) . . . a warning sign.

DISSECTION OF CAROTID AND VERTEBRAL ARTERIES

- Dissection develops when a tear occurs in the intima of the vessel and blood collects between the linings. This not only creates an occlusion but also provides a source for microemboli to form along the tear.
- Numerous tiny infarcts in a hemisphere are a clue that carotid artery dissection may be present.
- Vertebral artery dissection is less common but does occur.
- Both types of dissection are more prevalent in young people and in the presence of trauma to the head or neck but can occur spontaneously (Figure 4.1).

■ Horner's syndrome may be seen with carotid dissection. It is characterized by this triad of symptoms on the same side as the dissection:
  ● Ptosis—droopy eyelid
  ● Anhidrosis—absence of hemifacial sweating
  ● Meiosis—pupil constriction
  ● A simple way to remember may be to think of PAM Horner (from the first three letters of the symptoms).

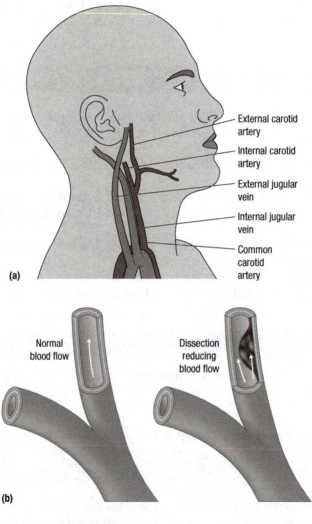

Figure 4.1 Carotid dissection.

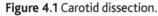

CLINICAL PEARL

Hyperextending the neck at a wash sink in a hair salon, lifting weights at a gym (increases in chest pressure/blood pressure), and chiropractic manipulation have been reported to be related to carotid artery and vertebral artery dissection. However, the majority of dissections are considered "spontaneous" with no known cause.

ARTERIOVENOUS MALFORMATION

- Arteriovenous malformations (AVMs) are abnormal vascular beds in which blood flows directly from arteries (with muscular walls) into veins (walls without muscles). The result is weakening and eventual rupture of the venous wall, causing intracerebral hemorrhage (ICH).
- AVMs vary in size and can be found anywhere in the nervous system.
- Unruptured AVMs cause few physical symptoms; thus, they are often undetected.

MOYAMOYA DISEASE

- Moyamoya is a rare and progressive disease caused by arterial occlusion in the basal ganglia.
- Its name means *puff of smoke* due to the characteristic appearance of a tangle of tiny vessels formed to compensate for the occlusion.
- Moyamoya primarily occurs in children and presents as an ischemic stroke or TIA.
- In adults, this disease presents as an ICH due to recurring clots in the fragile vessels.

HYPERCOAGULABLE CONDITIONS

- Hypercoagulable conditions are clotting disorders in which the blood clots under conditions in which it normally would not.
- Most common hypercoagulable conditions are factor V Leiden, protein S and C deficiencies, prothrombin gene mutation, and elevated homocysteine levels.
- The presence of cancer and numerous chemotherapy agents are known to be prothrombotic as well.

CLINICAL PEARL

It is sad, but not uncommon, for patients who come to the hospital with acute stroke symptoms to also learn that they have cancer. The prothrombotic nature of the cancer creates the potential for clots to form, and, if the clots reach the brain, they cause a stroke.

AMYLOID ANGIOPATHY

- Amyloid angiopathy is an accumulation of abnormal proteins (amyloid) in small cerebral arteries over the surface of the hemispheres.
- Progressive arterial narrowing leads to ischemia.
- This accumulation also weakens vessels, which leads to ICH.
- This condition is frequently associated with Alzheimer's disease.
- A definitive diagnosis requires a brain tissue sample; however, a probable diagnosis can be made based on imaging and clinical symptoms.

VASCULITIS

- Vasculitis is inflammation of the blood vessels, which can result in narrowing or occlusion of the blood vessels, and, in some cases, aneurysm formation and hemorrhage.
- Possible causes are immune system abnormalities, infections, cancer, and rheumatoid arthritis.

CEREBRAL VENOUS THROMBOSIS

- Cerebral venous thrombosis is caused by the presence of a clot in the dural venous sinuses, resulting in blocked drainage from the brain; the blocked drainage results in increased vascular pressure in the venous system and the potential for rupture of the vessel; 40% of patients present with ICH (Ulivi et al., 2020).
- This is an uncommon and frequently unrecognized type of stroke that mostly affects young people, with the most common symptom being headache.
- Most common causes are hypercoagulable conditions and oral contraceptive use.

CAVERNOUS ANGIOMA

- A cavernous angioma is a blood vessel abnormality characterized by large, adjacent capillaries with little or no intervening brain. The blood flow through these vessels is slow, and the vessels typically hemorrhage in small amounts, with bleeding episodes separated by months or years.

Mr. Hernandez is a 32-year-old primary care physician who had his wife drive him to the ED. He had been at the gym earlier today, doing his usual Tuesday routine of treadmill running, weight-lifting, and deep squats. He has no past medical history and takes no regular medications. While he was lifting, he felt a weird popping sensation in his right neck, but otherwise the workout was uneventful. He finished and went home. By the time he got there, he noticed that his left arm seemed heavy, and he had to use his right arm to use the turn signal. When he told his wife about it, he had trouble finding the words to describe what happened. He told her she better get him to the hospital.

1. What was he concerned that these symptoms represented?

    A. Acute arteriovenous fistula rupture
    B. Acute sternocleidomastoid hemorrhage
    C. Acute ischemic stroke
    D. Acute jugular vein occlusion

2. The vascular neurologist noted a pattern of several small areas of infarct on the left side of the brain. What clue does this provide as to the etiology of Mr. Hernandez's condition?

    A. Amyloid angiopathy protein accumulation in small vessels
    B. New brain tumor causing hypercoagulable state
    C. Clustered cerebral venous thromboses
    D. Arterial dissection with shower of small clots

3. Which of the cerebral vessels is involved based on Mr. Hernandez's symptoms?

    A. Internal carotid artery
    B. Vertebral artery
    C. Middle cerebral artery
    D. Anterior communicating artery

1. C) Acute ischemic stroke from a carotid dissection

Mr. Hernandez was concerned that his symptoms represented acute ischemic stroke from a carotid dissection. These symptoms are not indicative of arteriovenous fistula, sternocleidomastoid hemorrhage, or jugular vein occlusion.

2. D) Arterial dissection with shower of small clots

Arterial dissection can result in small clots traveling upstream in the same vascular bed. There is a pattern of small infarcts on one side of the brain or one vascular territory. Amyloid angiopathy deposits are within small vessels. The carotid artery is a large vessel. While brain tumors can cause hypercoagulable states, there is no pattern of tending to one hemisphere or another, it would be simply scattered throughout. Cerebral venous thromboses are rarely clustered and are almost always accompanied by a severe headache, which Mr. Hernandez did not present with.

3. A) Internal carotid artery

The popping sensation Mr. Hernandez felt in his right neck followed by the weakness on left side accompanied by expressive aphasia indicates internal carotid artery involvement. The vertebral artery, middle cerebral artery, or anterior communicating artery dissection would not induce symptoms involving a popping sensation in the neck.

1. Why do arteriovenous malformations (AVMs) result in hemorrhagic stroke?

   A. Arteries and veins are connected directly rather than the usual route of arteries to arterioles, to capillaries, to venules, to veins
   B. Connection of arteries to veins is underdeveloped in individuals with chromosomal disorders
   C. Anomalies of the vessels of the circle of Willis
   D. Chronic hypertension causes fistulas between arteries and veins

2. Which of the following statements would be correct when educating your patient?

   A. "You just had a ministroke; there was only a small infarct on your CT scan"
   B. "You just had a ministroke; there was no evidence of infarct on your CT scan"
   C. "You just had a ministroke, also known as moyamoya"
   D. "You just had a ministroke, not a transient ischemic attack (TIA)"

3. A patient presents with an intracerebral hemorrhage (ICH) and is treated with anticoagulants. This makes sense in which of the following conditions?

   A. Subacute bacterial endocarditis
   B. Horner's syndrome
   C. Vertebral dissection
   D. Venous sinus thrombosis

4. A nurse is told that one of their four patients had a stroke at lunch, which of them is it most likely to be?

   A. A patient with a urinary tract infection (UTI)
   B. A patient with prostate cancer
   C. A patient with a hot gall bladder
   D. A patient with heart failure

5. Multiple tiny infarcts in the same hemisphere are a clue to which condition?

   A. Binswanger's disease
   B. Incomplete circle of Willis
   C. Vertebral dissection
   D. Carotid dissection

1. A) Arteries and veins are connected directly rather than the usual route of arteries to arterioles, to capillaries, to venules, to veins

AVMs are direct connections between arteries and veins that are not normal in human anatomy. The normal blood flow path is from arteries to arterioles to capillaries to venules, and finally to veins. Arteries have muscular walls to handle the pulsing blood as it is pumped from the heart, but veins do not have muscular walls. Therefore, if arterial blood flows directly into a vein via an AVM, the veins are likely to rupture under the pressure. There is no known connection between chromosomal disorders and AVMs. The circle of Willis only contains arteries. Chronic hypertension is not known to cause fistulas between arteries and veins.

2. B) "You just had a ministroke; there was no evidence of infarct on your CT scan"

Ministrokes are also known as TIAs, which are not strokes and do not leave any evidence on imaging. Ministrokes do not damage brain tissue permanently, thus are not seen on imaging. Moyamoya is a condition in which tiny blood vessels are formed in an attempt to meet perfusion needs with blocked or narrowed anterior circulation; it is not the same as ministroke.

3. D) Venous sinus thrombosis

Venous sinus thrombosis is the presence of a clot in the venous sinuses, blocking drainage from the brain; the blocked drainage results in increased vascular pressure in the venous system and the potential for rupture of the vessel. Congestion results in petechial hemorrhage 40% of the time. Subacute bacterial endocarditis is an infection within the heart. Horner's syndrome and vertebral dissection are symptoms of ischemic stroke, not hemorrhagic.

4. B) A patient with prostate cancer

Cancer and some chemotherapies are known to be prothrombotic, putting people at risk for stroke. UTI is associated with stroke as an outcome, but not as a risk. Cholecystitis and heart failure are not considered stroke risks.

5. D) Carotid dissection

Carotid dissection is the tearing of the intima of the carotid artery. Commonly, tiny clots form along the torn, rough edges of the tear. As they break off and migrate up to the brain, multiple tiny infarcts can occur, and because each carotid artery supplies only one side of the brain, dissection would result in infarcts on only one side. Incomplete circle of Willis would not result in multiple tiny infarcts. Binswanger's disease is the name for multiple infarcts in the deep subcortical white matter. It is not related to hemispheric strokes. In vertebral dissection, the clots that break off and migrate would be joined in the basilar artery, which supplies the posterior brain, not the brain hemispheres.

6. Rheumatoid arthritis is associated with which of the following disorders?

   A. Vasculitis
   B. Moyamoya
   C. Amyloid angiopathy
   D. Venous thrombosis

7. Improved imaging technology has had what impact on diagnosis of associated stroke disorder?

   A. It has made it possible to get a definitive diagnosis of amyloid angiopathy
   B. It has resulted in changing the name from transient ischemic attack (TIA) to ministroke
   C. It has resulted in changing the definition of TIA to a tissue-based from a time-based
   D. It has resulted in a 50% increase in venous thrombosis diagnoses

8. A nurse is caring for a patient with Alzheimer's disease who has just had a stroke. Which associated stroke disorder is suspected to have contributed to the patient's stroke risk?

   A. Vasculitis
   B. Moyamoya
   C. Cavernous angioma
   D. Amyloid angiopathy

9. How is it possible for cavernous angiomas to remain undiagnosed in a patient for many years?

   A. Slow blood flow means leakage takes a long time to accumulate enough to create symptoms
   B. They occur in Alzheimer's disease patients who don't remember to report the symptoms
   C. They occur in the falx cerebri, a structure with no sensory input
   D. They only produce a symptom of sinus congestion, which is mistaken for a viral infection

10. Protein S and protein C are examples of which associated stroke disorder?

    A. Vasculitis conditions
    B. Hypercoagulable states
    C. Arterial dissections
    D. Moyamoya

(See answers next page.)

6. A) Vasculitis
Rheumatoid arthritis is a chronic inflammatory condition and creates a higher risk of stroke due to systemic inflammation. It is related to vasculitis, an associated stroke disorder. Moyamoya is a condition in which tiny blood vessels are formed in an attempt to meet perfusion needs with blocked or narrowed anterior circulation. Amyloid angiopathy is a condition with amyloid beta-peptide deposits within small blood vessels. Venous thrombosis is formation of stationary blood clots within veins. Moyamoya, amyloid angiopathy, and venous thrombosis are not related to rheumatoid arthritis.

7. C) It has resulted in changing the definition of TIA to a tissue-based from a time-based
Better imaging has made it possible to see strokes that occurred, even in patients with symptoms lasting less than 24 hours, thus invalidating the old time-based definition. It has had no real impact on diagnosis of amyloid angiopathy; TIA is the same as a ministroke. The name was never changed from TIA to ministroke. Imaging technology did not result in a 50% increase in venous thrombosis diagnoses.

8. D) Amyloid angiopathy
The accumulation of abnormal proteins in amyloid angiopathy is frequently associated with Alzheimer's disease. The accumulation of these abnormal proteins also impacts vascular integrity and is a risk for stroke. Vasculitis, moyamoya, and cavernous angioma are not associated with Alzheimer's disease.

9. A) Slow blood flow means leakage takes a long time to accumulate enough to create symptoms
Cavernous angiomas are the result of leakage from capillary beds with slow flow. They are not specific to Alzheimer's patients, they do not occur in the falx cerebri, and they do not produce sinus congestion.

10. B) Hypercoagulable states
Hypercoagulable states are conditions that include protein S and protein C, which make patients more likely to form clots. Protein S and protein C are not associated with vasculitis, arterial dissection, or moyamoya.

REFERENCES

Easton, J. D., Saver, J. L., Albers, G. W., Alberts, M. J., Chaturvedi, S., Feldmann, E., Hatsukami, T. S., Higashida, R.T., Johnston, S. C., Kidwell, C. S., Lutsep, H. L., Miller, E., & Sacco, R. L. (2009). Definition and evaluation of transient ischemic attack: A scientific statement for healthcare professionals from the American Heart Association/American Stroke Association Stroke Council; the Council on Cardiovascular Surgery and Anesthesia; the Council on Cardiovascular Radiology and Intervention; the Council on Cardiovascular Nursing; and the Interdisciplinary Council on Peripheral Vascular Disease. *Stroke, 40*(6), 2276–2293. https://doi .org/10.1161/STROKEAHA.108.192218

Ulivi, L., Squitieri, M., Cohen, H., Cowley, P., & Werring, D. J. (2020). Cerebral venous thrombosis: A practical guide. *Practical Neurology, 20*(5), 356–367. https://doi .org/10.1136/practneurol-2019-002415

Hyperacute Stroke Care

Prehospital care is the critical first step in the hyperacute stroke care continuum and has seen significant change since 1996, the year that intravenous (IV) tissue plasminogen activator (tPA) was approved by the U.S. Food and Drug Administration (FDA). In 2015, when mechanical clot retrieval was established as a standard of care, the role of the emergency medical services (EMS) provider grew and became even more critical. There are numerous stroke severity assessment tools for use by EMS providers to predict whether large-vessel occlusion (LVO) is present in a suspected stroke patient, along with routing plans and algorithms to guide them in selecting the most appropriate stroke center to which to take the patient.

The ED personnel, already well trained to multitask, need to be able to receive, identify, evaluate, treat, and obtain access to stroke expertise within a very short time frame. EMS and ED professionals represent the first care stroke patients receive in the continuum; they have the opportunity and responsibility to get it right.

◗ PREHOSPITAL

As always, the prehospital professional is first committed to rapid evaluation and stabilization of the ABC's—airway, breathing, and circulation—as well as rapid transport. Second is determining suspicion for stroke.

- Brief, standardized neurological assessment: Cincinnati Prehospital Stroke Scale or Los Angeles Prehospital Scale to determine stroke suspicion
- For patients who screen positive for suspected stroke, a standard severity assessment tool is be utilized to check for LVO:
  - LAMS: Los Angeles Motor Scale
  - VAN: Stroke Vision, Aphasia, Neglect Scale
  - RACE: Rapid Arterial oCclusion Evaluation Scale
  - sNIHSS-EMS: Shortened NIHSS for EMS Scale
  - CP-SSS: Cincinnati Prehospital Stroke Severity Scale
  - FAST-ED: Field Assessment Stroke Triage for Emergency Destination

Key components of effective prehospital stroke care are outlined in Box 5.1.

Box 5.1 Prehospital Management Recommendations

Assess airway, breathing, circulation; do not treat high blood pressure unless recommended
Implement cardiac monitoring
Maintain oxygen saturation >94%
Assess blood glucose and treat if <60 mg/dL
Do not administer excessive intravenous fluids or solutions containing glucose
Do not give any fluids or medication by mouth

(continued)

Box 5.1 Prehospital Management Recommendations (*continued*)

Establish intravenous access, two 18 gauge if possible
Determine LKN
Document medical history and medication use
Obtain family/friend/bystander phone numbers
Provide rapid transport to the most appropriate hospital capable of stroke emergency treatment

Source: Reprinted with permission. *Stroke.2021;52e1-e15.* @2021 American Heart Association, Inc.
LKN, last known normal.

- Use a standardized algorithm, such as the Mission Lifeline® algorithm, to guide which level of stroke center to take the patient to (Figure 5.1).
  - Provides step-by-step directions for evaluation of acute stroke and detailed description of on-scene responsibilities
  - Recommends bypass of LVO patients to comprehensive stroke center (CSC) unless it will add more than 30 minutes to the transport time; if so, go to the closest certified stroke center according to regional stroke system of care plan
  - Directs collection of both last known well (LKW, or LKN) time and time of symptom discovery

CLINICAL PEARL

LKW time is the time the patient was last known to be at baseline, with no stroke symptoms. Time of symptom discovery is the time the stroke symptoms were noted by someone else. These two terms are often mistakenly used interchangeably, so explicit capture of both will avoid confusion.

- Prearrival notification to receiving hospital of all suspected stroke patients; this has been shown to shorten treatment times by 16% (Powers et al., 2019).
- Mobile stroke units (MSUs) have been developed by several stroke centers across the country.
  - Purpose is to perform the stroke workup usually done in the ED, but in an ambulance outfitted with CT capability, IV thrombolytic, point-of-care laboratory, and a provider who can make treatment decisions
  - Outcomes: faster door-to-needle (DTN) as well as faster door-to-puncture (DTP) as these patients can bypass the ED and go directly to intervention, saving time and brain

CLINICAL PEARL

Progress has been made: An analysis of the National Health Interview Survey (NHIS) demonstrated that awareness of stroke symptoms and signs among U.S. adults improved from 2009 to 2014. In 2014, 68.3% of the survey respondents were able to recognize five common stroke symptoms, and 66.2% demonstrated knowledge of all five stroke symptoms and the importance of calling 911 (Virani et al., 2021).

Unfortunately, only 60% of stroke patients arrive at the hospital via EMS. Racial/ethnic minorities have been shown to be much less likely to call 911 (Adeoye et al., 2019).

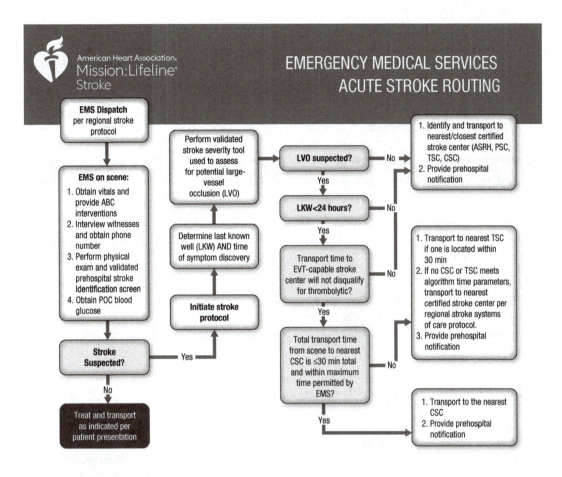

Figure 5.1 EMS acute stroke routing algorithm.

Source: Reprinted with permission from the American Heart Association. (2020). *Mission: Lifeline® Stroke: Emergency medical services acute stroke routing.* American Heart Association. https://www.heart.org/-/media/Files/Professional/Quality-Improvement/Mission-Lifeline/2_25_2020/DS15698-QI-EMS-Algorithm_Update-2142020.pdf

ABC, airway, breathing, circulation; ASRH, acute stroke–ready hospital; CSC, comprehensive stroke center; EMS, emergency medical services; EVT, endovascular treatment; LKW, last known well; LVO, large-vessel occlusion; POC, point-of-care; PSC, primary stroke center; TSC, thrombectomy-capable stroke center.

■ Prehospital involvement in stroke systems of care is recommended:
   ● Representatives of the area's EMS serve as members of the stroke center multidisciplinary stroke team
   ● Stroke educational programs provided to EMS personnel at least annually
      ○ Latest best practice standards
      ○ New developments in medications or interventions
      ○ Changes in stroke center requirements that impact prehospital
      ○ Opportunities to participate in community outreach activities
      ○ Review of quality metrics compliance
■ Suggested stroke quality metrics for EMS to track and report:
   ● Percent of cases with on-scene time of <15 minutes
   ● Percent of prehospital stroke screen completed
   ● Percent of prearrival notification done
   ● Percent of LKW time documented
   ● Percent of correct stroke diagnoses by EMS

- Percent of incorrect diagnoses by EMS
- DTN times comparing those with and without prearrival notification
- Percent of response time less than 8 minutes (time elapsed from receipt of call by the dispatch entity to arrival on scene of a properly equipped and staffed ambulance)
- Percent of dispatch time less than 1 minute
- Percent of turnout time (length of time from receipt of call to the unit being en route) less than 1 minute

CLINICAL PEARL

Measurement and sharing of quality metrics compliance with prehospital colleagues have been shown to increase prehospital personnel or EMS engagement with stroke program initiatives as well as improve their compliance. As always, if you tell them why, they're much more likely to comply.

Detailed recommendations for EMS care can be found in the Guidelines for Early Management of Patients with Acute Ischemic Stroke from the American Heart Association/ American Stroke Association (Powers et al., 2019). Box 5.2 outlines the use case for various stroke centers.

Box 5.2 Stroke Centers and Their Capabilities

Stroke Center Primer
Acute Stroke–Ready Hospital (ASRH) Rapid evaluation of acute stroke and administration of IV thrombolytic; neurological evaluation is often provided via telemedicine and teleradiology; transfer of intervention candidates to a CSC or TSC, complex cases to a CSC, with other stroke patients going to a PSC
Primary Stroke Center (PSC) Rapid evaluation of acute stroke and administration of IV thrombolytic; admitting and treating most stroke patients, with transfer agreement for sending intervention candidates and complex cases to a CSC; compliance with STK measures
Thrombectomy-Capable Stroke Center (TSC) Same as PSC, but with additional capability of performing emergent mechanical clot retrieval; requirement for minimum of 12 thrombectomies/provider annually; compliance with STK measures and five of the CSTK measures
Comprehensive Stroke Center (CSC) Treat the most complex stroke patients, including hemorrhagic strokes; mechanical clot retrieval for ischemic strokes; research protocols in various aspects of stroke care; dedicated neuro intensive care unit; and compliance with STK and CSTK measures

CSC, comprehensive stroke center; CSTK, comprehensive stroke quality measures; IV, intravenous; PSC, primary stroke center; STK, stroke quality measures; TSC, thrombectomy-capable stroke center.

There has been continued debate over whether to bypass to a CSC from acute stroke–ready hospitals (ASRHs) or primary stroke centers (PSCs). The pros and cons of bypass to a CSC have been identified (Southerland et al., 2016):

Pros	Cons
Bypass would save time and brain—the median delay of onset to reperfusion as a consequence of drip and ship compared with mothership was ≈2 hours. (Drip and ship refers to patients receiving IV tPA [drip] at one hospital and being transferred to another hospital for further care [ship]. Mothership refers to patients being taken to the hospital that provides advanced care right away.)	In rural areas where a CSC is very distant, bypass represents a significant treatment delay. Without a tool that has high sensitivity and specificity, there is risk that patients without LVO could have scored positive and been sent to a CSC, potentially overburdening the CSC.
IV tPA is not that effective in LVO, so bypass to CSC is the best option even if it means delay in IV tPA.	Bypass to CSC eliminates or delays the administration of IV tPA.

CSC, comprehensive stroke center; EMS, emergency medical services; IV tPA, intravenous tissue plasminogen activator; LVO, large-vessel occlusion.

▶ STROKE MIMICS

- Refers to conditions that can look like stroke on initial presentation
- Education and experience help EMS personnel to differentiate
- Examples of stroke mimics:
  - Seizure—either an absence-type seizure or postictal phase of a tonic-clonic seizure
  - Bell's palsy
  - Complex migraine
  - Hypo- or hyperglycemia
  - Brain tumor
  - Multiple sclerosis
  - Conversion disorder

● CLINICAL PEARL

Except for the headache associated with hemorrhagic stroke, symptoms of stroke do not hurt. Pain is a great motivator for seeking treatment, and its absence makes it possible for stroke patients to adopt a "wait and see" and "hope this goes away" mentality. Precious time is lost, limiting the acute treatment options available.

● PREHOSPITAL CERTIFICATIONS RELATED TO STROKE CARE

▶ ADVANCED STROKE LIFE SUPPORT (ASLS®)

- Released in 1998, uses a train-the-trainer format, with an 8-hour curriculum
- Utilizes the Miami Emergency Neurologic Deficit (MEND) exam

- Twelve-item score to gauge both the probability and the severity of a stroke
- Certification is good for 4 years (Michael S. Gordon Center for Research in Medical Education, 2017)

▶ EMERGENCY NEUROLOGICAL LIFE SUPPORT (ENLS)

- Developed in 2012 by the Neurocritical Care Society, uses a train-the-trainer format, with a 15-hour curriculum
- Involves 14 protocols, two of which are related to stroke—acute ischemic stroke (AIS) and intracerebral hemorrhage (ICH)
- Certification is good for 2 years

CLINICAL PEARLS

Many nurses do not understand the difference between an emergency medical technician (EMT) and a paramedic. There are significant differences: An EMT receives 120 to 150 hours of training and cannot start IVs or give injections. A paramedic receives 1,200 to 1,800 hours of training, with many earning a 2-year degree; paramedics can start IVs and give injections. In many communities, the majority of the EMTs are volunteers.

IN THE EMERGENCY DEPARTMENT: STROKE-ALERT PROCESS

▶ THE GOLDEN HOUR

- This refers to the time from patient arrival until IV tPA is administered (Figure 5.2).
- Critical steps to be accomplished during that time were established by the National Institute of Neurological Disorders and Stroke (NINDS).
- Administration of tPA should be accomplished within 60 minutes for 80% or more of treated patients.
- As a result of successful quality improvement initiatives like Target: Stroke, the American Heart Association recommendations indicate a new goal of under 30 minutes, and many stroke centers are meeting this quality benchmark (American Heart Association, 2019).

CLINICAL PEARL

The golden hour was first described by R. Adams Cowley, MD, in the 1960s. From his observations in post–World War II Europe, and then in Baltimore, Dr. Cowley recognized that the sooner trauma patients reached definitive care—particularly if they arrived within 60 minutes of being injured—the better their chance of survival. The term has come to represent the critical first 60 minutes for many populations, with stroke being one of them.

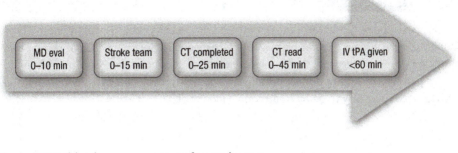

Figure 5.2 Golden hour components for stroke care.
IV, intravenous; tPA, tissue plasminogen activator.

In 1996, NINDS established ED-based stroke care time recommendations that have provided guidance and metrics for process improvement ever since. Some of the metrics have been adjusted since then as imaging and process improvement resulted in faster capabilities.

- Door to physician <10 minutes
- Door to stroke team <15 minutes
- Door to CT initiation <25 minutes, now <20 minutes
- Door to CT interpretation <45 minutes, now <30 minutes
- Door to drug (80%, now 85%) <60 minutes
- Door to stroke unit admission <3 hours

▶ INITIAL EVALUATION

The primary goal is to identify patients with possible stroke as well as to exclude stroke mimics. These steps are often accomplished as a team effort in the hallway or CT suite; in other words, the efforts undertaken during the golden hour do not follow a linear process.

- ABCs
- Stroke team notification—with prenotification by EMS, the stroke team is ready in the ED when the patient arrives
- Stat head CT
- Hand-off report from EMS
- Patient history—confirm LKW time, review medical history, particularly related to eligibility for therapeutic interventions
- Neurological assessment using a standardized tool such as National Institutes of Health Stroke Scale (NIHSS)
  - Standardized assessment tools can be performed rapidly and ensure consistency among healthcare providers.
- ECG to assess for concurrent myocardial ischemia or arrhythmias
- Oxygen saturation to assess for hypoxia and treatment if <94%
  - Blood tests are ideally drawn by EMS shortly before arrival to ED; otherwise, blood is drawn as early as possible in the ED without delaying treatment decisions (see Chapter 6 for the standard list of the blood tests).

● CLINICAL PEARL

Blood glucose is the only laboratory test required prior to thrombolytic treatment in AIS patients. Hypoglycemia is a common mimic of stroke, and correcting it alleviates the need for thrombolytic; hyperglycemia in stroke is an indicator of poor outcomes with thrombolytic. Abnormal platelets or international normalized ratio (INR) results are rare enough that they are not deemed necessary to delay treatment (Jauch et al., 2013).

▶ BLOOD PRESSURE MANAGEMENT

Numerous published studies have failed to demonstrate a consensus on a specific systolic blood pressure (SBP) or mean arterial pressure (MAP) for ischemic stroke, ICH, and subarachnoid hemorrhage (SAH). The following are general recommendations from the respective guidelines, but all agree that individual patient condition and comorbidities will affect optimal blood pressure (BP) parameters for each patient. See Chapter 8 for further discussion about BP management and cerebral autoregulation.

- Ischemic stroke:
  - Upper limit = 220/105 mmHg; antihypertensive medications should be given as ordered with close monitoring to determine whether goal was met, if there is need for more medication, or there is a need to address hypotension
  - Lower limit is based on patient's premorbid BP and current condition; care should be taken when administering an antihypertensive to not "overshoot" the goal, causing hypotension; swelling accompanies ischemic stroke, and perfusion of the ischemic penumbra is dependent on adequate BP
- Hemorrhagic stroke:
  - Upper limit for SBP:
    - SAH = 160 mmHg
    - ICH = 140 mmHg
  - Lower limit is based on patient's premorbid BP and current condition; care should be taken when administering an antihypertensive to not "overshoot" the goal, causing hypotension and decreased cerebral perfusion

▶ BLOOD SUGAR MANAGEMENT

- Recommendations vary as to specific target values for upper and lower limits.
- In ischemic stroke patients, optimum glucose range is 150 to 180 mg/dL.
  - This is especially important in patients who have received thrombolytics.
- Evidence indicates that sustained blood sugar levels greater than 200 mg/dL during the first 24 hours are associated with worse outcomes. See Chapter 8 for further discussion of effects/management of glucose levels.

▶ TEMPERATURE MANAGEMENT

- A temperature higher than 38 °C (100.4 °F) should be considered for treatment to achieve normothermia, as increased temperature is associated with worse outcomes. See Chapter 8 for discussion of effects/management of hyperthermia.

▶ THROMBOLYTIC ADMINISTRATION

Alteplase, also known as tissue plasminogen activator (tPA), was approved for use in AIS by the FDA in 1996. Tenectaplase (TNKase), a modified form of tPA, was approved for use in acute myocardial infarction in 2000 but not for stroke. It is being used by numerous stroke centers for their AIS patients due to it being a single IV push, with no hour-long infusion needed as with alteplase.

● CLINICAL PEARL

It has been estimated that each 15-minute reduction in DTN time results in an additional month of disability-free life after stroke (Middleton et al., 2015).

▶ INTRAVENOUS ADMINISTRATION

Eligibility criteria should be reviewed by the team. For a detailed list, see table 8 in Powers et al., 2019 (see references). The patient and/or family members should be informed of risks/benefits of thrombolytic therapy. Consider using a fact sheet to augment the verbal discussion.

- BP must be less than 185/110 mmHg prior to administration; consider having a second nurse to assist during the initial hour of stroke alert:
  - Ensures rapid setup, dose check, and administration of thrombolytic.
  - Rapid acquisition and administration of antihypertensive medication is needed if indicated.
  - Quicker establishment of a second IV site.
- Frequent neurological checks and vital sign documentation ensure early detection of any change in patient status; see Chapter 8 for the schedule to follow. If bleeding is noted, or angioedema is evident, discontinue the infusion, notify the provider, and monitor the patient for anaphylaxis.
- Alteplase administration guide
  - Dosage calculation: 0.9 mg/kg infused over 1 hour; 10% of dose to be administered as initial bolus over 1 minute
  - Total dose must never exceed 90 mg regardless of patient weight
- Tenecteplase administration guide
  - Dosage calculation: 0.25 mg/kg as IV bolus over 5 seconds
  - BP must be maintained <180/105 for first 24 hours postthrombolytic administration

● CLINICAL PEARL

Many terms are being used to refer to thrombectomy, or clot removal, in the cerebral arteries. Mechanical thrombectomy (MT) and endovascular thrombectomy (EVT) are the most common, but mechanical clot retrieval/removal, intra-arterial thrombectomy, and mechanical endovascular reperfusion (MER) are also used.

LVO refers to clots in either the carotid artery, the middle cerebral artery (MCA) including branches M1 and M2, or the vertebral and basilar arteries. No other cerebral arteries are reachable with the current devices.

▶ ACUTE ENDOVASCULAR INTERVENTION

In 2015, the positive outcomes of several clinical trials established MT as standard of care for AIS patients. With 30% of AIS patients in the United States having LVO, MT has become a valuable treatment option for prevention of severe disability and death.

- All patients with LVO should be considered for endovascular intervention regardless of whether they received IV thrombolytic or not
- Advanced imaging such as CT angiogram (CTA) or MR angiogram (MRA) provides location of the thrombus in the proximal portion of one of the major cerebral arteries
- Informed consent is needed, and having a fact sheet about endovascular intervention to augment the discussion with the patient and/or the family may be helpful
  - If the patient cannot consent and there is no legally authorized patient representative available, the procedure can be done as a current standard of care under the premise of emergency consent (Ashcraft et al., 2021)
- Time frame to begin the start of the procedure is within 24 hours from LKW
- Team members accompany the patient to the intervention suite; with the intervention team, they assess/document neurovascular check of limb intended for access to provide baseline for postprocedure checks
- After an endovascular intervention, the schedule for frequent neurological and vital sign checks is restarted from the time of the end of the procedure whether IV thrombolytic had been given or not
- Time goals have been established for ED arrival (door time) to skin puncture to drive efforts to expedite transport and decision times (Ashcraft et al., 2021)
  - 90 minutes for patients in the ED of intervention hospital
  - 60 minutes for patients transferred from another stroke center
- See Chapter 8 for more information regarding nursing care during and postendovascular intervention

▶ MECHANICAL RETRIEVAL DEVICES

- Penumbra system
  - Clot disruption and suction device in which a "separator" is threaded through the suction device and used to disrupt the clot; as pieces are broken loose, they are pulled back into the suction catheter; this process is repeated until the clot is removed
  - Recanalization success rate 52% to 86%
  - Received FDA approval in 2008

- Stent retrievers
  - Recommended by the American Heart Association/American Stroke Association Guidelines (Powers et al., 2019)
  - Mechanism is a self-expanding, stent-like device that is inserted into the blockage through a sheath; once the sheath is through the clot, it is withdrawn, releasing the stent, which expands, compressing the clot against the arterial wall; after several minutes (time allowed for the clot to become more engaged with the stent filaments), the device is collapsed and withdrawn, pulling the clot with it
  - Recanalization success rates reported as 70% to 92%
  - Received FDA approval in 2012

● CLINICAL PEARL

The Thrombolysis In Cerebral Infarction (TICI) grading system was described in 2003 by Higashida et al. as a tool to measure the success of the endovascular intervention for ischemic stroke and correlates with prognosis. Only grades 2B and 3 are considered to be successful outcomes.

Grade 0: No perfusion
Grade 1: Penetration with minimal perfusion
Grade 2: Partial perfusion
Grade 2A: Only partial filling (less than two-thirds) of the entire vascular territory is visualized
Grade 2B: Complete filling of all of the expected vascular territory is visualized, but the filling is slower than normal
Grade 3: Complete perfusion

▶ INTRA-ARTERIAL ADMINISTRATION

Intra-arterial thrombolytic therapy is not recommended as a first-line, stand-alone therapy by the American Heart Association/American Stroke Association Guidelines (Powers et al., 2019). It is still sometimes used as an adjunct therapy following mechanical retrieval.

▶ DOOR IN, DOOR OUT

- *Door in, door out (DIDO)* refers to the time from when a stroke patient arrives at a hospital until that patient is transferred out to a higher level of care, usually for thrombectomy or advanced stroke care like a hemicraniectomy.
  - This includes recognition of stroke symptoms, acute workup, consultation, and treatment with IV tPA if warranted, and preparation for transfer: arrange transportation, copy of records/imaging, family contact info
- Goal of 120 minutes has been identified by The Brain Attack Coalition (Alberts et al., 2013); STK-OP-1 (stroke measure, outpatient -1) is the reporting metric for PSCs and ASRHs.

▶ DYSPHAGIA SCREEN

A nursing bedside dysphagia screen differs from full evaluation performed by a speech and language pathologist (SLP).

- Aspiration pneumonia incidence is reduced when a screen is performed prior to any oral intake and nothing-by-mouth (NPO) status until a full evaluation can be performed by an SLP (Hinchey et al., 2005).
- Use of numerous tools has been reported with varying results.
  - The dysphagia screening measure was removed from the Get With the Guidelines stroke measures and retired from The Joint Commission performance standards in 2012 due to lack of clinical trials identifying an optimal screening tool.
- All experts agree that screening for dysphagia is important and *should* still be done to prevent aspiration and inadequate hydration/nutrition.
- The American Speech–Language–Hearing Association (ASHA) supports the utilization of a nursing screening process.
- Use of a water swallow trial has been found to be valid, but more research is needed.
- In the meantime, experts recommend that multidisciplinary teams continue to implement continuous quality improvement (CQI) processes to ensure optimal training for nurses who perform the dysphagia screens and to review outcomes data in their organization (Donovan et al., 2013).

▶ USE OF TELESTROKE (TELEMEDICINE)

- The term *telestroke* was first used in the 1990s to describe interactive telemedicine in acute stroke evaluation and intervention.
- Telestroke is recommended to increase access to acute stroke care in underserved areas.
  - A stroke–neurology expert can view and interact with the patient and the patient can view the care provider via two-way audio–video technology.
  - This technology provides expert consultation without "being there."
- Telestroke also facilitates initiation of interventions proven to reduce complications and stroke recurrence.
  - It is proven to shorten DTN time in patients receiving IV thrombolytic.
- Reduces transportation costs by providing remote specialty consultation while still in the patient's home community hospital and eliminates unnecessary transfers.

CLINICAL PEARL

Telestroke technology not only facilitates rapid identification and treatment/transport but also facilitates identification of patients for whom transfer is not indicated. Examples are stable, small-territory ischemic strokes that can be managed by the community hospital and devastating hemorrhagic strokes for which there is no acute intervention; comfort measures can be provided to these patients in the community hospital. Telestroke eliminates unnecessary, expensive transport, which has the benefit of controlling healthcare costs as well as saving the family from traveling a distance.

Ben Rowe, a 70-year-old man, is eating lunch with his wife at an outdoor café. He is telling her about his recent fishing trip and his biggest catch ever. He is excited, talking fast, and stumbling over his words. His wife asks him to slow down and notes that he's hesitating and some of the words don't make sense. They have had lemonade with their meal. His medical history includes hypertension and chronic obstructive pulmonary disease (COPD) for which he takes Lisinopril and uses an Albuterol inhaler. Against his wishes, she dials 911 and reports that his speech isn't right. It is 12:15 p.m.

1. What response can be expected from emergency medical services (EMS)?

    A. Recommendation that she call their primary care provider (PCP) for a same-day appointment
    B. Rapid arrival, quick exam using the Glasgow Coma Scale (GCS), and transport to the nearest stroke center
    C. Quick telehealth evaluation by the dispatcher to determine insurance and triage priority
    D. Rapid dispatch of Advanced Life Support (ALS), quick Cincinnati Prehospital Stroke Scale exam, and determination of last known well (LKW) time

2. The emergency medical services (EMS) personnel have also conducted a screen using the RACE tool, and it is positive. Which of the following actions is indicated next?

    A. Determine patient preference and expedite transport to that hospital
    B. Explain the need for advanced stroke intervention capability and transport them to the nearest acute stroke–ready hospital (ASRH), knowing that if imaging is positive, they can be transferred to a comprehensive stroke center (CSC)
    C. Explain the need for advanced stroke intervention capability and transport them to the nearest CSC or thrombectomy-capable stroke center (TSC)
    D. Explain that the RACE tool is not 100% accurate but offer to take them to a CSC if they wish

3. On arrival to hospital at 12:40 p.m., emergency medical services (EMS) find that the ED is busy, and they must wait 8 minutes until someone can take report. What did they fail to do that would have expedited treatment time?

    A. Use of lights and sirens that alerts receiving team of impending arrival
    B. Prearrival notification that alerts receiving team of expected arrival
    C. Prearrival survey of which hospital has shortest wait time
    D. Prearrival review of hospital capabilities to determine who is likely to have staff ready

1. D) Rapid dispatch of Advanced Life Support (ALS), quick Cincinnati Prehospital Stroke Scale exam, and determination of last known well (LKW) time

The use of a prehospital neurological assessment tool to rule out stroke as well as the determination of LKW time are proven to be critical actions by EMS. Same-day appointments with a PCP are not appropriate for people with new stroke symptoms. The use of the GCS provides no benefit in an emergent stroke evaluation. Insurance eligibility should be done prior to the hyperacute evaluation and transport, not through a telehealth evaluation.

2. C) Explain the need for advanced stroke intervention capability and transport them to the nearest CSC or thrombectomy-capable stroke center (TSC)

Even though none of the stroke severity assessment tools for large-vessel occlusion (LVO) determination have proven to be 100% accurate, it is recommended that a positive score warrants transport to a CSC or TSC, if available. With suspicion of LVO, a patient's preference toward a CSC or TSC should not take precedence. The use of LVO tools is designed to eliminate multiple stops/transfers; patients should be given clear guidance based on available evidence and not have it left up to them to decide.

3. B) Prearrival notification that alerts receiving team of expected arrival

The prearrival notification alerts the receiving ED team to be ready to expedite evaluation and treatment. Lights and sirens are not the appropriate mechanism to alert the receiving team. Wait times in the ED are not a concern with a prearrival notification, as these patients are expedited. ED staffing concerns are not the EMS providers' responsibility.

4. The ED personnel, on receiving report from emergency medical services (EMS) at 12:48 p.m., make the determination that which of treatment options are available for Mr. Rowe?

A. Intravenous (IV) thrombolytic only

B. IV thrombolytic and endovascular intervention

C. Endovascular intervention only

D. None of the above since the patient is on Lisinopril

5. What conditions need to be present for endovascular intervention to be an option?

A. Last known well (LKW) time under 24 hours and patent foramen ovale (PFO) noted on CT of head

B. LKW time under 4 hours and large-vessel occlusion (LVO) noted on CT angiogram (CTA)

C. LKW time under 24 hours and LVO noted on CTA

D. LKW time under 6 hours and arteriovenous malformation (AVM) noted on CTA

6. Mr. Rowe has a dry cough, and his wife brought over a bottle of water from the vending machine nearby, which the nurse finds her offering to him. The nurse's best action is which of the following?

A. Stop her, explaining that it must first be determined that he can swallow safely

B. Watch him take several big swallows, counting that as the dysphagia screen

C. Ask her if he choked on his beverage at lunch and, if not, let him drink the water

D. Stop her, explaining that she could have caused him to get pneumonia if he choked

(*See answers next page.*)

4. B) IV thrombolytic and endovascular intervention

Both IV thrombolytic and endovascular intervention are options for Mr. Rowe with a last known well (LKW) time under 60 minutes. Lisinopril has no impact on a patient's eligibility for acute stroke treatment.

5. C) LKW time under 24 hours and LVO noted on CTA

For patients with LVO noted on the CTA, endovascular intervention is considered for up to 24 hours from LKW time. Presence of a PFO or AVM has no impact on endovascular intervention eligibility.

6. A) Stop her, explaining that it must first be determined that he can swallow safely

A water swallow exam involves small sips with patient sitting as high as possible and only after careful evaluation by the nurse. Large swallows are not part of a nursing bedside swallow evaluation and put patients at risk for aspiration. Basing a patient's ability to swallow safely on a previous meal is not recommended. It is important to educate the wife on the necessity of having a screening done before the husband can drink safely while avoiding making the wife feel guilty.

1. The first patient of the day arrives with a blood pressure (BP) of 226/132 on presentation. Emergency medical services (EMS) report it had been 180's/90's enroute to the hospital. After double checking, the nurse can anticipate which orders?

   A. Monitor and notify provider if BP exceeds 220 systolic

   B. Stat continuous infusion of intravenous (IV) nicardipine, with rechecks within 5 to 10 minutes

   C. Stat administration of an oral angiotensin-converting enzyme (ACE) inhibitor, with rechecks every 5 to 10 minutes

   D. Stat administration of single-dose IV beta blocker, with recheck in 30 minutes

2. The benefit of telemedicine for smaller hospitals without neurology support would be which of the following?

   A. Support during infusion of IV tissue plasminogen activator (tPA) to monitor for vasospasm

   B. For communication with the family

   C. For remote neurology/neurosurgery evaluation and treatment recommendation

   D. For continuing education lectures by neurologists

3. The golden hour was first described in the trauma population. It is used in the stroke population with which purpose?

   A. Emergent stroke care should take 60 minutes for thorough evaluation

   B. To represent the first hour of patient symptoms

   C. To represent the best practice transport time for emergency medical services (EMS)

   D. To represent critical first 60 minutes of ED care

4. A patient's husband reports that she went to bed before him at 10 p.m. He went to bed at 2 a.m. and she was sleeping peacefully, but he was awakened by her at 6 a.m., mumbling something about her arm not working right. What is her last known well (LKW) time?

   A. 10 p.m.

   B. 6 a.m.

   C. 2 a.m.

   D. Unable to determine

5. Prehospital notification by emergency medical services (EMS) has been credited with which of the following?

   A. Improved relationship between EMS and ED

   B. Reduced incidence of misdiagnosis

   C. Reduced treatment time

   D. All of the above

(See answers next page.)

1. B) Stat continuous infusion of intravenous (IV) nicardipine, with rechecks within 5 to 10 minutes

IV antihypertensive is the quick action needed with such a high BP, and checks should be within 5 to 10 minutes. In case there is any acute treatment planned, allowing a BP up to 220 is inadvisable. ACE inhibitors are not recommended in the hyperacute treatment phase. Thirty minutes is too long an interval between dose and recheck; therefore, it is not advised to administer a single dose of an IV beta blocker, then recheck after 30 minutes.

2. C) For remote neurology/neurosurgery evaluation and treatment recommendation

For remote neurology/neurosurgery evaluation and treatment recommendation. Telemedicine refers to a two-way audio and video connection between two different locations. In stroke care, it is used to provide neurology/neurosurgery consult expertise to hospitals that do not have onsite consultants experienced with diagnosing and treating acute stroke. It is not used to monitor for vasospasm; telemedicine does enhance communication between the specialist and the family—if present—but it is not as valuable as evaluation and treatment recommendations; continuing education has been provided through telemedicine, but again the main benefit is the timely evaluation and treatment recommendation.

3. D) To represent critical first 60 minutes of ED care

The golden hour represents the critical first hour of ED care. It is not a guideline for how long an evaluation should take, it does not represent the first hour of symptoms, nor does it represent transport time for EMS.

4. A) 10 p.m.

The LKW time is the time the patient was awake and normal, so even though the husband was awake at 2 a.m., the patient was asleep, so there is no way of knowing if the stroke had occurred. Thus, her LKW time at the time she went to bed. 6 a.m. is the time her condition was discovered, but not the LKW time.

5. Reduced treatment time

Prehospital notification by EMS has been recognized as contributing to reduced door-to-imaging, reduced door-to-needle (DTN) time, and reduced interfacility transport times (Higashida et al., 2003), thus reducing overall treatment time. There is no evidence to support that it has improved relationships or reduced incidence of misdiagnosis.

6. Which of the following is a validated and standardized instrument for prehospital stroke screening?

    A. FAST (Face, Arm, Speech, Time)
    B. LAPSS (Los Angeles Prehospital Stroke Scale)
    C. CPSS (Cincinnati Prehospital Stroke Scale)
    D. All of the above

7. The difference between an emergency medical technician (EMT) and a paramedic is:

    A. An EMT is a volunteer, while a paramedic is a paid employee
    B. A paramedic receives roughly 10 times the training hours as an EMT
    C. An EMT can start intravenous fluids and give injections, while a paramedic cannot
    D. A paramedic can do the prehospital severity scale scoring, while an EMT cannot

8. Mrs. Brown's husband came in from milking the cows at 8:15 a.m. and found her unable to move her left arm and looking bewildered. He called 911 and reported she was fine when he had left the house at 7:00 a.m. He was shocked when a helicopter landed in his yard. Why would the dispatcher have sent a helicopter?

    A. All strokes are air transport–level now
    B. They suspected a large-vessel occlusion (LVO) from the husband's information
    C. The farm is located 50 miles from the closest hospital
    D. Roads were icy

9. Which of the following statements is true about the emergency medical services (EMS) system in the United States?

    A. All state EMS agencies follow a single stroke protocol
    B. All prehospital personnel are paid and regulated regarding education and competencies
    C. Stroke is a high-urgency call in all areas of the country
    D. Most state EMS are divided into regions/districts that function independently

10. Each 15-minute decrease in intravenous (IV) thrombolytic treatment delay results in:

    A. Better reimbursement for the hospital
    B. Lower risk of platelet deficiency
    C. More stable blood pressure over 24 hours
    D. One month of additional disability-free life after stroke

6. D) All of the above

FAST (Face, Arm, Speech, Time), LAPSS (Los Angeles Prehospital Stroke Scale), and CPSS (Cincinnati Prehospital Stroke Scale) are all tools that are validated and standardized instruments used by prehospital personnel.

7. B) A paramedic receives roughly 10 times the training hours as an EMT

Paramedics receive more education and can perform more critical care functions than an EMT. Not all EMTs are volunteers. Paramedics can start IVs and give injections, not EMTs. Both paramedics and EMTs can perform the prehospital stroke severity score.

8. C) The farm is located 50 miles from the closest hospital

Many state protocols have wording indicating that if travel and transport time will exceed 30 minutes, air transport should be considered. It is no longer just for interfacility transport. Not all strokes are transported by air. There was not enough information to warrant suspicion of LVO. Icy roads could be a factor; however, the distance and time to treatment are the chief considerations that warrant air transport.

9. D) Most state EMS are divided into regions/districts that function independently

Regions and districts usually divide EMS, and they tend to function independently of one another. Unfortunately, prehospital policies vary from one state to another, and most states even have regional variations. Some prehospital personnel are unpaid or underpaid. There are still some areas of the country where stroke is not a high-urgency call.

10. D) One month of additional disability-free life after stroke

Based on multiple research study data, it has been estimated that each 15-minute reduction in door-to-needle time results in an additional month of disability-free life after stroke. Reimbursement is not tied to treatment time. Timeliness of thrombolytic treatment is not associated with more stable blood pressure after treatment.

11. Which diagnostic study is the only required test prior to thrombolytic treatment in a 32-year-old female who has arrived 1 hour after onset of stroke symptoms, with a National Institutes of Health Stroke Scale (NIHSS) score 7 (arm weakness and sensory loss, aphasia) and no medical history?

   A. Chest x-ray (CXR)
   B. Head CT angiogram (CTA)
   C. Glucose
   D. Serum electrolytes

12. The air medical transport team's main responsibility when transporting an intracerebral hemorrhage (ICH) patient to a comprehensive stroke center is which of the following?

   A. Monitoring blood pressure (BP) and titration of antihypertensive drip to maintain systolic blood pressure (SBP) under 185 mmHg
   B. Monitoring neurological status and vitals for early signs of rising intracerebral pressure (ICP)
   C. Monitoring peripheral pulses in preparation for possible intervention
   D. Monitoring swallow ability and preparation for early antithrombotic dose

13. A patient dropped off at the ED by his husband, who then goes to park the car, is identified in triage as a suspected acute stroke. The CT scanner is occupied, and it takes 11 minutes until it is cleared, followed by another 8 minutes for three tries to get the intravenous (IV) site established. This is a perfect example of which of the following?

   A. The importance of spouses staying with the patient in the ED
   B. The need for a second CT scanner in the ED
   C. The need for a closer parking area for spouses
   D. The benefit of calling 911 and expediting the acute stroke workup process through prearrival notification

14. A patient tests positive for possible stroke using the Cincinnati Prehospital Stroke Scale. The nurse's next step will be which of the following?

   A. Provide prearrival notification to nearest hospital
   B. Raise head of the bed to 45 degrees and perform dysphagia screen
   C. Screen for possible large-vessel occlusion (LVO) utilizing the Cincinnati Prehospital Stroke Severity Scale
   D. Assess lung sounds to rule out atrial fibrillation (Afib)

15. A patient's CT angiography reveals aneurysmal subarachnoid hemorrhage (aSAH). A recheck of their blood pressure (BP) shows a rise to 178/86. What is the nurse's next action?

   A. Continue to monitor, knowing that 185/110 is the top limit
   B. Notify the provider and anticipate an order to administer labetalol 10 mg and repeat once with the goal of lowering the systolic blood pressure (SBP) to under 140
   C. Administer labetalol 40 mg every 15 minutes until SBP is below 160
   D. Notify the provider and anticipate an order to administer labetalol 10 mg and repeat once with the goal of lowering the SBP to under 160

11. C) Glucose
Glucose is the only test required prior to thrombolytic treatment. A CXR is no longer a standard part of most acute stroke workups. A head CTA is not done on all stroke patients and should not delay intravenous (IV) thrombolytic.

12. B) Monitoring neurological status and vitals for early signs of rising intracerebral pressure (ICP)
With a hemorrhagic stroke, the most important thing for the transport team is to monitor for signs of increasing ICP. The BP parameter for ICH is 140 mmHg systolic or lower. Peripheral pulses are to be noted, but not continually monitored. The swallow evaluation is important, but it is not as important as neurological monitoring. Early antithrombotic therapy is only for ischemic stroke patients.

13. D) The benefit of calling 911 and expediting the acute stroke workup process through prearrival notification
It has been proven in numerous studies that the quickest way to get a neurological evaluation for suspected acute stroke is through the emergency medical services (EMS) system. The spouse staying with the patient or having a closer parking spot serves no time benefit. While a second scanner would be beneficial, it is usually cost prohibitive.

14. C) Screen for possible large-vessel occlusion (LVO) utilizing the Cincinnati Prehospital Stroke Severity Scale
The Cincinnati Prehospital Stroke Severity Scale is one of several LVO tools used by emergency medical services (EMS) to determine presence of LVO that would further guide which hospital to transport the patient to. More information is needed to know which hospital to prenotify. Dysphagia screening is not an EMS priority, so it would be unnecessary to raise the head of the bed to 45 degrees. Afib is not detected through lung assessment.

15. D) Notify the provider and anticipate an order to administer labetalol 10 mg and repeat once with the goal of lowering the SBP to under 160
For aSAH, the goal is to keep the SBP under 160. The BP parameters of 185/110 are for ischemic stroke. Keeping the SBP below 140 is for intracerebral hemorrhage (ICH). A dose of 40 mg of labetalol is too high (Connolly et al., 2012).

16. The quality metrics for a hospital's stroke population have not improved over the past 2 years despite providing annual educational programs. What else could the nurse do to improve prehospital stroke care?

A. Mandatory monthly stroke education for all prehospital personnel

B. Allowance of blood pressure (BP) control measures in all ambulances and helicopters

C. Support for paramedics administering intravenous (IV) thrombolytic prior to CT in select patients

D. Patient-specific feedback and quality metrics compliance provided to transport teams

17. Door in, door out (DIDO) is a concept that requires quality improvement measures and reporting for which level of stroke center?

A. Acute stroke–ready hospital (ASRH) and primary stroke center (PSC)

B. ASRH only since they seldom admit stroke patients

C. PSC only since ASRH seldom get stroke patients

D. Thrombectomy-capable stroke center (TSC) and comprehensive stroke center (CSC)

18. Tenecteplase has gained favor over alteplase among some stroke centers for what reason?

A. It is more cost-effective due to saving the cost of tubing and intravenous (IV) pump

B. It is reimbursed at twice the amount of alteplase

C. It simplifies and expedites transfer to higher level of care

D. It has demonstrated no side effects or complications

19. For what reason would a nurse not treat a blood pressure (BP) of 190/90 in an ischemic stroke patient in the ED?

A. Aggressive treatment could cause hypotension, which could threaten the penumbra

B. Inability to find a manual cuff to confirm accuracy of monitor readings

C. Aggressive treatment could cause hypotension and severe headache

D. Inability to secure drug from pharmacy within 30 minutes

20. Which endovascular intervention has the greatest likelihood of resulting in Thrombolysis In Cerebral Infarction (TICI) 3 outcome?

A. Intra-arterial thrombolysis

B. Merci device

C. Penumbra system

D. Stent retriever

16. D) Patient-specific feedback and quality metrics compliance provided to transport teams

Prehospital personnel have reported that getting patient-specific feedback on outcomes and compliance with quality metrics has provided them valuable information on which to base expectations and accountability. It has also raised the level of interest in stroke. Mandatory stroke education has not been found to improve engagement. BP control measures allowed by emergency medical services (EMS) vary considerably from state to state. IV thrombolytic is never administered without a CT.

17. A) Acute stroke–ready hospital (ASRH) and primary stroke center (PSC)

DIDO refers to the time spent in the ED of either ASRH or PSC prior to transfer to higher level of care such as a TSC or CSC.

18. C) It simplifies and expedites transfer to higher level of care

As a single bolus, tenecteplase does not require an IV pump, which makes preparation for transfer by emergency medical services (EMS) much simpler and quicker. The costs of tubing and IV pump are minimal compared to the cost of the drug. Tenecteplase has not yet been approved for use in stroke, even though tenecteplase shows slightly fewer side effects and complications when compared to alteplase (Zitek et al., 2020).

19. A) Aggressive treatment could cause hypotension, which could threaten the penumbra

In acute ischemic stroke management without thrombolytic or thrombectomy, allowing systolic blood pressure (SBP) up to 220 is recommended in order to avoid hypotension, particularly in patients with a history of hypertension. It is not acceptable for the inability to find a manual cuff or inability to secure the drug from pharmacy to be a reason to not treat a BP of 190/90 in an ischemic stroke patient. A severe headache would not result from lowering the BP.

20. D) Stent retriever

Stent retrievers have shown superior outcomes compared to intra-arterial thrombolysis, merci devices, and penumbra systems, and are specifically recommended in the American Heart Association/American Stroke Association guidelines.

⬤ REFERENCES

Adeoye, O., Nystrom, K., Yavagal, D., Luciano, J., Nogueira, R., Zorowitz, R., Khalessi, A. A., Bushnell, C., Barsan, W. G., Panagos, P., Alberts, M. J., Tiner, A. C., Schwamm, L. H., & Jauch, E. (2019). Recommendations for the establishment of stroke systems of care: A 2019 update. *Stroke*, *50*(70), e187–e210. https://doi.org/10.1161/STR.0000000000000173

Alberts, M. J., Latchaw, R. E., Jagoda, A., Wechsler, L. R., Crocco, T., George, M. G., Connolly, E. S., Mancini, B., Prudhomme, S., Gress, D., Jensen, M. E., Bass, R., Ruff, R., Foell, K., Armonda, R. A., Emr, M., Warren, M., Baranski, J., & Walker, M. D. (2011). Revised and updated recommendations for the establishment of primary stroke centers: A summary statement from the Brain Attack Coalition. *Stroke*, *42*(9), 2651–2665. https://doi.org/10.1161/STROKEAHA.111.615336

Alberts, M., Wechsler, L., Jensen, M., Latchaw, R., Crocco, T., George, M., Baranski, J., Bass, R. R., Ruff, R. L., Huang, J., Mancini, B., Gregory, T., Gress, D., Emr, M., Warren, M., & Walker, M. (2013). Formation and function of acute stroke–ready hospitals within a stroke system of care: Recommendations from the Brain Attack Coalition. *Stroke*, *44*(12), 3382–3393. https://doi.org/10.1161/STROKEAHA.113.002285

American Heart Association. (2019). *Target: Stroke Phase III suggested time intervals goals.* https://www.heart.org/-/media/files/professional/quality-improvement/target-stroke/target-stroke-phase-iii/9-17-update/final-door-to-device-best-practice-one-pager

American, Heart Association. (2020). *American Heart Association Mission Lifeline: Stroke Severity-based Stroke Triage Algorithm for EMS.* https://www.heart.org/HEARTORG/Professional/MissionLifelineHomePage/MissionLifeline-Stroke_UCM_491623_SubHomePage.jsp

Ashcraft, S., Wilson, S., Nystrom, K., Dusenbury, W., Wira, C., & Burrus, T. (2021). on behalf of the American Heart Association Council on Cardiovascular and Stroke Nursing and the Stroke Council. Care of the patient with acute ishemic stroke (prehospital and acute phase of care): update to the 2009 comprehensive nursing care scientific statement: a scientific statement from the American Heart Association. *Stroke*, *52*(5), e1–e15. https://doi.org/10.1161/STR.0000000000000356

Connolly Jr, E. S., Rabinstein, A. A., Carhuapoma, J. R., Derdeyn, C. P., Dion, J., Higashida, R. T., Hoh, B. L., Kirkness, C. J., Naidech, A. M., Ogilvy, C. S., Patel, A. B., Thompson, G., & Vespa, P. (2012). Guidelines for the management of aneurysmal subarachnoid hemorrhage: A guideline for healthcare professionals from the American Heart Association/American Stroke Association. *Stroke*, *43*(6), 1711–1737. https://doi.org/10.1161/STR.0b013e3182587839

Donovan, N. J., Daniels, S. K., Edmiaston, J., Weinhardt, J., Summers, D., & Mitchell, P. H. (2013). Dysphagia screening: State of the art: Invitational conference proceeding from the State-of-the-Art Nursing Symposium, International Stroke Conference 2012. *Stroke*, *44*(4), e24–e31. https://doi.org/10.1161/STR.0b013e3182877f57

Higashida, R. T., Furlan, A. J., & the Technology Assessment Committees of the American Society of Interventional and Therapeutic Neuroradiology and the Society of Interventional Radiology. (2003). Trial design and reporting standards for intra-arterial cerebral thrombolysis for acute ischemic stroke. *Stroke*, *34*(8), e109–e137. https://doi.org/10.1161/01.STR.0000082721.62796.09

Hinchey, J., Shephard, T., Furie, K., Smith, D., Wang, D., & Tonn, S. (2005). Formal dysphagia screening protocols prevent pneumonia. *Stroke*, *36*(9), 1972–1976. https://doi.org/10.1161/01.STR.0000177529.86868.8d

Jauch, E. C., Saver, J. L., Adams, H. P., Bruno, A., Connors, J. J., Demaerschalk, B. M., Khatri, P., McMullan Jr, P. W., Qureshi, A. I., Rosenfield, K., Scott, P. A., Summers, D. R., Wang, D. Z., Wintermark, & Yonas, H, M. (2013). Guidelines for the early management of patients with acute ischemic stroke: A guideline for healthcare professionals from the American Heart Association/American Stroke Association. *Stroke, 44*(3), 870–947. https://doi.org/10.1161/STR.0b013e318284056a

Michael S. Gordon Center for Research in Medical Education. (2017). *Advanced stroke life support.* http://www.asls.net/about_introduction.php

Middleton, S., Grimley, R., & Alexandrov, A. (2015). Triage, treatment, and transfer: Evidence-based clinical practice recommendations and models of nursing care for the first 72 hours of admission to hospital for acute stroke. *Stroke, 46*(2), e18–e25. https://doi.org/10.1161/STROKEAHA.114.006139

Powers, W. J., Rabinstein, A. A., Ackerson, T., Adeoye, O. M., Bambakidis, N. C., Becker, K., Biller, J., Brown, M., Demaerschalk, B. M., Hoh, B., Jauch, E. C., Kidwell, C. S., Leslie-Mazwi, T. M., Ovbiagele, B., Scott, P. A., Sheth, K. N., Southerland, A. M., Summers, D. V., & Tirschwell, D. L. (2019). Guidelines for the early management of patients with acute ischemic stroke: A guideline for healthcare professionals from the American Heart Association/American Stroke Association. 2019 update to the 2018 guidelines for the management of acute ischemic stroke. *Stroke, 50*(12), e344–e418. https://doi.org/10.1161/STR.0000000000000211

Southerland, A. M., Johnston, K. C., Molina, C. A., Selim, M. H., Kamal, N., & Goyal, M. (2016). Suspected large vessel occlusion: Should emergency medical services transport to the nearest primary stroke center or bypass to a comprehensive stroke center with endovascular capabilities? *Stroke, 47*(7), 1965–1967. https://doi.org/10.1161/STROKEAHA.115.011149

Virani, S. S., Alonso, A., Aparicio, H. J., Benjamin, E. J., Bittencourt, M. S., Callaway, C. W., Carson, A. P., Chamberlain, A. M., Cheng, S., Delling, F. N., Elkind, M. S. V., Evenson, K. R., Ferguson, J. F., Gupta, D. K., Khan, S. S., Kissela, B. M., Knutson, K. L., Lee, C. D., Lewis, T. T., & ... Tsao, C. W. (2021). Heart disease and stroke statistics—2021 update: A report from the American Heart Association. *Circulation, 143*(8), e254–e743. https://doi.org/10.1161/CIR.0000000000000950

Zitek, T., Ataya, R., & Brea, I. (2020). Using tenecteplase for acute ischemic stroke: What is the hold up? *Western Journal of Emergency Med, 21*(2), 199–202. https://doi.org/10.5811/westjem.2020.1.45279

Stroke Diagnostics

Time is brain, so during an acute stroke workup, diagnostic tests must be prioritized carefully in order to maximize their value without compromising brain tissue viability. Blood glucose, tested via a finger stick by prehospital personnel, is a valuable diagnostic test that can differentiate hypoglycemia-induced symptoms from those produced by cerebral ischemia. Brain imaging is the first line of diagnostics once the patient arrives in the ED in order to clarify the cause of neurological symptoms. For most organizations, a noncontrast computed tomographic (NCCT) scan is the imaging done emergently to rule out hemorrhage, detect and measure the ischemic tissue, and exclude other possible mimics of stroke (neoplasm, multiple sclerosis, etc.). The emergence of artificial intelligence (AI) software has significant potential to reduce decision-making time, thus speeding up treatment processes. An ECG and blood tests are done soon after to provide other critical information to facilitate rapid treatment decisions. An echocardiogram is done during the first 24 to 48 hours of hospitalization, and, depending on the patient's presentation, other diagnostics, such as lumbar puncture, transcranial Doppler (TCD), chest x-ray, EEG, and hypercoagulable lab tests, may be performed.

● BRAIN IMAGING

- **CT scan**
  - The first CT scans were done in 1971; *tomography* is from the Greek words *tomos*, meaning *slice* or *section*, and *graphia*, meaning *describing*.
  - **CT without contrast (noncontrast CT, also known as NCCT)**
    - This is a first-line diagnostic due to its speed and availability as compared to an MRI (Latchaw et al., 2009).
    - NCCT is the gold standard for detection of intracerebral hemorrhage and is superior to lumbar puncture in detection of subarachnoid hemorrhage (SAH).
  - **CT angiography**
    - CT angiography (CTA) depicts the occlusion site and vessel details, helps grade collateral blood flow, and helps characterize carotid atherosclerotic disease.
    - **CTA is used for patients with acute ischemic stroke (AIS) within 6 hours last known well (LKW) time.**
    - Requires use of contrast material.
  - **CT perfusion**
    - CT perfusion (CTP) delineates the ischemic tissue (penumbra) from infarcted tissue (core) by showing decreased cerebral blood flow (CBF), increased mean transit time, and normal or increased cerebral blood volume (CBV).
    - CTP is used for patients with AIS within a 6- to 24-hour window with large-vessel occlusion (LVO) in anterior circulation.
    - Requires use of contrast material.

> ### ⬤ CLINICAL PEARL
>
> Due to the emergent nature of AIS and the value of rapid imaging, it is recommended that if LVO is suspected and patient has no history of renal impairment, to proceed with CTA before obtaining serum creatinine (Powers et al., 2018).

- **MRI**
  - MRI was first done in 1977; it uses an intense magnetic field to produce images rather than the radiation used in traditional radiographic studies.
  - Patients with metal implants (pacemakers, pumps, or shunts) or history of welding are not able to have magnetic resonance tests.
  - **Diffusion weighted imaging**
    - Diffusion weighted imaging (DWI) measures changes in diffusion properties of water in brain tissue.
    - Restricted diffusion generally indicates unsalvageable brain tissue that is destined for infarction.
    - DWI is accurate for detecting ischemia within minutes of occurrence.
    - It differentiates acute infarcts from older infarcts.
    - DWI does not require contrast material.
  - **Magnetic resonance angiography**
    - Magnetic resonance (MR) angiography (MRA) is similar to CTA; both the blood flow and the condition of the blood vessel walls can be seen with this study.
    - MRA is useful in detecting carotid artery dissection, intracranial aneurysms, and arteriovenous malformations (AVMs).
    - Does not require contrast material.
  - **MR perfusion**
    - Similar to CTP, MR perfusion (MRP) demonstrates CBF, mean transit time, and CBV.
    - Requires use of contrast material.
  - **MR venography**
    - MR venography (MRV) is similar to MRA, but the technology is used only to visualize veins.
    - Requires use of contrast material.
  - **High-resolution or vessel-wall MRI**
    - This provides visualization of the plaque components in vessels.
  - **Susceptibility-weighted imaging**
    - Susceptibility-weighted imaging (SWI) assesses oxygen saturation and the presence of cerebral microbleeds.

> ### ⬤ CLINICAL PEARL
>
> In brain imaging, the term *angio* refers to blood vessels, so a CTA or MRA utilizes contrast agents and visualizes the vasculature. The term *perfusion* refers to the adequacy of the blood supply to the brain tissue.

ARTIFICIAL INTELLIGENCE

The term *artificial intelligence (AI)* refers to the use of computer software to perform tasks usually done by humans, often completed more quickly with AI facilitation. With brain imaging being the most critical tool in acute treatment decisions, time delays associated with human processes and interpretation can be costly to the patients. The following are some of the positive impacts AI has had on the field of stroke care:

- Detection of key imaging characteristics such as LVO, hemorrhage, and salvageable and unsalvageable tissue.
- Makes images available via app-based technology, allowing multiple team members to view images simultaneously from their smartphone or tablet.
- Valuable for nonthrombectomy-capable stroke centers like acute stroke–ready hospitals (ASRHs) and primary stroke centers (PSCs) in quickly identifying those with LVO who warrant transfer out:
  - Provides better selection of high-risk patients who need higher level of care, so fewer transfers out; able to keep more stroke patients without LVO.
- Studies have shown a significant 45% reduction in door-in door-out (DIDO) time, and a 11.4% improvement in modified Rankin Scale (mRS) scores (Duraes, 2021).
- Useful in predicting long-term functional outcomes based on acute imaging (Mouridsen et al., 2020).

CEREBRAL ANGIOGRAPHY, AKA DIGITAL SUBTRACTION ANGIOGRAPHY

- Cerebral angiography visualizes the blood vessels using fluoroscopy and contrast material.
- It requires access through a large artery—usually the femoral artery; a catheter is threaded up past the heart to the cerebral vasculature.
- Cerebral angiography is the standard against which all noninvasive assessments are compared.

CAROTID DUPLEX

- Carotid duplex is a noninvasive ultrasound technology used for assessment of the carotid artery.
- It uses no contrast material.
- It has a lower sensitivity for detection of abnormality than CTA, MRA, or digital subtraction angiography (DSA), and so has essentially been replaced in acute stroke care.

TRANSCRANIAL DOPPLER

- TCD is a noninvasive ultrasound technology used to assess most large cerebral arteries (middle cerebral artery [MCA], anterior cerebral artery [ACA], carotid siphon, vertebral artery, basilar artery, and ophthalmic artery).

- It is approached mainly via the temporal bone acoustic window (the area of thin bone above the zygomatic arch).
- It is used to detect and quantify intracranial stenosis, occlusion, collateral flow, embolic events, and cerebral vasospasm (particularly after SAH), as well as the response to thrombolytic therapy.

LUMBAR PUNCTURE

- Lumbar puncture is used in cases of suspected SAH in which imaging does not show blood.
- Cerebrospinal fluid (CSF) is analyzed for the presence of blood products.
- Headache is experienced by 10% to 30% of patients due to leakage of CSF from the dura.

ECHOCARDIOGRAM

- Cardioembolic sources are responsible for up to 30% of all strokes, hence the need for echocardiography.
- **Transthoracic echocardiogram**
  - This is done on most ischemic stroke patients.
  - Transthoracic echocardiogram (TTE) is excellent for identifying ventricular abnormalities such as dyskinetic wall segment.
- **Transesophageal echocardiogram**
  - Transesophageal echocardiogram (TEE) is done in those patients in whom a cardiac source is strongly suspected.
  - It requires passage of a transducer catheter down the esophagus.
  - TEE's visualization of the heart is superior because there is no impedance from chest muscles or the rib cage.
  - TEE is superior at identifying atrial and aortic abnormalities, such as patent foramen ovale or aortic arch atherosclerosis.

ECG

- ECG is done on all stroke patients as part of the initial workup, but not prior to acute treatment decision.
- It is used to identify atrial fibrillation, coexisting acute myocardial infarction (MI), cardiac arrhythmias, or chronic cardiac disease that may predispose to embolic sources.

CHEST RADIOGRAPHY

- Chest radiography (CXR) may be done during the initial workup but should not interfere with rapid evaluation and treatment decisions.

EEG

- EEG measures brain waves through several electrical leads attached to the scalp.
- EEG is not routinely used for stroke diagnosis but may be done to rule out or monitor seizure activity.

LABORATORY TESTS

- Glucose is the only lab result that must precede the initiation of intravenous thrombolytic. It is often obtained through point-of-care (POC) finger stick, either by prehospital personnel or by ED personnel.
- For those patients on anticoagulants, the international normalized ratio (INR) must also be determined. It can be measured in many EDs.
- All acute stroke patients should have the following tests:
  - Blood glucose, electrolytes, blood urea nitrogen (BUN), creatinine, complete blood count (CBC) with platelets, troponin, INR, and partial thromboplastin time (PTT).
- Select patients may also require the following tests:
  - Liver function panel, toxicology screen, blood alcohol level, pregnancy test, HIV test, and arterial blood gas.
- During the hospital stay, all acute stroke patients should have the following tests: hemoglobin A1C and lipid profile (Powers et al., 2018).

Ms. Achebe is traveling with her partner from out of state and has arrived at the ED at 6 p.m. with symptoms of facial droop, aphasia, and right arm weakness. Emergency medical services (EMS) reports her last known well (LKW) time to be 5:20 p.m., blood pressure (BP) 170/87, heart rate (HR) 98, temp 36 °C (96.8 °F), and positive large-vessel occlusion (LVO) using the RACE tool (Rapid Arterial oCclusion Evaluation). She is 44 years old with no past medical history. She proudly tells the nurse that she does not take any medications and has no drug allergies.

1. The diagnostic test that would be reported by emergency medical services (EMS) is which of the following?

   A. Serum creatinine
   B. CT angiography (CTA)
   C. Blood glucose
   D. Partial thromboplastin time (PTT)

2. The next diagnostic test to be done in Ms. Achebe workup would be which of the following?

   A. Noncontrast CT (NCCT)
   B. Complete blood count (CBC)
   C. ECG
   D. Chest radiography (CXR)

3. The neurologist agrees with emergency medical services (EMS) that there is likely a large-vessel occlusion (LVO) in the proximal middle cerebral artery (MCA). What is the next step diagnostically?

   A. Proceed with CT angiography (CTA) and notify the intervention suite team
   B. Stat point-of-care (POC) creatinine prior to contrast for CTA
   C. Proceed with magnetic resonance angiography (MRA) and notify the intervention suite team
   D. Check with the partner to determine if she really has no past medical history

1. C) Blood glucose

Blood glucose is the only lab required prior to thrombolysis and resulted by EMS. EMS may draw lab specimens for a variety of labs, including serum creatinine and PTT, but they would not be resulted for report on arrival. Even if she were brought on a mobile stroke unit that has a CT scanner, a CTA would not have been completed.

2. A) Noncontrast CT (NCCT)

NCCT is the priority over a CBC, an ECG, and a CXR because it is the only diagnostic test that will expedite treatment decisions, given the patient presentation.

3. A) Proceed with CT angiography (CTA) and notify the intervention suite team

With no history of renal insufficiency, it is recommended to proceed with a CTA without checking renal status. MRA is not indicated for emergent LVO evaluation. A negative past medical history does not impact an emergent treatment decision.

1. The benefits of artificial intelligence (AI) in acute stroke care include everything except which of the following?

   A. Information on which thrombectomy device to use
   B. Ability to view images from wherever the team member is
   C. Information on amount of salvageable tissue
   D. Ability to keep more stroke patients at primary stroke centers

2. In reviewing a patient's progress notes, the nurse knows that they must have had a CT angiogram (CTA) by which statement?

   A. Evidence of hypodensity involving 40% of the right frontal lobe
   B. Evidence of hemorrhage in left basal ganglia
   C. Evidence of 70% stenosis distal left internal carotid
   D. Evidence of uncal herniation

3. A 28-year-old female has arrived at the ED having been found at the gym with severe aphasia and right-sided weakness; there is no one to provide a medical history at this time. Which diagnostic tests would be added to her workup?

   A. Glucose tolerance and liver function
   B. Sedimentation rate and specific gravity
   C. Pregnancy and tox screen
   D. Arterial blood gas and pituitary hormone level

4. An inadequate temporal bone acoustic window might be a barrier for which diagnostic test?

   A. Transesophageal echocardiogram (TEE)
   B. Positron emission tomography (PET)
   C. Magnetic resonance venography (MRV)
   D. Transcranial Doppler (TCD)

5. For carotid imaging, name a circumstance in which a carotid duplex would be done rather than a CT angiogram (CTA).

   A. Patient has multiple contrast allergies
   B. Patient has severe cervical dystonia
   C. Patient has complex carotid vascular anatomy
   D. Patient has limited time available for test

(See answers next page.)

1. A) Information on which thrombectomy device to use

AI software does not make recommendations of type of device to use for thrombectomy, only that there is a large-vessel occlusion (LVO) along with salvageable tissue. The benefits of AI include the ability to view images from anywhere, detailed information on the salvageable tissue, and the ability to better select who would benefit from transfer to a higher level.

2. C) Evidence of 70% stenosis distal left internal carotid

A CTA uses contrast to view vessel details, like the degree of stenosis. Therefore, an evidence of 70% stenosis distal left internal carotid would indicate that a CTA was used. Evidence of hypodensity involving 40% of the right frontal lobe, evidence of hemorrhage in left basal ganglia, and evidence of uncal herniation would all be visible from a noncontrast CT (NCCT) and would not prove that a CTA was used.

3. C) Pregnancy and tox screen

Considering the patient's age and inability to provide information, a pregnancy test and toxicology screen are most likely. In the hyperacute setting, glucose tolerance, liver function, sedimentation rate, specific gravity, arterial blood gas, and hormone level are not useful.

4. D) Transcranial Doppler (TCD)

TCD involves ultrasound technology through the temporal bone acoustic window; if inadequate (common in older women), it may affect ability to perform the test as well as accuracy of results. A TEE, PET scan, and MRV are not done through the temporal window; therefore, an inadequate temporal bone acoustic window will have no effect on the diagnostic test.

5. A) Patient has multiple contrast allergies

A CTA requires contrast material, whereas a carotid duplex does not; therefore, allergies are to be considered when conducting a CTA, posing as a potential barrier to the test. Cervical dystonia would be more of a barrier for carotid duplex than a CTA. The complexity of vascular anatomy would likely indicate the need for a CTA rather than a carotid duplex. A CTA is quicker than carotid duplex; thus, it would be more likely in the event of a time constraint.

6. Which vascular imaging test is the "gold standard" against which others are compared?

   A. Transcranial Doppler (TCD)
   B. Magnetic resonance angiography (MRA)
   C. CT angiography (CTA)
   D. Digital subtraction angiography (DSA)

7. Which diagnostic test would not be done for a patient with a pacemaker?

   A. CT scan
   B. MRI
   C. EEG
   D. Chest radiography (CXR)

8. A lumbar puncture has been ordered for a stroke patient whose CT scan showed no abnormality. What are they looking for?

   A. Blood in the cerebrospinal fluid (CSF)
   B. Air in the CSF
   C. Cloudy CSF
   D. Reduced CSF pressure

9. CT perfusion (CTP) is useful in differentiating which of the following?

   A. Gray matter from white matter
   B. Penumbra from core
   C. Hyperperfused from hemorrhagic
   D. Hypodense from hyperdense

10. Would a patient teaching differ between transthoracic echocardiogram (TTE) and transesophageal echocardiogram (TEE)? If so, how?

   A. No, they both involve lying flat for 6 hours afterwards
   B. Yes, TTE usually requires premedication with antihistamine
   C. Yes, TEE usually involves copious use of conduction gel
   D. Yes, TEE usually results in sore throat

(See answers next page.)

6. D) Digital subtraction angiography (DSA)

DSA, also known as cerebral angiography, continues to be the most highly regarded vascular imaging tool; however, its invasive nature, and the relative ease of the CTA, limits its use in the emergent setting. The CTA, MRA, and TCD are not considered the gold standard of vascular imaging.

7. B) MRI

MRI involves strong magnets that could cause damage to the implanted device or displace it. There are no contraindications for patients with pacemakers to have CT scan, EEG, or CXR.

8. A) Blood in the cerebrospinal fluid (CSF)

If the stroke is suspected to be subarachnoid hemorrhage (SAH), but not visualized on the CT scan, a lumbar puncture is done to look for blood in the CSF. Air in the CSF, a cloudy CSF, and reduced CSF pressure would all be noted with lumbar puncture, but they are not the reason it is done in the hyperacute phase.

9. B) Penumbra from core

CTP delineates the ischemic area (penumbra) from the already infarcted area (core). Gray/white matter differentiation and density are seen on noncontrast CT (NCCT). There is no such thing as hyperperfusion from hemorrhage. Hypo- versus hyperdense tissue is measured on an NCCT.

10. D) Yes, TEE usually results in sore throat

Because of passing the transducer down the esophagus in a TEE, patients often experience a sore throat postprocedure. Neither test requires lying flat afterward or premedication with antihistamine. It is a TTE, not a TEE, that would involve conduction gel.

⬤ REFERENCES

Duraes, J. (2021). *New data on stroke care show the impact of Viz.ai's artificial intelligence-powered platform on patient outcomes.* Viz.ai. https://www.viz.ai/press-release/new -data-on-stroke-care-show-the-impact-of-viz-ais-artificial-intelligence-powered -platform-on-patient-outcomes

Latchaw, R. E., Alberts, M. J., Lev, M. H., Connors, J. J., Harbaugh, R. E., Higashida, R. T., Hobson, R., Kidwell, C. S., Koroshetz, W. J., Mathews, V., Villablanca, P, Warach., S, & Walters, B. (2009). Recommendations for imaging of acute ischemic stroke: A scientific statement from the American Heart Association. *Stroke, 40*(11), 3646–3678. https://doi .org/10.1161/STROKEAHA.108.192616

Mouridsen, K., Thurner, P., & Zaharchuk, G. (2020). Artificial intelligence applications in stroke. *Stroke, 51*(8), 2573–2579. https://doi.org/10.1161/STROKEAHA.119.027479

Powers, W. J., Rabinstein, A. A., Ackerson, T., Adeoye, O. M., Bambakidis, N. C., Becker, K., Biller, J., Brown, M., Demaerschalk, B. M., Hoh, B., Jauch, E. C., Kidwell, C. S., Leslie-Mazwi, T. M., Ovbiagele, B., Scott, P. A., Sheth, K. N., Southerland, A. M., Summers, D. V., & Tirschwell, D. L. (2018). 2018 guidelines for the early management of patients with acute ischemic stroke: A guideline for healthcare professionals from the American Heart Association/American Stroke Association. *Stroke, 49*(3), e46–e99. https://doi.org/10.1161/STR.0000000000000158

Neurological and Functional Assessment and Severity Scores

The ability to do a thorough neurological assessment is a key skill of a stroke-certified nurse. The combination of these abilities enables the nurse to (a) correlate the findings on the assessment with the areas of the brain affected and (b) anticipate what changes to be vigilant for in the assessment over the next 24 to 48 hours.

The neurological status of a patient with a new stroke can change in an instant and often fluctuates. Close monitoring is essential, but inconsistencies in terminology and assessment technique can make it difficult to track patient status. The use of standardized neurological examination and documentation tools ensures that major components of the neurological examination are accomplished efficiently and consistently.

Severity scores impact healthcare more than most bedside nurses realize. Hospital quality indicators, such as mortality rate, complication rate, and length of stay, have been difficult to compare among various levels of stroke centers and all other hospitals that do not have essential details about the severity of the stroke. Comprehensive stroke centers (CSCs), by design, will care for the most complex stroke patients who may not meet the criteria for higher "severity of illness" under the current system. Therefore, when unadjusted outcomes are compared, comprehensive centers may appear to provide inferior care due to higher complication and mortality rates in the more complex patients.

Clinically, the use of standardized severity scores provides an efficient, consistent assessment method that produces a score that can be utilized in handoff reports, in daily progress monitoring, and in discharge planning.

● CLINICAL PEARL

A good stroke-relevant neurological assessment starts at the head and progresses down to the feet. This consistent pattern facilitates accuracy and completeness. While the Glasgow Coma Scale (GCS) is simpler than the National Institutes of Health Stroke Scale (NIHSS), it provides minimal information and its use is NOT recommended in acute stroke (Green et al., 2021). With the GCS, it is possible for an awake patient with hemiplegia to earn a "perfect 15" while unable to move half of their body.

● STROKE-RELEVANT NEUROLOGICAL ASSESSMENT

▶ NATIONAL INSTITUTES OF HEALTH STROKE SCALE

The NIHSS has become the standard for nursing stroke assessment (Green et al., 2021).
- It was created in 1983 by the National Institute of Neurological Disorders and Stroke (NINDS; Exhibit 7.1).
- It provides a quantifiable score that is more objective than the GCS.

- It is used in eligibility consideration for thrombolysis and endovascular therapy.
- It is used for both ischemic and hemorrhagic stroke patients.
- Score range is 0 to 42; points are earned for deficits: the higher the score, the greater the deficits.
- NIHSS predicts the severity of injury and correlates with patient outcome.
  - Eighty percent of patients with an NIHSS less than 12 to 14 have good or excellent outcomes; only 20% of patients with an NIHSS score greater than 20 to 26 have good or excellent outcomes.
    - An NIHSS score greater than 22 on admission indicates a 17% higher risk of hemorrhagic conversion after administration of intravenous (IV) thrombolytic.
- NIHSS predicts discharge disposition.
  - Score less than or equal to 5 indicates likely discharge to home.
  - Score of 6 to 13 indicates likely discharge to acute rehabilitation facility.
  - Score greater than 13 indicates likely discharge to nursing home.
- Use of the full version is recommended—use of the shortened version, the modified NIHSS (mNIHSS), increases risk of false-negative results.

There is no standard schedule for when the NIHSS should be done; many organizations do it at the following transitions: change of shift, transition to another unit, or in response to a new neurological change. It is done as a joint assessment between the nurse handing off the patient and the nurse accepting the patient.

Exhibit 7.1 National Institutes of Health Stroke Scale Sheet.

NIH STROKE SCALE	Neuro A&P Correlation
LOC: 0 = Alert 1 = Drowsy 2 = Obtunded 3 = Unresponsive	LOC
LOC to questions: *Ask patient month and age.* 0 = Both correct 1 = One correct 2 = Neither correct	LOC
LOC to commands: *Open, close eyes; make fist, let go; substitute other one step command if needed.* 0 = Obeys both correctly	LOC
Best gaze: *Eyes open, patient follows examiner's fingers or face horizontally. Only test horizontal gaze.* 0 = Normal 1 = Partial gaze palsy 2 = Forced deviation	CN III, VI

NIH STROKE SCALE	Neuro A&P Correlation
Visual: *Face patient, hold hand out at edge of visual field, display 1, 2, or 5 fingers. Have patient report how many fingers he or she sees. Do this in all 4 visual-field quadrants. Use your visual field as baseline for normal. Alternative: wiggle finger at edge of visual field and bring in until patient sees it.* 0 = No visual loss 1 = Partial hemianopsia 2 = Complete hemianopsia 3 = Bilateral hemianopsia	CN II
Facial palsy: *Show teeth, raise eyebrows, and squeeze eyes shut.* 0 = Normal 1 = Minor asymmetry 2 = Partial (lower face paralysis) 3 = Complete unilateral paralysis	CN VII/Motor
Motor arm—left: *Elevate extremity 45 degrees for 10 seconds and score drift/movement.* 0 = No drift 1 = Drift before 10 seconds 2 = Falls before 10 seconds 3 = No effort against gravity (falls immediately) 4 = No movement	Motor
Motor arm—right: *Elevate extremity 45 degrees for 10 seconds and score drift/movement.* 0 = No drift 1 = Drift before 10 seconds 2 = Fails before 10 seconds 3 = No effort against gravity (falls immediately) 4 = No movement	Motor
Motor leg—left: *Elevate extremity 30 degrees for 5 seconds and score drift/movement.* 0 = No drift 1 = Drift before 5 seconds 2 = Falls before 5 seconds 3 = No effort against gravity (falls immediately) 4 = No movement	Motor
Motor leg—right: *Elevate extremity 30 degrees for 5 seconds and score drift/movement.* 0 = No drift 1 = Drift before 5 seconds 2 = Falls before 5 seconds 3 = No effort against gravity (falls immediately) 4 = No movement	Motor

(*continued*)

Exhibit 7.1 National Institutes of Health Stroke Scale Sheet (*continued*).

NIH STROKE SCALE	Neuro A&P Correlation
Limb ataxia: *Finger to nose: Hold your finger up for patient to see, have patient take his or her finger and touch his or her nose, then touch your finger, and repeat a few times. Heel down shin: Help patient place heel of unaffected side on upper shin of affected side and slide heel down shin. Do same on both sides. Score only if inability to perform task is out of proportion to patient's weakness. If score >1 on motor, do not score ataxia for that limb.* 0 = Absent 1 = Present in upper or lower 2 = Present in both upper and lower	Cerebellar
Sensory: *Sensation or grimace to pinprick to face, arm, trunk, and leg compared side to side. Use proximal portion of limbs. Score only sensory loss attributable to stroke, not preexisting loss (diabetic neuropathy, etc.). Alternative method: Use cold sensation like metal of stethoscope, pen, penlight, etc.* 0 = Normal 1 = Mild—Patient feels pinprick/coldness, but it is dull compared to other side 2 = Patient not aware of being touched	Sensory
Best language: *Name items, describe a picture, or read sentences. Can have patient name simple items like pen, neck tie, glasses, TV, and so on; looking for inability to name objects or inability to comprehend.* 0 = No aphasia 1 = Mild to moderate aphasia 2 = Severe aphasia 3 = Mute	Speech/Language
Dysarthria: *Evaluate speech clarity by patient repeating words; ask intubated patients to write words.* Suggested words: Mama, Tip-top, Fifty-fifty, Thanks, Huckleberry, Baseball player. Sentences: You know how. Down to earth. I got home from work. Near the table in the dining room. 0 = Normal articulation 1 = Mild to moderate slurring—can be understood with some difficulty 2 = Severe—near unintelligible or mute	Cerebellar

NIH STROKE SCALE	Neuro A&P Correlation
Extinction and inattention (neglect): *Have patient close eyes. Touch one side at a time, have patient indicate which side is being touched. Touch both sides simultaneously and assess patient's response. Next, hold hands out at edge of visual fields, wiggle fingers, have patient say when he or she sees fingers wiggle.* 0 = Normal, no neglect 1 = Partial neglect (mild hemi-attention) 2 = Profound neglect (does not recognize stimulation, or orients to only one side)	Sensory
Key: Score 1–5: Anticipate discharge to home—patient may require outpatient services 6–13: Anticipate discharge to acute rehab >13: Anticipate discharge to extended care facility	

A&P, anatomy and physiology; CN, cranial nerve; LOC, level of consciousness; NIH, National Institutes of Health; NIHSS, National Institutes of Health Stroke Scale.
Source: Adapted from National Institute of Neurological Disorders and Stroke. (2013). *NIH Stroke Scale.* Retrieved from https://stroke.nih.gov/documents/NIH_Stroke_Scale.pdf

⬤ CLINICAL PEARL

Although studies have shown that an increase or decrease of 4 points in the NIHSS indicates important changes in the patient's neurological status, it is the content of the neurological exam changes that determines the necessity for notification of the provider. Therefore, nursing care protocols should NOT base notification of the provider on the 4-point change alone. A patient with loss of arm strength, with no other changes, will only have an increase of 3 points but warrants action by the healthcare team.

▶ NEURO CHECKS

For the more frequent routine neurological checks done post thrombolytic or endovascular intervention, or on an hourly basis in the ICU, the NIHSS is not used. Instead, an abbreviated group of assessments is done that is generally referred to as a neuro check. The most basic checks involve reviewing the status of the presenting symptoms and the previous neuro checks. Unfortunately, there is still no evidence-based standardized content for neuro checks. The following is a neuro check that is generally used but which varies between institutions:

- Level of consciousness and cognition—This is the first to change when there is trouble and includes the appropriateness of patient's responses, as well as orientation to person, place, and time.
- Pupils—Size, symmetry, reactivity to light, and whether consistent with prior exam; abnormalities are due to cranial nerve (CN) II involvement.

- Arm and leg strength—Abnormalities are due to motor fiber involvement, either cortical (motor strip) or subcortical (basal ganglia).
- Coordination and balance—Ataxia is utilized in most assessments with finger-to-nose test for upper extremities and heel-to-shin test for lower extremities; abnormalities are due to cerebellar involvement.
- Sensation—Test ability to feel a stimulation (pin prick, cold metal pen, firm touch, noxious stimuli for minimally conscious or unconscious patient) as well as comparing right to left side (patient's eyes are closed); abnormality is due to sensory fiber involvement, either cortical (sensory strip) or subcortical (basal ganglia).

Extinction is sometimes included in a neuro check and is part of the NIHSS. It is the toughest aspect of neuro assessment for nurses to reliably score. Extinction is a result of dysfunction of the right parietal lobe, characterized by an inability to be aware of stimulation on the affected side when the stimulation is presented simultaneously on right and left sides. It can be tactile, visual, auditory, or spatial.

- Tactile: Assessment can be accomplished during the sensation assessment by applying stimulation simultaneously to both sides (patient's eyes are closed); if the patient had reported normal sensation when each side had been individually stimulated, but then only reports feeling one side when simultaneously stimulated, the patient has tactile extinction.
- Visual: Assessment can be accomplished during visual field assessment by presenting visual stimulation simultaneously to both sides.
- Auditory: Assessment is accomplished by providing simultaneous sound stimulation to both ears.
- Spatial: Assessment is accomplished by (a) asking the patient to describe what they see in their surroundings, (b) observing the patient's eating pattern (do they only eat food on the right side of the plate?), (c) having the patient read (do they only read the right half of the page?), or (d) having the patient draw a clock (do they only draw the right side of the clock face?).

▶ CRANIAL NERVE ASSESSMENT

CN assessment can seem daunting and has been identified as a barrier to nurses working in neuroscience roles. Table 7.1 details practical tips to assess the CN in a few minutes.

There are many mnemonics to help us remember the names of the 12 CNs. One of the most common—and socially acceptable—is **O**n **O**ld **O**lympus **T**owering **T**op **a** **F**inn **a**nd **G**erman **V**iewed **S**ome **H**ops.

- **O**lfactory
- **O**ptic
- **O**culomotor
- **T**rochlear
- **T**rigeminal
- **A**bducens
- **F**acial
- **A**uditory (vestibulocochlear)
- **G**lossopharyngeal
- **V**agus
- **S**ensory
- **H**ypoglossal

Table 7.1 The Cranial Nerve Assessment

Cranial Nerve	Function	Testing Technique
I. Olfactory	Sensory—smell	Can you smell this? Use coffee or mint.
II. Optic	Sensory—visual acuity, visual fields, pupillary reactions	Can you see this? Use Snellen chart or visual confrontation.
III. Oculomotor	Motor—extraocular movement	Follow my finger. Test extraocular movement.
IV. Trochlear	Motor—extraocular movment	Look down and in toward your nose.
V. Trigeminal	Both—facial sensation, jaw movement, corneal reflexes	Touch each cheek. Clench your teeth. Touch cornea with wisp of cotton.
VI. Abducens	Motor—extraocular movement	Look out to the side.
VII. Facial	Both—facial movement, sense of taste	Smile, raise your eyebrows, keep eyes and lips closed while you try to open them.
VIII. Vestibulocochlear (acoustic)	Sensory—hearing and balance	Can you hear this? Crinkle paper at the ear.
IX. Glossopharyngeal	Both—swallowing, gag reflex, sense of taste	Depress back of tongue with tongue depressor. Ask them to swallow.
X. Vagus	Both—swallowing, gag reflex voice and speech	Hoarse? Open up and say "ahh."
XI. Spinal accessory	Motor—shrugging shoulders, turning head	Shrug the shoulders and turn head from side to side.
XII. Hypoglossal	Motor—movement and protrusion of tongue	Stick out the tongue, look for deviation.

But how do we remember what each of them does? The answer is the CN face (Figure 7.1; Bolek, 2006).

⬤ FUNCTIONAL ASSESSMENT

In addition to the NIHSS, other examples of functional scores are the modified Rankin Scale (mRS) and Barthel Index (BI).

▶ MODIFIED RANKIN SCALE

- The mRS is ideally done at admission, basing the score on pre-event status, and at discharge from acute care; it is also done at strategic points along the recovery continuum.
- The purpose of the preadmission status score is to provide a functional baseline for discharge planning.
- The purpose of the discharge score is to establish functional status.
- The calculation of change from prehospital score indicates the effect of the stroke.

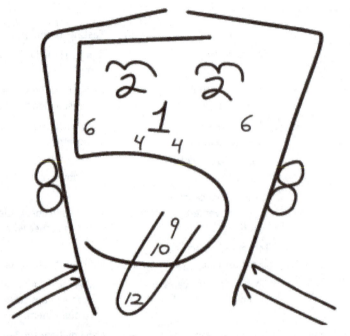

Figure 7.1 Cranial nerve face.

The next time you're trying to remember the locations and functions of the cranial nerves, picture this drawing. All 12 cranial nerves are represented, though some may be a little harder to spot than others. For example, the shoulders are formed by the number "11" because cranial nerve XI controls neck and shoulder movement. If you immediately recognize that the sides of the face and the top of the head are formed by the number "7," you're well on your way to using this memory device.

Source: Copyright © 2021. HealthCom Media. Used with permission. All rights reserved. myamericannurse.com

- Population scores (mean, median, and range) are representative of each stroke-type outcome.
- It continues to be the most widely used outcomes measure.
- Score range is 0 (fully independent) to 6 (dead).
  - Score of 5: Indicates severe disability; patient is bedridden, incontinent, and requires constant nursing care and attention.
    - This is the highest possible score for patients being discharged alive.
  - Score of 4: Indicates moderately severe disability; patient is unable to walk without assistance and unable to attend to activities of daily living (ADLs) without assistance.
  - Score of 3: Indicates moderate disability; patient requires some help but can walk without assistance.
  - Score of 2: Indicates slight disability; patient is unable to carry out all of their previous activities but can look after their affairs without assistance.
  - Score of 1: Indicates no significant disability despite symptoms; patient can carry out all usual duties and activities.
  - Score of 0: Indicates no symptoms are present.

▶ BARTHEL INDEX

- The BI is ideally done close to hospital discharge and then at intervals during the post-discharge period.
- It measures the patient's performance in 10 ADLs: feeding, bathing, grooming, dressing, bowels, bladder, toilet use, transfers, mobility, and stairs.
  - Each category is scored as 0, 5, or 10, with 0 = dependent and 10 = independent.
    - Total score range is 0 (totally dependent) to 100 (fully independent).
  - Score of more than 60 is considered compatible with good outcomes/ability to live at home.

⬤ CLINICAL PEARL

Functional scores differ from severity scores in that they have been demonstrated to provide a measure of functional ability, or independence, whereas the severity scores are utilized to determine not only the amount of deficit but also the risk for mortality. The NIHSS and mRS are unique in that they have been utilized as both a severity score and a functional score.

⬤ SEVERITY SCORES

Severity scores are considered required reporting for CSCs and thrombectomy-capable stroke centers (TSCs). Both the NIHSS and the mRS are utilized both as functional scores and severity scores. The other severity scores are described below. While the remaining scores are generally scored by providers, stroke nurses who understand what the scores indicate will have a better idea of prognosis for their patients.

▶ INTRACEREBRAL HEMORRHAGE SCORES

- Original intracerebral hemorrhage (ICH) score and modified ICH (mICH) score (Table 7.2).

Table 7.2 Intracerebral Hemorrhage and Modified Intracerebral Hemorrhage Components

ICH	mICH
Glasgow Coma Scale 3–4 = 2 points 5–12 = 1 point 13–15 = 0 points	NIHSS
Age >80 = 1 point	Admission temperature
ICH volume ≥30 = 1 point	Pulse pressure
IVH = 1 point	IVH
Infratentorial origin of hemorrhage = 1 point	Subarachnoid extension of hemorrhage

ICH, intracerebral hemorrhage; IVH, intraventricular hemorrhage; mICH, modified ICH; NIHSS, National Institutes of Health Stroke Scale.

- Utilized for ICH patients (Cheung & Zou, 2003).
- Research has found the ICH and mICH are equivalent in predicting outcomes.
- Recent research suggests that a score at 24-hours posthemorrhage may be more accurate than the admission score.

▶ SUBARACHNOID HEMORRHAGE SCORES

- Hunt and Hess score (Table 7.3)
  - Most used severity scale for the subarachnoid hemorrhage (SAH) population (Rosen & MacDonald, 2005).
  - Based on patient's level of consciousness and accompanying symptoms.
  - Initially established for surgical risk prediction.
  - Eighty percent correlation with outcomes at 6 months poststroke.
- Fisher Scale score (Table 7.4)
  - Based on amount/location of blood present on initial CT scan.
  - Correlation to outcomes has been demonstrated.
- World Federation of Neurosurgical Societies (WFNS) score (Table 7.5)
  - Based on GCS score and presence/absence of motor deficit.
  - Correlation to outcomes is less well demonstrated than Hunt and Hess.

Table 7.3 Hunt and Hess Score Components

Asymptomatic, mild headache, slight nuchal rigidity	1
Moderate to severe headache, nuchal rigidity, no neurological deficit other than cranial nerve palsy	2
Drowsiness/confusion, mild focal neurological deficit	3
Stupor, moderate to severe hemiparesis	4
Coma, decerebrate posturing	5

Table 7.4 Fisher Scale Score Components

No hemorrhage evident	1
SAH less than 1 mm thick	2
SAH more than 1 mm thick	3
SAH of any thickness with intraventricular hemorrhage or parenchymal extension	4

SAH, subarachnoid hemorrhage.

Table 7.5 World Federation of Neurosurgical Societies Score Components

Grade	GCS	Motor Deficit
I	15	−
II	14–13	−
III	14–13	+
IV	12–7	+/−
V	6–3	+/−

GCS, Glasgow Coma Scale.

▶ ABCD2 SCORE

- Acronym stands for:
  - <u>A</u>ge
  - <u>B</u>lood pressure (BP)
  - <u>C</u>linical features
  - <u>D</u>uration of symptoms
  - <u>D</u>iabetes
- Established to predict short-term risk of stroke in patients with transient ischemic attack (TIA; 7 days post TIA; Johnston et al., 2007).
- Effective in distinguishing true TIAs from mimics such as dizziness and altered level of consciousness.
- Utilized in the ED to determine whether admission is advised (score 4 or higher) or patient may be discharged with outpatient workup (score <4); range of score is 0 to 7 (Table 7.6).
  - 1 to 3 = low risk
  - 4 to 5 = moderate risk
  - 6 to 7 = high risk

Table 7.6 ABCD2 Score Components

Age >60 years	1
Elevated BP systolic ≥140; diastolic ≥90	1
Diabetes	1
Unilateral weakness	2
Speech impairment	1
Symptom duration	
≥60 minutes	2
10–59 minutes	1
<10 minutes	0
Total possible score	7

ABCD2, Age, Blood pressure, Clinical features, Duration of symptoms, and Diabetes; BP, blood pressure.

▶ CHA₂DS₂-VASc SCORE

- Acronym stands for:
  - <u>C</u>ardiac failure
  - <u>H</u>ypertension history
  - <u>A</u>ge >75—gets 2 points, therefore the subtext 2
  - <u>D</u>iabetes history
  - <u>S</u>troke/TIA/thromboembolism history—gets 2 points, therefore the subtext 2
  - <u>V</u>ascular disease history (prior myocardial infarction [MI], peripheral artery disease, or aortic plaque)
  - <u>A</u>ge 65 to 74
  - <u>S</u>ex <u>c</u>ategory—female

- Used for atrial fibrillation stroke risk assessment to guide medical therapy.
  - Score 0: All patients with atrial fibrillation will be prescribed at least an antithrombotic.
  - Score of 1 or greater: Strong consideration for oral anticoagulation.
    - If the score of 1 is due to gender alone, anticoagulant therapy is not warranted.
- More inclusive of common stroke risk factors and modifiers than previous version, $CHADS_2$, which only included the first five components of the CHA_2DS_2-VASc score— Cardiac failure, Hypertension history, Atrial fibrillation history, Diabetes history, and Stroke/TIA/thromboembolism history.

Dr. Shah is a 32-year-old veterinarian with no known prior medical history (PMH). He was admitted 3 days ago with sudden onset left-sided weakness and difficulty finding the right words to say; modified Rankin Scale (mRS) was 0 and National Institutes of Health Stroke Scale (NIHSS) score was 8 on admission. He received intravenous (IV) thrombolytic within 90 minutes of last known well (LKW) time. He is one of the nurse's four patients on the stroke unit.

1. During daily rounds, the social worker asks what his prestroke functional status was. Which score provides this information?

   A. Modified Rankin Scale (mRS)

   B. National Institutes of Health Stroke Scale (NIHSS)

   C. Hunt and Hess

   D. World Federation of Neurosurgical Societies (WFNS)

2. During the National Institutes of Health Stroke Scale (NIHSS) assessment, the nurse notes partial gaze palsy. Which cranial nerve (CN) would be involved with this?

   A. CN XI

   B. CN IX

   C. CN III

   D. CN I

3. Which of the following would be consistent with him having had a stroke, rather than a transient ischemic attack (TIA)?

   A. Documented ABCD2 score of 2

   B. Heart rhythm monitoring

   C. Order for hemoglobin (Hgb) A1C

   D. Barthel Index (BI) score of 85

1. A) Modified Rankin Scale (mRS)
The mRS score done on admission reflects the pre-event functional status. The NIHSS represents deficits resulting from the event. Hunt and Hess and WFNS are only scored on subarachnoid hemorrhage (SAH) stroke patients.

2. C) CN III
CN III controls extraocular movements, and dysfunction would result in gaze palsy. CN XI, the accessory nerve, is involved in shoulder shrug. CN IX, the glossopharyngeal nerve, is involved in the gag reflex. CN I, the olfactory nerve, is responsible for the sense of smell.

3. D) Barthel Index (BI) score of 85
BI is a functional assessment score. A score of 100 indicates full independence, and a score of 85 indicates deficit, which would not be present in a TIA. ABCD2 score indicates the risk of a TIA patient having a subsequent stroke. Heart rhythm does not provide diagnostic information regarding TIA versus stroke. Hgb A1C is important in secondary prevention of both TIA and stroke.

1. While performing the q 12 hours National Institutes of Health Stroke Scale (NIHSS) on a patient, the nurse finds that they continue to have right arm and leg weakness, for which 3 points each are scored. The patient's left arm and leg are normal, as are the previous areas tested so far. What is the most appropriate next action?

   A. Skip ataxia portion, as the patient's weakness is so great as to make the ataxia exam untestable
   B. Stop the scoring session immediately and notify the provider that the patient's NIHSS score has risen from 4 to 6 since last exam 12 hours ago
   C. Get second opinion from fellow nurse to see if they agree with the finding
   D. Proceed to ataxia portion, testing only the left arm and leg

2. What is the rationale for Bell's palsy to be considered a mimic of acute stroke?

   A. It is a dysfunction of cranial nerve (CN) XIII and results in dysphagia
   B. It is a dysfunction of CN VII and results in facial droop
   C. It is a dysfunction of CN VII and results in tactile extinction
   D. It is a dysfunction of the basal ganglia and results in diplopia

3. The Glasgow Coma Scale (GCS) score is utilized in calculating which of the following scores?

   A. Intracerebral hemorrhage (ICH) score
   B. Fisher Scale score
   C. Barthel Index (BI) score
   D. Hunt and Hess score

4. An ICU patient is 36 hours postthrombectomy. Their blood pressure (BP) is 155/80, their heart rate (HR) is 76, and they are awake and alert. What form of neuro assessment would the nurse be performing and on what schedule?

   A. National Institutes of Health Stroke Scale (NIHSS) q 30 minutes
   B. Neuro check q 1 hour
   C. Glasgow Coma Scale (GCS) q 1 hour
   D. Neuro check q 30 minutes

5. The content of which of the following is not an evidence-based tool, but is used widely in stroke assessment?

   A. Barthel Index (BI)
   B. World Federation of Neurosurgical Societies (WFNS) score
   C. Modified Rankin Scale (mRS) score
   D. Neuro check

(See answers next page.)   **115**

1. D) Proceed to ataxia portion, testing only the left arm and leg

NIHSS ataxia testing rules indicate that ataxia is scored only if the inability to perform the task is out of proportion to the weakness. If weakness is >2 on motor exam, ataxia of that limb cannot be scored. The patient scored 3 on their right limbs. The ataxia portion should be skipped entirely, only in their affected limbs. The weakness is not new, and so does not warrant stopping and notifying the provider. A second opinion is not necessary, as the exam hasn't changed.

2. B) It is a dysfunction of CN VII and results in facial droop

Bell's palsy results from damage to CN VII, which would result in facial droop. Dysphagia could be the result of dysfunction of five of the CNs (V, VII, IX, X, and XI), but not CN VIII, which brings sound information to the brain. Tactile extinction is the result of dysfunction of the right parietal lobe. Diplopia is the result of CN III or IV dysfunction, not basal ganglia, which controls speech, movement, and posture.

3. A) Intracerebral hemorrhage (ICH) score

The GCS is one of the components of the ICH score and the World Federation of Neurosurgical Societies (WFNS) score. The Fisher Scale is based on imaging. The BI is based on components of activities of daily living (ADLs). The Hunt and Hess is based on presenting symptoms.

4. B) Neuro check q 1 hour

This patient is >24 hours postthrombectomy and is stable; the schedule including every (q) 30 mini assessments has passed. Stable ICU patients are assessed q 1 hour or q 2 hours. The GCS is not recommended for routine neurological assessments in stroke.

5. D) Neuro check

There has been no established evidence-based content for neuro checks; however, they are a recognized integral part of poststroke frequent assessments. The BI, WFNS, and mRS have been well established through research.

6. Which of these statements regarding admission National Institutes of Health Stroke Scale (NIHSS) scores is NOT true?

   A. Admission score of ≤5 indicates likely discharge to rehab
   B. Admission score >22 indicates a 17% higher risk of hemorrhagic conversion after administration of intravenous (IV) thrombolytic
   C. Admission score is done on both ischemic and hemorrhagic patients
   D. Admission score is used in determining eligibility for intervention

7. A patient is being discharged home. Their modified Rankin Scale (mRS) score changed from 0 on admission to 4 at discharge. What discharge instructions does the nurse anticipate providing?

   A. Outpatient information for driving evaluation
   B. Homecare and PT/OT consult information
   C. List of area nursing homes
   D. Vocational rehab consult information for return to work

8. Besides the extinction portion of the National Institutes of Health Stroke Scale (NIHSS) exam, in what other portion might the nurse pick up on extinction?

   A. Motor leg
   B. Visual fields
   C. Limb ataxia
   D. Dysarthria

9. Which hemorrhagic severity score was initially developed to determine surgical risk but has become a reliable tool for estimating outcomes?

   A. Modified intracerebral hemorrhage (mICH) score
   B. Fisher Scale
   C. Hunt and Hess score
   D. World Federation of Neurosurgical Societies (WFNS) score

10. Which treatment would be warranted for Elaine Wells, a 74-year-old woman with new-onset atrial fibrillation and a history of heart failure and diabetes?

    A. Antithrombotic with score of 4
    B. Anticoagulant with score of 7
    C. None is warranted
    D. Anticoagulant with score of 4

(See answers next page.)

6. A) Admission score of ≤5 indicates likely discharge to rehab

An admission NIHSS score of ≤5 indicates likely discharge to home, not rehab. An admission score is used in determining eligibility for intervention and is done on both ischemic and hemorrhagic patients. A score of above 22 indicates a 17% higher risk of hemorrhagic conversion after the administration of IV thrombolytic.

7. B) Homecare and PT/OT consult information

An mRS score of 4 indicates moderate to severe disability, with inability to walk unassisted or take care of activities of daily living (ADLs) without help. Driving and return to work will be much later in recovery. Since the patient had a prearrival mRS score of 0, the nurse would anticipate an acute rehab hospital stay rather than a nursing home.

8. B) Visual fields

When assessing the visual fields, the nurse can observe visual extinction. An example of this is if the patient does not notice one side during a simultaneous simulation (wiggle fingers, etc.). Motor exam, limb ataxia, and dysarthria assessments do not provide evidence of extinction.

9. C) Hunt and Hess score

The Hunt and Hess score is the most used subarachnoid hemorrhage (SAH) score and was developed to help stratify surgical risk. The mICH is an intracerebral hemorrhage (ICH) severity score, and with virtually no emergent surgery being done on ICH, it is not used to determine surgical risk. The Fisher Scale is used to predict vasospasm after SAH. The WFNS score is utilized as a severity tool and is not correlated as successfully with surgical risk as the Hunt and Hess score.

10. D) Anticoagulant with score of 4

Using the CHA_2DS_2-VASc tool, she scores 4 (heart failure, diabetes, age 74, female). A score greater than 2 warrants anticoagulant.

REFERENCES

Bolek, B. (2006). Facing cranial nerve assessment. *American Nurse Today*, 1(2), 21–22. https://www.myamericannurse.com/wp-content/uploads/2006/11/ant11-CranialNerves-1026.pdf

Cheung, R. T. F., & Zou, L.-Y. (2003). Use of the original, modified, or new intracerebral hemorrhage score to predict mortality and morbidity after intracerebral hemorrhage. *Stroke*, 34(7), 1717–1722. https://doi.org/10.1161/01.STR.0000078657.22835.B9

Green, T. L., McNair, N. D., Hinkle, J. L., Middleton, S., Miller, E. T., Perrin, S., Power, M., Southerland, A. M., Summers, D. V., the American Heart Association Stroke Nursing Committee of the Council on Cardiovascular and Stroke Nursing, & the Stroke Council. (2021). Care of the patient with acute ischemic stroke (posthyperacute and prehospital discharge): Update to 2009 comprehensive nursing care scientific statement: A scientific statement from the American Heart Association. *Stroke*, 52(5), e179–e197. https://doi.org/10.1161/STR.0000000000000357

Johnston, S. C., Rothwell, P. M., Nguyen-Huynh, M. N., Giles, M. F., Elkins, J. S., Bernstein, A. L., & Sidney, S. (2007). Validation and refinement of scores to predict very early stroke risk after transient ischaemic attack. *Lancet*, 369(9558), 283–292. https://doi.org/10.1016/S0140-6736(07)60150-0

National Institute of Neurological Disorders and Stroke. (2013). *NIH Stroke Scale*. https://stroke.nih.gov/documents/NIH_Stroke_Scale.pdf

Rosen, D. S., & MacDonald, R. L. (2005). Subarachnoid hemorrhage grading scales: A systematic review. *Neurocritical Care*, 2, 110–118. https://doi.org/10.1385/NCC:2:2:110

Acute Stroke Care

Since 1997, stroke units—where the nurses and providers are educated and competent in providing the unique care required by stroke patients—have proven to produce better outcomes: patients who received care there are more likely to be alive, independent, and living at home 1 year after their stroke. A stroke unit is not necessarily a geographically distinct hospital unit, but an area with a defined group of beds, staff, equipment, and protocols that are used for the care of acute stroke patients and is the location where the majority of stroke patients are cared for in that facility. The stroke unit may or may not have an ICU incorporated within it—many operate as step-down units. This chapter focuses on the care aspects of all stroke patients in the hospital—whether in the stroke unit or the ICU.

Neuroscience nursing in the ICU is focused on identifying subtle changes in a patient's condition that can have a significant impact on patient outcome. Frequent bedside assessments are often supplemented with advanced neurological monitoring and testing capabilities. Neuroscience nurses in the ICU are detectives who piece together a puzzle by relying on accurate assessments and monitored values to identify changes that may negatively impact the patient. Neurological changes can be quite subtle, and neuroscience nurses at all levels must be knowledgeable, competent, keenly observant, and responsive to subtle changes.

CLINICAL PEARL

Every neurological assessment done should not just be recorded but also compared to the previous assessment as well as to the patient's baseline. This best nursing practice will facilitate trending and pattern identification.

ASSESSMENT

- There is no specific guideline outlining assessment schedules other than for postintravenous (IV) thrombolysis and acute endovascular intervention patients. The schedule for the rest of the stroke patients is determined by each organization and is usually based on care level.
  - ICU—every hour
  - Transitional or intermediate care unit—every 2 hours
  - Stroke unit or general neuroscience unit—every 4 hours
- Bedside handoff is essential and should include a joint neurological assessment to ensure consistency.
  - Cranial nerve assessment should be included in nurses' neurological assessments (see Chapter 7), especially for patients with a posterior fossa stroke since most of the cranial nerves originate in the brainstem.
- Continuous cardiac monitoring along with frequent vital sign checks and nursing assessments are routine expectations.
  - Increased frequency of assessments may be used to monitor for signs of deterioration related to conditions such as increasing cerebral edema or reperfusion syndrome.

- Level of consciousness (LOC) is the first indicator of a neurological change.
- Tips for assessing the unconscious patient:
  - Before interacting with the patient, take a minute to observe them.
    - Note any spontaneous movements and whether the patient's movements appear to be intentional, like pulling at the nasogastric (NG) tube, monitor leads, or endotracheal tube.
    - Note the patient's breathing pattern and, if ventilated, look for spontaneous breathing.
    - Note whether they appear restless even without being stimulated.
  - Pause sedation if possible; this is sometimes called a *sedation vacation* and is done with provider order.
    - This allows for accurate assessment of the patient's actual neurological status.
  - When noxious stimulation is warranted to determine response level, consider varying the methods to produce the least amount of bruising.
    - Sternal pressure instead of sternal rub
    - Trapezius pinch, not a twist
    - Supraorbital pressure

BLOOD PRESSURE MANAGEMENT

Close blood pressure (BP) management is a nursing responsibility with great potential to positively impact the patient's ultimate functional recovery. Conversely, if BP is not well managed, it will likely pose a detriment to the recovery process.

- When systemic BP is too high, the blood–brain barrier may be disrupted, resulting in increasing cerebral edema, hemorrhagic transformation, or expansion of hemorrhagic stroke.
  - Patients with chronic hypertension and sustained hypertension are especially predisposed to these complications.
- When systemic BP is too low or reduced dramatically, perfusion pressure may be inadequate for the penumbra, resulting in extension of the infarct or loss of the penumbra.
  - Patients with chronic hypertension are especially susceptible and are at risk even with BP levels that are "normal."
- BP outside the specified parameters may not produce immediate clinical changes and the patient may look "fine," but this has been shown to impact functional recovery down the road.
- Constipation should be avoided; a stool softener should be ordered to minimize straining, which can cause spikes in BP.
  - In a normal brain, a mean arterial pressure (MAP) of about 60 mmHg is necessary to perfuse coronary arteries, brain, and kidneys, but may not be adequate to perfuse an injured, swollen brain.
- Nursing considerations:
  - High and low alarm limits in bedside monitoring equipment should be set to patient-specific goals; parameters will vary according to the patient's history and type and size of the stroke.
  - A BP reading outside the ordered goals should be reassessed before action is taken—do not treat an isolated BP.

- Consider other causes for increased BP:
  - ○ Agitation—A raise in BP could be caused by fear, confusion, overstimulation, anger, or feeling cold/hot/pain
  - ○ Pain—May be caused by the bladder catheter or occur at the IV site or arterial line, external ventricular drain (EVD), surgical site, or puncture site
- If antihypertensives are administered, BP is reassessed in 15 to 30 minutes to determine whether BP goals are being reached in a timely manner.

CLINICAL PEARL

In addition to BP management, three clinical protocols have become standard of care for acute stroke: temperature, blood sugar, and dysphagia. These collectively have become known as the fever, sugar, and swallow (FeSS) protocols. The Quality in Acute Stroke Care Trial (QASC) demonstrated that monitoring and managing these in stroke patients reduced 90-day death and dependency by 16%, further proof that "routine" nursing care can result in significantly improved stroke recovery (Middleton et al., 2018).

TEMPERATURE MANAGEMENT

- Fever (body temperature ≥38.3 °C [100.94 °F]) increases metabolic demand on the already injured brain; it also accelerates the ischemic cascade, thus contributing to the conversion of penumbra to infarct.
  - For each degree increase, the normal metabolic demand increases by 10%.
- Fever is the most common complication of subarachnoid hemorrhage (SAH), occurring in up to 72% of SAH patients (Boling & Groves, 2019).
- Fever within the first 24 hours has been associated with a twofold increase in mortality.
  - Normothermia is the goal and may require acetaminophen or a cooling blanket to accomplish.
- Nursing considerations:
  - Acetaminophen or ibuprofen should be administered as needed.
  - Use of blankets should be limited; temperature of room should not be excessively warm.
    - ○ Family member and visitor education is important so that they do not add blankets.
  - If cooling blanket is used, assess and manage shivering, which increases the body's metabolic demand and decreases brain tissue oxygenation (Boling & Groves, 2019).
  - Medications like meperidine, magnesium, and buspirone may be beneficial.
  - Counter warming with hand warmers and surface warming may be beneficial and do not raise the patient's body temperature.
  - Performing skin care every 2 to 4 hours is a priority to monitor for breakdown or frostbite.

CLINICAL PEARL

Hyperglycemia monitoring is important in all stroke patients—not just diabetic stroke patients. Hyperglycemia after stroke results in threefold higher risk of mortality and poor functional recovery, regardless of past medical history (Green et al., 2021).

BLOOD SUGAR MANAGEMENT

- Hyperglycemia increases anaerobic metabolism, lactic acidosis, and free-radical production.
  - Hyperglycemia leads to infarct expansion, hemorrhagic transformation, and reduced recanalization with thrombolytics, associated with increased length of stay and increased mortality.
- FeSS protocol recommends treatment with insulin for blood sugar >180 mg/dL in ischemic stroke; for hemorrhagic stroke, hyper- and hypoglycemia are to be avoided, but no specific metric has been identified.
- IV solutions containing glucose should not be used.
- Insulin drips are often utilized to ensure tighter control than intermittent injections; use of goal range of 140 to 180 mg/dL will ensure tight control and prevent hypoglycemia.
- Nursing considerations:
  - Measure blood sugar a minimum of four times per day for 3 days (Middleton et al., 2018).
  - If a sliding-scale method is utilized, ensure that a schedule is followed and that treatment is punctual to avoid peaks and valleys.
  - Alternate fingers to prevent discomfort and infection.

CLINICAL PEARL

Cerebral reperfusion injury, also referred to as reperfusion syndrome, may occur in stroke patients following an intervention procedure. It is a deterioration of the ischemic, but salvageable, brain tissue (penumbra) as a result of reperfusion. It may lead to a cerebral edema, intracranial hemorrhage (ICH), or an increase in the size of the initial stroke. A breakdown of the blood–brain barrier as a result of reperfusion injury may lead to vasogenic edema.

POSTINTRAVENOUS THROMBOLYSIS AND ENDOVASCULAR THROMBECTOMY MANAGEMENT

- Vital signs and neurological assessment:
  - Assess every 15 minutes for 2 hours (starting at completion of procedure).
  - Assess every 30 minutes for 6 hours.
  - Assess every hour for 16 hours, then according to level of care.
  - If IV thrombolysis was administered before the thrombectomy, restart the schedule at the end of the thrombectomy.
- Check the groin puncture site and perform neurovascular checks of the extremity used for the procedure.
  - Best practice for extremity assessment is every 15 minutes for 1 hour, every 30 minutes for the following hour, then every hour for the next 4 hours (Rodgers et al., 2021).
  - To keep things simple, many organizations do these checks on the same schedule as the vital signs and neuro checks for the first 24 hours.

- Nursing considerations:
  - Assess frequent vital signs, taking action to maintain BP <180/105 for first 24 hours.
  - Ongoing neuro assessments monitoring for deterioration that could result from reperfusion injury.
  - Monitor for bleeding from any site or angioedema.
  - Assess the patient, puncture site, and extremity for the following signs:
    - Hematoma development at the puncture site
    - Swelling, bleeding, or drainage at the puncture site
    - Development of a pseudoaneurysm, dissection of the artery, or clot formation
      - Monitor for complaint of increasing back or thigh pain
      - Monitor pallor, pain, and paresthesia in the sheath extremity
  - Hemodynamic instability: hypotension and tachycardia related to blood loss.
  - Neurovascular checks:
    - Pulses distal to arterial puncture site.
    - Capillary refill, skin color, temperature, sensation, and motor function (Rodgers et al., 2021).
    - Plethysmography or a pulse oximetry probe on the toe of the extremity can be used to monitor limb blood flow.

POSTSTROKE COMPLICATIONS

▶ SPECIFIC TO HEMORRHAGIC STROKE PATIENTS

- Seizures
  - About 20% to 25% of SAH patients will have seizures, most often after middle cerebral artery (MCA) rupture.
  - Blood irritating the parenchymal tissue or an increased intracerebral pressure (ICP) can cause seizures.
  - Antiseizure medications are no longer a Class A recommendation as side effects outweigh the benefit.
    - Continuous bedside EEG monitoring may be utilized.
- Hydrocephalus
  - Usually presents in the first 24 hours after injury.
  - Watch for a decrease in LOC due to rising ICP.
  - A ventricular catheter may be placed to drain cerebrospinal fluid (CSF); see the "Cerebral Edema and Intracerebral Pressure Management" section for catheter care and nursing considerations.
- Rebleeding
  - Symptoms of rebleeding are related to an increase in ICP.
  - IV vasoactive medications are used to decrease BP or maintain hemodynamic parameters to limit risk of rebleeding or poor cerebral perfusion.
- Hyponatremia
  - Occurs in up to 50% of SAH patients.
  - Results from cerebral salt wasting (CSW) or syndrome of inappropriate antidiuretic hormone (SIADH).
    - CSW = hypovolemia; treatment is mild hypertonic saline solution or mineral corticoids
    - SIADH = euvolemia or hypervolemia; treatment is fluid restriction or mild hypertonic saline solution

- Treatment is for sodium (Na) less than 135 mEq/L or clinical deterioration attributable to hyponatremia.
- Vasospasm
  - A common cause of neurological deterioration after an SAH patient is initially stabilized; results in delayed cerebral ischemia (DCI).
  - Usually occurs between days 4 and 10 following the original bleed.
    - Can be seen up to 21 days post-SAH
  - Transcranial Doppler (TCD) is useful in monitoring for vasospasm as well as CT perfusion study to detect areas of hypoperfusion treatment.
    - Maintain euvolemia (triple H therapy: hypertension, hemodilution, and hypervolemia is no longer recommended; Connolly et al., 2012).
    - Induction of hypertension is only for patients with DCI (Connolly et al., 2012).
    - Oral nimodipine should be administered to patients with aneurysmal SAH; it does not reduce vasospasm as initially thought but has been shown to improve neurological outcomes (Connolly et al., 2012).
- DCI
  - Term is used interchangeably with vasospasm, but they are not the same; vasospasm can be a cause of DCI.
  - DCI refers to acute neurological deterioration, including but not limited to new hemiparesis, aphasia, and altered LOC (Boling & Groves, 2019).
- Nursing considerations:
  - Close BP, temperature, and glucose management.
  - Ongoing neurological assessments, being alert for new deficits that may indicate DCI.
  - Anticipate sensory depression or drowsiness.
  - Seizure precautions:
    - Assess/document seizure duration, body parts involved, and results of medical intervention.
    - Prevent injury due to change in LOC: pad side rails and institute safety measures, such as using a low bed, and institute fall precautions.
    - Protect airway: supplemental oxygen, functioning wall suction, and an oral suction tube should be readily available in the patient's room.
  - ECG changes, which frequently occur after SAH; although most abnormalities are benign, cardiac ischemia should be ruled out before assuming the change is of neurological origin.
  - Cardiac markers and serial 12-lead ECGs may be warranted.

CLINICAL PEARL

Patients with SAH often have hyponatremia due to CSW or SIADH. Clinical symptoms of CSW include hyponatremia and polyuria. The low sodium state in CSW is caused by excessive removal of salt by the kidneys and is not a dilutional low sodium level as seen in SIADH. Healthcare providers must be cognizant of the reasoning behind presenting symptoms and treat CSW with oral sodium replacement and/or hypertonic saline rather than fluid restriction, which would be detrimental to the SAH patient's outcome.

▶ SPECIFIC TO ISCHEMIC STROKE PATIENTS

- Hemorrhagic conversion (also known as hemorrhagic transformation)
  - The natural hemorrhagic conversion rate is 1.5% in the absence of reperfusion therapy (Green et al., 2021).
  - In the National Institute of Neurological Disorders and Stroke (NINDS) trial, patients who received IV thrombolysis had a 6.4% rate of hemorrhagic conversion.
    - Petechial hemorrhage, also referred to as hemorrhagic infarct (HI): patchy hemorrhage often found on routine 24-hour imaging but without space-occupying effect, so patients are usually asymptomatic
      - HI 1 is along the margins of the infarct
      - HI 2 is within the infarcted area
    - Parenchymal hemorrhage (PH): hemorrhage with mass effect; patient is usually symptomatic
      - PH 1 is a clot not exceeding 30% of the infarcted area, with mild space-occupying effect
      - PH 2 is dense clot(s) exceeding 30% of the infarct volume with significant space-occupying effect (von Kummer et al., 2015)
  - Hemorrhagic transformation has been considered a marker of successful reperfusion therapy and is considered a good sign as long as it is not clinically significant (Molina et al., 2002).
  - Clinical significance is determined by the presence of any of the following conditions: patient is symptomatic, requires a change in treatment, or results in disability or death.
  - BP control is a significant factor as the penumbra is vascular and ischemic, making it susceptible to conversion.
  - For every 10-mmHg elevation in BP after tissue plasminogen activator (tPA) is given, the odds of hemorrhage increase 59% (Butcher et al., 2010).
  - Vasoactive medications may be administered as continuous infusions as needed if antihypertensive dosing is not effective.

● CLINICAL PEARL

Classification of hemorrhagic transformation can be quite confusing. But it is important for the stroke nurse to understand that not all hemorrhagic transformation is bad. It is the clinical significance that matters—in other words, the condition of the patient. Whether the patient received reperfusion therapy or not, in the presence of any hemorrhagic transformation, close assessment of the stroke patient is prudent.

● CEREBRAL EDEMA AND INTRACEREBRAL PRESSURE MANAGEMENT

- Cerebral edema is seen with large territory ischemic stroke and hemorrhagic strokes and is the primary reason for decompressive craniectomy.
- Isotonic fluids (0.9% normal saline or lactated Ringer) are preferred; as the body uses up the glucose content in IV fluid containing dextrose, the water that remains crosses the blood–brain barrier and increases cerebral edema.

- Mannitol (osmotic diuretic) and hypertonic saline (23.4%) decrease ICP by pulling fluid out of the cerebral cell and back into the intravascular space.
- An EVD, or ventriculostomy, in the nondominant ventricle is used to drain CSF, which can lower ICP.
- Nursing considerations:
  - Close monitoring of vital signs and neuro assessment, with prompt treatment of fever and hypertension; decreased LOC is an early sign of rising ICP.
  - Strict aseptic technique is essential to limit risk of hospital-acquired central nervous system (CNS) infection.
    - Dressings must remain dry and intact.
  - Monitor daily weights and for signs and symptoms of dehydration.
  - Limit visitors/physical stimulation; use low lighting.
  - Position patient properly.
    - Place head of the bed at 30 degrees unless contraindicated.
    - Maintain neck in midline position to allow venous drainage.
    - Avoid hip flexion; this will increase ICP.
  - Monitor elimination.
    - Administer stool softeners daily; prevent urinary distension.

CLINICAL PEARL

Treatment of increased ICP is based on the Monro–Kellie doctrine. The skull is a closed box that contains roughly 80% brain matter, 10% blood, and 10% CSF. If one of the contents increases, then one of the other two must decrease. Treatment decisions are based on what item in the box can be altered to lower the pressure in the cranial vault.

RESPIRATORY COMPONENT

- Cerebral oxygenation monitoring facilitates assessment of brain tissue perfusion and oxygenation.
  - Jugular saturation ($SjvO_2$) catheter—jugular venous oximetry measures jugular venous oxygen saturation
- Hyperventilation should be avoided, as hypocapnia is a potent vasoconstrictor.
- Nursing considerations:
  - Ongoing chest/lung auscultation
  - Diligent oral care decreases the risk of ventilator-associated pneumonia (VAP)
  - Epiglottis-level suctioning prevents oral flora from contaminating the lungs
  - Keeping the head of the bed at 30 degrees is effective in the prevention of VAP
  - Perform dysphagia screening postextubation and prior to any oral intake; older age and duration of intubation are associated with dysphagia

DECOMPRESSIVE CRANIECTOMY

- Partial bone flap removal allows the size of the cranial vault to be altered, providing the brain room to swell, decreasing the threat of herniation.
  - Often seen in malignant MCA strokes with a large ischemic area

- Nursing considerations:
  - ○ Ensure use of a protective helmet when out of bed (OOB) because the skull is no longer intact.
  - ○ Optimal wound care is essential to limit skin flora exposure to the surgical site.
  - ○ If the bone flap is stored in subcutaneous tissue (abdomen or thigh), provide wound care and monitor for signs of infection.
  - ○ The bone flap (either the patient's own bone or prosthetic material) may be replaced in 6 to 8 weeks after the risk for swelling and increased ICP have passed.

MINIMALLY INVASIVE REMOVAL OF INTRACRANIAL HEMORRHAGE

ICH is considered the most costly and debilitating type of stroke. Historically, evacuation of ICH represented high-risk surgery as it required craniotomy and significant brain tissue manipulation. It was not recommended for early ICH evacuation.

Minimally invasive devices are being developed for use within the first 24 hours after ICH occurs, with some achieving U.S. Food and Drug Administration (FDA) clearance. This procedure is referred to as minimally invasive parafascicular surgery (MIPS). The proposed benefit is to achieve maximum clot evacuation through a smaller opening than traditional surgery and with far less brain tissue disruption. Research is ongoing to determine if the clinical outcomes are superior to medical management.

VENOUS THROMBOEMBOLISM PREVENTION, AKA DEEP VEIN THROMBOSIS

Box 8.1 Deep Vein Thrombosis (DVT) Assessment and Nursing Interventions

Assessment	Nursing Interventions
■ Redness, swelling, tenderness of extremities ■ Risk due to immobility and limb paralysis	■ Ongoing assessments ■ Early mobilization ■ Minimize dependent edema: position limb on pillow ■ Anticoagulants ■ Sequential compression devices (SCDs) ■ Patient and family education about SCDs

- Stroke patients spend more than 50% of their time in bed during the first 2 weeks.
- Use of sequential compression devices (SCDs) in combination with anticoagulants has been shown to be highly effective.
- Anticoagulation is contraindicated for hemorrhagic stroke and large territory ischemic stroke patients.
- Patients with pulmonary embolus from venous thromboembolism (VTE) in the lower extremity and a contraindication for anticoagulant treatment may benefit from placement of an inferior vena cava filter.
- The use of aspirin as prophylaxis in the acute setting has had mixed reviews; more studies are underway.

CLINICAL PEARL

Thromboembolic deterrent (TED) stockings should not be used for the stroke population. They are difficult to put on and are rarely put on by the patient who would know if they "felt right." Many stroke patients have sensory and/or communication deficits, or they may have an altered LOC. So, patients either are not aware of a bad fit or cannot tell anyone. Results from the CLOTS-1 trial (Clots in Legs or Stockings After Stroke), reported by the CLOTS Trials Collaboration (2009), indicated that although graduated compression stockings were effective in surgical patients, they were not effective in stroke patients, and the potential for harm made them something to avoid.

CARDIAC MONITORING

- Patients with large deficits and right hemispheric strokes are at increased risk for myocardial infarction, heart failure, and atrial fibrillation.
- Patients with SAH are at risk for "stunned myocardium" with cardiac dysrhythmias; cardiac monitoring is required for the first 24 hours, and extended monitoring may be indicated.
- Nursing considerations:
  - Ongoing assessment of patient as well as monitored rhythm
  - BP management within ordered parameters

NUTRITION MANAGEMENT

- Dehydration and malnutrition slow recovery, and dehydration is a potential cause of VTE; 50% of stroke patients develop dehydration during their hospital stay (Tamburri et al., 2020).
- Dysphagia screening is not just for the ED—any change in LOC should prompt the nurse to rescreen the patient for swallow competence.
- Older age and duration of intubation have been associated with risk of postextubation dysphagia (Green et al., 2021).
  - If unable to take orally, IV fluid support of Ringer solution or normal saline will maintain hydration.
- If the patient fails the bedside nursing dysphagia screen, consultation with a speech and language pathologist (SLP) is indicated.
  - A video barium swallow may be ordered to assess swallow competence.
  - Consultation with a dietitian will help determine calorie needs and appropriate nutritional support.
  - Enteral feeding should be considered within the first 72 hours to prevent undernourishment.
    - Presence of an NG feeding tube increases risk of aspiration by 38% due to increased incidence of reflux or vomiting (Green et al., 2021).
    - Consider a percutaneous endoscopic gastrostomy (PEG) tube if long-term (more than 6–8 weeks) nutritional support is anticipated; most long-term care facilities do not accept patients with an NG feeding tube.

- Nursing considerations:
  - Dysphagia screening postextubation and prior to oral intake.
  - Aggressive oral care will minimize the bacterial count in the mouth and decrease the risk of aspiration pneumonia.
  - Assess and maintain feeding in proper position.
  - For patients who can tolerate oral intake, basic principles of feeding include:
    - Sitting in a high Fowler position, preferably in a chair, and remaining seated upright for 30 minutes after meals.
    - Recommendations of the SLP should be followed: ensure proper head positioning during swallowing (chin tuck or neck extension) and thicken fluids.
    - Mouth care should be performed prior to feeding (facilitates sensation and production of saliva) as well as after eating to observe whether the patient is pocketing food.
    - Pulmonary status should be assessed after eating.

CLINICAL PEARL

Cerebral autoregulation is the ability of the brain to adjust to changes in systemic BP, ensuring steady cerebral perfusion despite extremes of systemic pressure. This is accomplished through a complex system of mechanisms acting to adjust the resistance of cerebral vascular beds. In an injured brain, these hemodynamics are impaired or abolished, leaving the cerebral blood flow at the mercy of systemic perfusion pressure. Ischemic brain tissue has increased metabolic demand and, along with increased ICP due to edema, makes the case for the importance of close BP management—not too high and not too low.

MOBILIZATION

- The rehabilitation team should be consulted early to develop a plan for rehabilitation.
- For patients unable to get OOB, range of motion exercises should be done to assist with daily stretching of the hemiparetic limb; families can be instructed on how to do this safely, providing an excellent opportunity to involve the family in the care of the patient.
- Resting ankle splints may be utilized at night and during standing to prevent ankle contracture.
- Early, frequent, but short sessions of mobility are recommended.
  - Reduces risk of postural hypotension, which could result in decreased cerebral perfusion.
- Nursing considerations:
  - When initially getting the patient OOB, monitor BP sitting and standing: If a significant increase or decrease is noted, the patient should be returned to bed and the healthcare provider notified.
    - If autoregulation has been impacted, patient will be dependent on systemic pressure for perfusion; be aware of change in neurological status while sitting OOB as it may be a sign of decreased perfusion. If this is noted, patient should be returned to bed and monitored for return to previous neurological status; if this does not occur, notify the healthcare provider.
  - If the patient is ambulatory, note the presence of visual field defect, gaze palsy, or neglect that may impact ability to transfer in and OOB or ambulate safely.

SAFETY MEASURES

- For patients with significant upper extremity weakness:
  - Shoulder subluxation is a common and painful complication that can inhibit recovery.
  - Avoid pulling on affected arm and shoulder when transferring or when repositioning in bed.
  - Position arm on a small pillow to minimize weight of limb pulling on shoulder joint, minimize dependent edema, and prevent limb slipping off the side of the bed and possibly getting caught between the side rail and mattress.
- For patients with significant lower extremity weakness, position the leg on a small pillow to minimize dependent edema, prevent external rotation of the hip, and prevent limb slipping off the bed and getting caught between the side rail and mattress.
- Fall prevention:
  - Motor, sensory, communication, visual, balance, and cognitive deficits put stroke patients at increased risk for falls.
  - Nursing considerations:
    - Frequent nursing rounds have demonstrated reduced fall rates.
    - Frequent orientation and reiteration of instructions are necessary.
    - Place call bell and bedside table within reach and on the patient's unaffected side.
    - Utilize safety belt around patient's waist to assist with ambulation and transfers.
    - Offer toileting at least every 2 hours while awake and every 4 hours at night.
    - Consider bed/chair alarms or video monitoring.
- Pressure injury prevention:
  - Stroke patients are at increased risk due to immobility, loss of sensation, incontinence, and impaired circulation; in addition, diabetes is a common comorbid condition that increases the risk of skin breakdown.
  - Nursing considerations:
    - Utilize a standardized skin assessment tool to evaluate and predict risk.
    - Patients should be repositioned regularly using proper techniques to avoid excessive friction; skin assessment should be done with each repositioning.
    - Skin should be kept clean and dry.
    - Consider specialized mattress and wheelchair cushion.

CLINICAL PEARL

Infections are common following stroke and adversely influence the outcome. Research evidence indicates that stroke leads to suppression of immune responses, which predisposes to infection. Poststroke immunodepression has been associated with increased susceptibility to infection—the most common being urinary tract infection (UTI) and pneumonia.

- Infection prevention:
  - Pneumonia is responsible for up to 37% of acute stroke patient deaths (Hannawi et al., 2013).
    - Pneumonia incidence is highest with mechanical ventilation, dysphagia, and prolonged immobility, which leads to atelectasis.
    - Pneumonia is associated with longer length of stay and poorer functional outcomes (Green et al., 2021).

- UTIs occur in ≤25% of stroke patients and are associated with poor outcomes.
  - Incidence of UTIs is highest with indwelling catheter placements.
  - Loss of sphincter control (incontinence) increases the risk for UTI.
- Nursing considerations:
  - Ongoing assessment of vital signs and lung sounds.
  - Early mobilization and frequent repositioning.
  - Dysphagia screening protocols should be implemented, as discussed in Chapter 5.
  - Regular, thorough pulmonary hygiene.
  - Intensive, regular oral hygiene.
  - Avoid indwelling catheters; if one is necessary, provide meticulous catheter care and removal as soon as possible.
  - Frequent handwashing—for both nurse and patient.
  - Education and reassurance for the patient/family regarding the need/care for an endotracheal tube and/or bladder catheter may reduce anxiety and facilitate cooperation.

KB is a 47-year-old intracranial hemorrhage (ICH) patient. A nurse ending the night shift is getting ready to give the handoff report on day 4. Overnight, KB has become much more alert, and her blood pressure (BP) has stabilized. The nurse was able to wean off the nicardipine drip and the nurse anticipates that she will be extubated after morning rounds. Her temperature remains 39 °C (102.2 °F) and her blood sugar at last check was 110. Prior to admission, she was a 1 pack/day smoker, on no routine medications, with two grown children, and lived alone in a two-story house.

1. Which medication would have been administered to KB during the previous shift?

   A. Propofol to facilitate good endotracheal tube care
   B. Metformin to maintain blood sugar control
   C. Phenytoin to prevent seizures
   D. Acetaminophen to lower her temperature

2. In the handoff report, the night-shift nurse and the day-shift nurse do a joint National Institutes of Health Stroke Scale (NIHSS) score, giving KB a 1 for best language. How is this possible with an intubated patient?

   A. Best language includes assessment of ability to write; she left off the first letter of most of the words
   B. The nurses were able to deflate her endotracheal tube cuff for a minute or two and had her speak; she had a lot of hesitation and said she couldn't find some words she wanted to say
   C. Best language is automatically scored as a 1 in intubated patients
   D. It is not possible; NIHSS cannot be done on an intubated patient

3. What information is needed that will impact KB's discharge plan?

   A. Notes from social worker on her relationship with her children
   B. Notes from physical, occupational, and speech therapy on functional ability
   C. Notes from vocational rehabilitation on her prestroke employment status
   D. Notes from care management on her insurance carrier/coverage

4. What nursing function will the day-shift nurse perform on her today that wouldn't necessarily be done on day 4 for all stroke patients?

   A. Assist her to take a shower postextubation
   B. Swallow screening postextubation
   C. Propofol dose preextubation
   D. Seizure precautions preextubation

(See answers next page.)

1. D) Acetaminophen to lower her temperature

Normothermia is the goal, and 39 °C (102.2 °F) is hyperthermia and is best addressed with acetaminophen. Sedation is not required for endotracheal tube care. KB's blood sugar is within normal range. Prophylactic seizure medications are not recommended.

2. A) Best language includes assessment of ability to write; she left off the first letter of most of the words

Best language does include the ability to write, and this should be used to assess intubated, alert patients. Without a provider order, deflation of the endotracheal tube cuff is not used in NIHSS scoring. There is no automatic scoring of 1 due to intubation. NIHSS can be done on intubated patients.

3. B) Notes from physical, occupational, and speech therapy on functional ability

Documented assessment of current functional abilities is critical in determining the best disposition at discharge. Notes regarding relationship with children and insurance coverage will be valuable once her functional ability is determined. Employment status does not impact discharge plans.

4. B) Swallow screening postextubation

Patients who have been intubated are at risk for dysphagia and should be screened postextubation and prior to oral intake. Assisting with showering would be a normal day 4 activity. Propofol would not be given preextubation, and there is no association with extubation and seizure risk.

1. Which of the following is not one of the common complications seen after a subarachnoid hemorrhage (SAH)?

   A. Hypercalcemia
   B. Hydrocephalus
   C. Cerebral vasospasm
   D. Seizure activity

2. A patient just returned from having endovascular embolization of an arteriovenous malformation (AVM). The nursing care for the next hour will include which of the following?

   A. Initiation of prophylactic seizure medications within 2 hours
   B. Vital signs and neurological checks q 15 minutes along with scalp incision checks
   C. Vital signs and neurological checks q 15 minutes along with groin site checks
   D. Education about the procedure and possible complications

3. Why would a nurse give their patient docusate (Colace) every day?

   A. Neurological ICU patients are prone to constipation secondary to cerebral edema
   B. Patients with constipation are more likely to develop Sundowner syndrome
   C. Straining as a result of constipation causes blood pressure (BP) spikes
   D. Both A and B

4. It is day 3 of an ICU patient's stay. Their oxygen saturation has been reading 90% since the start of the nurse's shift. Which of the following is suspected?

   A. Aspiration pneumonia
   B. Hypoventilation
   C. Airway obstruction
   D. All of the above

5. An intubated intracerebral hemorrhage patient is restless, despite sedation; the patient's blood pressure (BP) has risen to 176/90. What is the nurse's first action?

   A. Assess the patient for respiratory distress or other causes of pain
   B. Increase the dose of sedative within parameters and monitor for response
   C. Tell the patient care assistant (PCA) to notify another nurse on duty
   D. Document the change in the patient's notes so that if further deterioration occurs, there will be clear trending of events

1. A) Hypercalcemia
Imbalance of calcium is associated with cause of hemorrhagic strokes, not a complication. Hydrocephalus develops when the blood clots over the arachnoid villi, blocking flow of cerebrospinal fluid. Vasospasm develops because the blood is irritating the outer layer of the arteries, causing them to spasm. Seizure activity is the result of the irritation of the blood on the surrounding tissue—think of it as a short circuit of the brain's electrical system.

2. C) Vital signs and neurological checks q 15 minutes along with groin site checks
Endovascular embolization is done via an arterial approach, not transcranial, so groin checks, not scalp incision checks, would be done along with vitals and neurological checks every 15 minutes. Prophylactic seizure treatment is not recommended. The first hour post-procedure is likely too early for detailed education.

3. C) Straining as a result of constipation causes blood pressure (BP) spikes
Straining involves the Valsalva maneuver, which results in transient high BP. For new stroke patients, and possibly inactive autoregulation, BP spikes could be dangerous. Autoregulation is present in normal, healthy brains. It is the mechanism that keeps a steady intracerebral pressure, regardless of what is going on in the body. When the brain is injured, autoregulation may be temporarily inactivated, so the brain is particularly susceptible to highs and lows of systemic BP. There is no association between constipation and cerebral edema or Sundowner syndrome.

4. D) All of the above
Hypoxia could result from aspiration pneumonia, hypoventilation, and airway obstruction. Aspiration pneumonia can occur because the inflammatory process produces excess mucus and secretions that inhibit oxygen absorption and exchange. Hypoventilation is possible because inadequate inflation or low respiratory rate limits the amount of oxygen exchanged. Airway obstruction can be indicated because if oxygenated air cannot get into the lungs, it cannot get absorbed into the blood.

5. A) Assess the patient for respiratory distress or other causes of pain
If a restless patient is unable to communicate what is wrong, assessment of possible causes of distress, respiratory or pain, will help to determine the appropriate treatment. Increasing the dose of sedative without further assessment is dangerous because if the cause of the restlessness is found and resolved, there is risk of oversedation and hypotension, which is not good for the patient's injured brain. It is not advised to first notify another nurse on duty. Documentation of the issue is important, but it would not be the first action.

6. Why does a doctor order glucose checks every 4 hours for a 69-year-old ischemic stroke patient with no history of diabetes?

   A. This knowledge is outside of the scope of stroke nurse education
   B. Hyperglycemia is common in ischemic stroke, even without a diabetes history, and can worsen outcomes if not controlled
   C. Hypoglycemia can occur suddenly after ischemic stroke as a result of increased intracerebral pressure (ICP) and can worsen outcomes if not controlled
   D. Patients are known to deny a history of diabetes, so all stroke patients are tested

7. A patient's temperature has risen to 39.6 °C (103.28 °F). Which of the following fever-induced complications will the nurse monitor for?

   A. Urinary tract infection (UTI)
   B. Aspiration pneumonia
   C. Cerebral edema
   D. Hyperkalemia

8. Why would the provider have ordered buspirone for a patient whose temperature is being maintained with a cooling blanket?

   A. Persistent fever
   B. Constipation
   C. Shivering
   D. Decreasing level of consciousness (LOC)

9. A nurse is told that their stroke patient passed the swallow screening and swallowed a baby aspirin already. What might warrant repeating the swallow screening during this patient's hospital stay?

   A. Patient is newly noted to be drooling
   B. There is an increase in the National Institutes of Health Stroke Scale (NIHSS) or clinical deterioration
   C. There is no documentation of the swallow screening in the patient's medical record
   D. All of the above

10. Two ischemic stroke patients had repeat imaging done. Patient A's was scheduled; Patient B's was done as a result of new-onset headache and drowsiness. Both showed hemorrhagic transformation. Which of the following would most likely be true?

    A. Patient B had a reaction to a new antihypertensive
    B. Patient A had parenchymal hemorrhage, and Patient B had petechial hemorrhage
    C. Both had intraventricular hemorrhage
    D. Patient A had petechial hemorrhage, and Patient B had parenchymal hemorrhage

6. B) Hyperglycemia is common in ischemic stroke, even without a diabetes history, and can worsen outcomes if not controlled

Research has shown that sustained hyperglycemia after stroke is associated with worse outcomes, even in patients without diabetes. Provider orders should be followed; however, a stroke nurse must know why it is being done. There is no association between hypoglycemia and increased ICP. This practice is not done because patients tend to deny history of diabetes.

7. C) Cerebral edema

Fever results in cerebral edema owing to the breakdown of the blood–brain barrier. UTI and aspiration pneumonia are causes of fever, not results. High potassium may result in fever as a complication.

8. C) Shivering

Shivering is a common challenge with surface cooling. If not controlled, it can raise the patient's body temperature, thus negating the impact of the cooling therapy. Buspirone is given to control shivering, not to control fever, constipation, or a decreased LOC.

9. D) All of the above

Despite being told in the report that the patient passed a swallow screen, if it is not documented it is important repeat it. For a patient with a change in neurological status or an NIHSS increase, the ability to swallow safely may also have changed. For a patient who had been deemed safe to swallow but is drooling, repeating the swallow screen is essential, as new drooling is closely linked to swallow ability.

10. D) Patient A had petechial hemorrhage, and Patient B had parenchymal hemorrhage

Petechial hemorrhage is defined as patchy hemorrhage, and patients are usually asymptomatic. Thus, it is likely that Patient A's scheduled exam would reveal an asymptomatic hemorrhage. Parenchymal hemorrhage is defined as hemorrhage with mass effect, and patients are usually symptomatic. Drowsiness is not a common side effect of antihypertensive therapy unless their blood pressure dropped precipitously. Hemorrhagic transformation only occurs after ischemic stroke, so both having new intraventricular hemorrhage is highly unlikely.

11. What is the difference between cerebral salt wasting (CSW) and syndrome of inappropriate antidiuretic hormone (SIADH)?

   A. There is no difference; CSW is the older term for SIADH
   B. CSW symptom is hyponatremia; SIADH symptom is hypernatremia
   C. CSW is often seen with subarachnoid hemorrhage (SAH) patients, and SIADH is often seen with ischemic stroke patients
   D. CSW is treated with sodium replacement, and SIADH is treated with fluid restriction

12. Which of the following is NOT true about blood pressure (BP) management of stroke patients?

   A. Postintravenous (IV) thrombolysis patients need BP below 180/105 for the first 24 hours
   B. Recheck a BP outside the parameters before treating to ensure accuracy
   C. Systolic blood pressure (SBP) parameters for ischemic and intracerebral hemorrhage patients are 170 to 185 mmHg
   D. Recheck a BP after treatment with antihypertensive to ensure goal is met

13. Reperfusion syndrome is best described by which of the following?

   A. Acute neurological change after intravenous (IV) thrombolysis during second stroke event
   B. Deterioration of the penumbra as a result of removal/dissolution of clot
   C. Acute-onset hypotension following second pass of mechanical retrieval device
   D. Ipsilateral seizure following successful embolization of aneurysm

14. A 76-year-old male patient post–ischemic stroke has current vital signs of blood pressure (BP) 134/78, heart rate (HR) 98, respiratory rate (RR) 22, temperature 37 °C (98.6 °F), and pulse oxygen 88% on room air. What should be the nurse's next action?

   A. Replace pulse oxygen sensor and, if still showing 88%, document that patient is not feeling short of breath
   B. Recheck pulse oxygen and notify provider for oxygen order
   C. Recheck pulse oxygen with next scheduled check of vital signs and neurological status
   D. Place the patient on 2 L of oxygen by nasal cannula and document as standard of care

15. Subarachnoid hemorrhage (SAH) patients usually have length of stays averaging 10 days. What is the rationale?

   A. Adequate stroke education takes a minimum of 8 days
   B. There is a high risk of rebleed in the first few days
   C. There is a high risk of vasospasm between 4 and 10 days
   D. Anticoagulant has not yet reached therapeutic level

11. D) CSW is treated with sodium replacement, and SIADH is treated with fluid restriction

CSW is caused by excessive removal of salt by the kidneys and is treated with sodium replacement. SIADH is dilutional low sodium and is treated with fluid restriction. CSW and SIADH are not synonymous.

12. C) Systolic blood pressure (SBP) parameters for ischemic and intracerebral hemorrhage patients are 170 to 185 mmHg

The BP parameters for ischemic and hemorrhagic patients are not the same, with hemorrhagic patients having a lower range of acceptable BP than ischemic patients. Post-IV thrombolysis patients should be controlled below 180/105 for the first 24 hours. Treating isolated BP outside the parameter is not advised in case it is inaccurate. The stroke nurse must always recheck BP after treatment to ensure the goal was met.

13. B) Deterioration of the penumbra as a result of removal/dissolution of clot

Reperfusion syndrome is described as the inflammatory reaction to the restoration of blood flow to an ischemic area. It is associated with postprocedure hypertension, and the treatment is tight management of the blood pressure. It is not a result of IV thrombolysis during a second stroke event. Reperfusion would not result from hypotension due to the second pass of the retrieval device, nor would it result from an aneurysm embolization as that does not result in restored circulation to an ischemic area.

14. B) Recheck pulse oxygen and notify provider for oxygen order

This patient is showing signs of mild respiratory distress with increased pulse and respiratory rate. In addition, the injured brain needs better oxygenation than an 88% saturation provides, so notify the provider if that is what it is on recheck. More action than simple documentation is necessary for this patient. Waiting until the next scheduled assessment is not appropriate. Oxygen therapy of any amount requires a provider order.

15. C) There is a high risk of vasospasm between 4 and 10 days

The risk of vasospasm is highest in the first 10 days after an SAH. The risk of rebleed is highest in the first 24 hours after SAH. The need for anticoagulation in SAH patients would be rare, so it would not impact standard length of stay.

16. A patient with a left hemisphere ischemic stroke complains of 4:10 right arm pain. What would the nurse's next action be?

   A. Notify the provider and anticipate repeat CT scan of the head
   B. Reposition the patient, ensuring that the affected arm is well supported
   C. Document as new pain and include in report to next shift
   D. Notify provider and anticipate order for opioid analgesic

17. The stroke neurologist asks a patient about their family history of diabetes. What in the medical record would prompt this?

   A. Atherosclerosis on CT
   B. Fasting glucose of 115
   C. Hemoglobin (Hgb) A1C of 9%
   D. Documentation of extreme heat intolerance

18. Which of the following is *not* a recommended treatment for prevention of venous thrombosis?

   A. Low–molecular weight heparin
   B. Elastic compression stockings, also called thromboembolic deterrent (TED) stockings
   C. Intermittent pneumatic compression (IPC) devices, also called sequential compression devices (SCDs)
   D. Heparinoids

19. Use of anticoagulants for deep vein thrombosis (DVT) prophylaxis would warrant closer observation for which patient type?

   A. Basal ganglia lacunar stroke
   B. Secured aneurysmal subarachnoid hemorrhage (SAH)
   C. Brainstem lacunar stroke
   D. Subcortical intracerebral hemorrhage

20. What is the rationale for the high incidence of urinary tract infection (UTI) poststroke?

   A. Urinary incontinence and retention as a result of neurological injury
   B. Poor hygiene associated with hemiparesis
   C. Intolerance of prophylactic antibiotics due to dysphagia
   D. Inadequate bladder catheter care

16. B) Reposition the patient, ensuring that the affected arm is well supported

Patients with hemiparesis of the upper extremity can experience arm pain from weight of the arm pulling down. The best next action would be to reposition and ensure that the arm is properly supported and assess for possible relief of pain. Arm pain is not an indication of need for repeat imaging of the head. Documentation is important but not appropriate as a first action, as it does not address the patient's pain. Provider notification will be necessary if pain continues. Opioid analgesia is not warranted.

17. C) Hemoglobin (Hgb) A1C of 9%

Hgb A1C is an indicator of the average level of blood sugar over the past 2 to 3 months. A level greater than 6.5% meets the threshold for diagnosis of diabetes. A fasting blood sugar greater than 126 also meets the threshold. Atherosclerosis may result from long-term uncontrolled diabetes but is not as diagnostic as the high Hgb A1C. A fasting glucose of 115 is just slightly above normal. There is no association between family history of diabetes and extreme heat intolerance.

18. B) Elastic compression stockings, also called thromboembolic deterrent (TED) stockings

The benefits do not outweigh the risk of harm when using TED stockings. Thus, it is not a recommended aspect of the treatment plan. In the acute stroke population, there is a high likelihood of the stockings being applied by someone other than the patient, and with possible language or sensory deficits, the patient cannot always communicate, or be aware, if there is poor fit and compromised circulation or skin integrity. Low–molecular weight heparin, IPC devices, and heparinoids are all recommended treatments for the prevention of venous thrombosis.

19. D) Subcortical intracerebral hemorrhage

Anticoagulation during the acute phase of stroke recovery is most risky in subcortical intracerebral hemorrhage, unsecured aneurysms, and large territory ischemic stroke patients. A basal ganglia lacunar stroke, secured aneurysmal SAH, or brainstem lacunar stroke would not warrant closer observation following the use of anticoagulants for DVT.

20. A) Urinary incontinence and retention as a result of neurological injury

Patients with neurological injury, such as stroke, are at risk for incontinence and retention. Retention of urine in the bladder is a risk for a UTI, even with optimal hygiene. Poor hygiene and inadequate bladder catheter care can contribute to UTI poststroke, but not as much as urinary continence and retention. Prophylactic antibiotics are standard of care poststroke in the prevention of UTI.

REFERENCES

Boling, B., & Groves, T. R. (2019). Management of subarachnoid hemorrhage. *Critical Care Nurse, 39*(5), 58–67. http://doi.org/10.4037/ccn2019882

Butcher, K., Christensen, S., Parsons, M., De Silva, D. A., Ebinger, M., Levi, C., Jeerakathil, T., Campbell, B. C. V., Barber, P. A., Bladin, C., Fink, J., Tress, B., Donnan, A, G., & Davis, S. M. (2010). Postthrombolysis blood pressure elevation is associated with hemorrhagic transformation. *Stroke, 41*(1), 72–77. https://doi.org/10.1161/STROKEAHA.109.563767

CLOTS Trials Collaboration. (2009). Effectiveness of thigh-length graduated compression stockings to reduce the risk of deep vein thrombosis after stroke (CLOTS trial 1): A multicentre, randomised controlled trial. *Lancet, 373*(9679), 1958–1965. https://doi.org/10.1016/S0140-6736(09)60941-7

Connolly, E. S., Rabinstein, A. A., Carhuapoma, J. R., Derdeyn, C. P., Dion, J., Higashida, R. T. Hoh., L, B., Kirkness, C. J., Naidech, A. M., Ogilvy, C. S., Patel, A. B., Thompson, B. G., & Vespa, P. (2012). Guidelines for the management of aneurysmal subarachnoid hemorrhage: A guideline for healthcare professionals from the American Heart Association/American Stroke Association. *Stroke, 43*(6), 1711–1737. https://doi.org/10.1161/STR.0b013e3182587839

Green, T. L., McNair, N. D., Hinkle, J. L., Middleton, S., Miller, E. T., Perrin, S., Power, M., Southerland, A. M., & Summers, D. V. (2021). Care of the patient with acute ischemic stroke (posthyperacute and prehospital discharge): Update to 2009 comprehensive nursing care scientific statement: A scientific statement from the American Heart Association. *Stroke, 52*(5), e000–e000. https://doi.org/10.1161/STR.0000000000000357

Hannawi, Y., Hannawi, B., Venkatasubba, C., Suarez, J., & Bershad, E. (2013). Stroke-associated pneumonia: Major advances and obstacles. *Cerebrovascular Diseases, 35*(5), 430–443. https://doi.org/10.1159/000350199

Middleton, S., McElduff, P., Drury, P., D'Este, C., Cadilhac, D., Dale, S., Grimshaw, J. M., Ward, J., Quinn, C., Cheung, N. W., & Levi, C. (2018). Vital sign monitoring following stroke associated with 90 day independence: A secondary analysis of the QASC cluster randomized trial. *International Journal of Nursing Studies, 89*, 72–79. https://doi.org/10.1016/j.ijnurstu.2018.09.014

Molina, C. A., Alvarez-Sabina, J., Montaner, J., Abilleira, S., Arenillas, J. F., Coscojuela, P., Romero, F., & Codina, A. (2002). Thrombolysis-related hemorrhagic infarction: a marker of early reperfusion, reduced infarct size, and improved outcome in patients with proximal middle cerebral artery occlusion. *Stroke, 33*(6), 1551–1556. https://doi.org/10.1161/01.str.0000016323.13456.e5

Rodgers, M. L., Fox, E., Abdelhak, T., Franker, L. M., Johnson, B. J., Kirchner-Sullivan, C., Livesay, S. L., & Marden, F. A. (2021). Care of the patient with acute ischemic stroke (endovascular/intensive care unit-postinterventional therapy): Update to 2009 comprehensive nursing care scientific statement: A scientific statement from the American Heart Association. *Stroke, 52*(5), e198–e210. https://doi.org/10.1161/STR.0000000000000358

Tamburri, L. M., Hollander, K. D., & Orzano, D. (2020). Protecting patient safety and preventing modifiable complications after acute ischemic stroke. *Critical Care Nurse, 40*(1), 56–65. https://doi.org/10.4037/ccn2020859

von Kummer, R., Broderick, J. P., Campbell, B. C. V., Demchuk, A., Goyal, M., Hill, M. D., Treurniet, K. M., Majoie, C. B. L. M., Marquering, H. A., Mazya, M. V., Román, L. S., Saver, J. L., Strbian, D., Whiteley, W., & Hacke, W. (2015). The Heidelbert bleeding classification: Classification of bleeding events after ischemic stroke and reperfusion therapy. *Stroke, 46*(10), 2981–2986. https://doi.org/10.1161/STROKEAHA.115.010049

Medications

Ritu C. Light

This chapter provides more detailed information regarding the pharmacological agents referenced in this book. This chapter contains medication charts to help the neuroscience nurse in becoming more familiar with the agents being prescribed and administered in the acute management and secondary prevention of stroke. This includes both the generic and brand/trade names of common medications, their therapeutic classification, and the disease state for which they are utilized. Also noted are common side effects and/or clinical pearls to equip the bedside nurse.

An online drug information reference or pharmacist colleague may be consulted for more detailed information, including dosing, renal dosage adjustments, drug interactions, contraindications, formulations, institutional formularies, and administration guidelines.

Table 9.1 Antihypertensives

THERAPEUTIC CLASS	GENERIC NAME (ROUTE OF ADMINISTRATION)	BRAND/TRADE NAME	NOTEABLE SIDE EFFECTS
ACE inhibitor* *(generic name ends in -pril)*	benazepril	Lotensin	Angioedema Dry cough Hyperkalemia Renal insufficiency
	captopril	Capoten	
	enalapril (oral) enalaprilat (IV)	Vasotec	
	fosinopril	Monopril	
	lisinopril	Prinivil, Zestril	
	moexipril	Univasc	
	perindopril	Aceon	
	quinapril	Accupril	
	ramipril	Altace	
	trandolapril	Mavix	
ARB* *(generic name ends in -sartan)*	azilsartan	Edarbi	Hyperkalemia Renal insufficiency
	candesartan	Atacand	
	irbesartan	Avapro	
	losartan	Cozaar	
	olmesartan	Benicar	
	telmisartan	Micardis	
	valsartan	Diovan	

(continued)

Table 9.1 Antihypertensives (*continued*)

THERAPEUTIC CLASS	GENERIC NAME (ROUTE OF ADMINISTRATION)	BRAND/TRADE NAME	NOTEABLE SIDE EFFECTS
Beta blocker (*generic name often ends in –olol*)	acebutolol	Sectral	Bradycardia Fatigue Masking of hypoglycemia symptoms
	atenolol	Tenormin	
	betaxolol	Kerlone	
	bisoprolol	Zebeta	
	carvedilol	Coreg	
	esmolol (IV)	Brevibloc	
	labetalol	Trandate	
	metoprolol	Lopressor (tartrate) Toprol XL (succinate)	
	nadolol	Corgard	
	nebivolol	Bystolic	
	propranolol	Inderal	
	pindolol	Visken	
CCB	amlodipine	Norvasc	Dihydropyridine CCB (*generic name ends in -pine*): peripheral/pedal edema, flushing, tachycardia Nondihydropyridine CCB: heart block, bradycardia **Note:** nimodipine (Nimotop/ Nymalize) is an oral CCB that is only used short-term in SAH for improvement in neurological outcome
	clevidipine (IV)	Cleviprex	
	diltiazem	Cardizem, Tiazac	
	felodipine	Plendil	
	isradipine	Dynacirc	
	nicardipine	Cardene	
	nifedipine	Adalat, Procardia	
	nisoldipine	Sular	
	verapamil	Calan, Verelan	

(*continued*)

Table 9.1 Antihypertensives (*continued*)

THERAPEUTIC CLASS	GENERIC NAME (ROUTE OF ADMINISTRATION)	BRAND/TRADE NAME	NOTEABLE SIDE EFFECTS
Diuretic (*distinguished by the site on the nephron at which they act to impair sodium reabsorption [e.g., loop, thiazide, or potassium-sparing diuretics]*)	amiloride	Midamor	Electrolyte disturbances (hypokalemia, hypomagnesemia, hyponatremia)
	bumetanide	Bumex	
	chlorthalidone	Hygroton	
	eplerenone	Inspra	
	ethacrynic acic	Edecrin	
	furosemide	Lasix	
	HCTZ	Hydrodiuril	
	indapamide	Lozol	
	metolazone	Zaroxolyn	
	spironolactone	Aldactone	
	triamterene*	Dyrenium	
	torsemide	Demadex	
OTHER (LESS COMMONLY USED CLASSES)			
THERAPEUTIC CLASS	GENERIC NAME (ROUTE OF ADMINISTRATION)	BRAND/TRADE NAME	NOTEABLE SIDE EFFECTS
Alpha-2 adrenergic agonist	clonidine	Catapres	Clonidine: rebound hypertension (taper to avoid)
	methyldopa	Aldomet	
Alpha-1 blocker (*generic name ends in -zosin*)	doxazosin	Cardura	Orthostatic hypotension
	prazosin	Minipress	
	terazosin	Hytrin	
Renin inhibitor	aliskiren	Tekturna	
Dopamine-1 agonist	fenoldopam (IV)	Corlopam	
Vasodilator	hydralazine	Apresoline	
	minoxidil	Loniten	
	nitroglycerin (IV)	--	
	nitroprusside (IV)	Nipride, Nitropress	

*May be available in combination with HCTZ—this lessens pill burden but limits dosing flexibility/titration.
ACE, angiotensin-converting enzyme; ARB, angiotensin II receptor blocker; CCB, calcium channel blocker; HCTZ, hydrochlorothiazide; IV, intravenous; SAH, subarachnoid hemorrhage.

Table 9.2 Antiplatelets

GENERIC NAME	BRAND/ TRADE NAME	USUAL DOSING (ORAL)	COMMON SIDE EFFECTS	CLINICAL PEARLS
aspirin	—	LD: 162-325 mg MD: 81 mg daily	Minor bruising/ bleeding GI upset	"Baby aspirin" refers to 81-mg strength Take with food EC formulation: Swallow tablet whole Also has antipyretic, analgesic, and anti-inflammatory properties Assess therapeutic benefit with aspirin platelet function test
aspirin/ dipyridamole	Aggrenox	One capsule (25 mg aspirin/200 mg dipyridamole ER) twice daily	Minor bruising/ bleeding GI upset HA (tolerance develops)	To minimize HA: consume caffeine 30 minutes prior to dose
cilostazol	Pletal	100 mg twice daily	GI upset HA	Administer 30 minutes before—or 2 hours after—meals (breakfast and dinner)
clopidogrel*	Plavix	LD: 300-600 mg MD: 75 mg daily	Minor bruising/ bleeding	Requires activation in the liver to exert its effect Effectiveness may be decreased by some proton pump inhibitors Assess therapeutic benefit with P2Y12 platelet assay
ticagrelor*	Brilinta	LD: 180 mg MD: 90 mg twice daily	Minor bruising/ bleeding Dyspnea (occurs at rest, mild to moderate, transient)	

*Based on transient ischemic attack (TIA)/stroke severity and etiology, may be used with aspirin as part of short-term (21–90 days) dual antiplatelet therapy (DAPT) and then modified to monotherapy.

EC, enteric coated; ER, extended release; GI, gastrointestinal; HA, headache; LD, loading dose; MD, maintenance dose.

Table 9.3 Anticoagulation

GENERIC NAME	BRAND/ TRADE NAME	ROUTE OF ADMINISTRATION	CLINICAL PEARLS*
DOAC**			
apixaban	Eliquis	oral	Don't administer via feeding tube that is distal to the stomach
dabigatran	Pradaxa	oral	May cause dyspepsia/GI effects Don't open capsules
edoxaban	Savaysa	oral	
rivaroxaban	Xarelto	oral	Doses ≥15 mg: administer with a meal for proper absorption/effect Don't administer via feeding tube that is distal to the stomach
VKA**			
warfarin	Coumadin Jantoven	oral	Dosing individualized per PT/INR result Numerous medication and dietary interactions (foods that contain vitamin K) Nine tablet strengths, each is a different color Brand Coumadin no longer made
OTHER			
enoxaparin	Lovenox	subQ injection	Used for DVT prophylaxis, therapeutic anticoagulation, and bridging to warfarin Preferred if anticoagulation is indicated due to malignancy
fondaparinux	Arixtra	subQ injection	Used in patients with history of HIT
heparin (unfractionated)	—	IV infusion (continuous) or subQ injection	Follow institutional protocols for infusion rate, boluses, and PTT monitoring

*All anticoagulants can cause frequent bruising, minor and/or major bleeding; to reduce bleeding risk, avoid nonsteroidal anti-inflammatory drugs (NSAIDs) and products that contain aspirin.

**Benefits of DOAC (vs. VKA): fixed dosing, quick onset, no requirement for frequent bloodwork monitoring, fewer drug interactions, no dietary interactions, and not affected by acute illness; Caveats of DOAC: quick offset, high cost/copay.

DOAC, direct oral anticoagulant; DVT, deep vein thrombosis; GI, gastrointestinal; HIT, heparin-induced thrombocytopenia; IV, intravenous; PT/INR, prothrombin time/international normalized ratio; subQ, subcutaneous; PTT, partial thromboplastin time; VKA, vitamin K antagonist.

Table 9.4 Antipyretics and Analgesics

NONOPIOID ANALGESIC (both antipyretic [reduce fever] and analgesic [reduce pain]) Due to increased risk of bleeding and/or bruising, limit/avoid NSAID and aspirin-containing products in patients on anticoagulants or antiplatelets			
THERAPEUTIC CLASS	**GENERIC NAME**	**BRAND/TRADE NAME**	**CLINICAL PEARLS**
Acetaminophen	acetaminophen (APAP)	Tylenol Ofirmev (IV)	Inappropriate use may cause hepatotoxicity: ■ Do not exceed 4 g per day (lower limits may be warranted) ■ Multiple strengths and formulations exist ■ Found in combination with prescription and OTC medications
Salicylate	aspirin	Bayer Bufferin Ecotrin	"Baby aspirin" refers to 81-mg strength Chewable and coated formulations exist Oral (take with food) and rectal routes of administration Used for antithrombotic purposes Also has NSAID/ anti-inflammatory properties

(*continued*)

Table 9.4 Antipyretics and Analgesics (*continued*)

NONOPIOID ANALGESIC (*continued*)			
THERAPEUTIC CLASS	**GENERIC NAME**	**BRAND/TRADE NAME**	**CLINICAL PEARLS**
NSAID	celecoxib	Celebrex	Also has anti-inflammatory properties Take with food
	ibuprofen	Advil, Motrin, Caldolor (IV)	
	ketorolac	Toradol	
	meloxicam	Mobic	
	naproxen	Aleve, Anaprox, Naprosyn	
OPIOID ANALGESIC			
	GENERIC NAME	**BRAND/TRADE NAME**	
	fentanyl	Actiq, Duragesic, Fentora, Lazanda, Subsys	
	hydrocodone	Hysingla ER, Zohydro ER; Lortab, Norco, and Vicodin are in combination with APAP	
	hydromorphone	Dilaudid	
	methadone	Dolophine, Methadose	
	morphine	Duramorph, Infumorph, MS Contin, Roxanol	
	oxycodone	OxyCONTIN, Roxicodone, Xtampza ER; Endocet and Percocet are in combination with APAP	
	tramadol	ConZip, Qdolo, Ultram; Ultracet is in combination with APAP	

APAP, acetaminophen; IV, intravenous; NSAID, nonsteroidal anti-inflammatory drug; OTC, over-the-counter.

Table 9.5 Antidepressants*

THERAPEUTIC CLASS	GENERIC NAME	BRAND/TRADE NAME
SSRI	citalopram	Celexa
	escitalopram	Lexapro
	fluoxetine	Prozac
	fluvoxamine	Luvox
	paroxetine	Paxil
	sertraline	Zoloft
SNRI	desvenlafaxine	Pristiq
	duloxetine	Cymbalta
	levomilnacipran	Fetzima
	milnacipran	Savella
	venlafaxine	Effexor
DNRI	bupropion	Aplenzin, Forfivo XL, Wellbutrin
Norepinephrine serotonin modulator	mirtazapine	Remeron
OTHER (LESS COMMONLY USED)		
THERAPEUTIC CLASS	GENERIC NAME	BRAND/TRADE NAME
Serotonin modulator	nefazodone	Serzone
	trazodone	Desyrel
	vilazodone	Viibryd
	vortioxetine	Trintellix
Tricyclic/tetracyclic antidepressant	amitriptyline	Elavil
	amoxapine	Asendin
	clomipramine	Anafranil
	desipramine	Norpramin
	doxepin	Silenor
	imipramine	Tofranil
	maprotiline	Ludiomil
	nortriptyline	Pamelor
	protriptyline	Vivactil
	trimipramine	Surmontil
MAOI	isocarboxazid	Marplan
	phenelzine	Nardil
	selegiline (transdermal patch)	Emsam
	tranylcypromine	Parnate

*Clinical Pearls: *There is a lag (2–4 weeks) to experience benefit; monitor for increased suicidal thoughts; continue medication when feeling better; and taper may be needed when discontinuing.*

DNRI, dopamine norepinephrine reuptake inhibitor; MAOI, monoamine oxidase inhibitor; SNRI, serotonin norepinephrine reuptake inhibitor; SSRI, selective serotonin reuptake inhibitor.

Table 9.6 Cerebral Edema Management

AGENTS*	MANNITOL (IV) (OSMOTIC DIURETIC)	HYPERTONIC SALINE (IV) (HYPEROSMOLAR AGENT)
Dosing	Varies between institutions; typically, intermittent doses every 4 to 6 hours	Varies
Concentration	20% to 25% primarily used for cerebral edema; frequent crystallization can occur—requires 0.22 micron in-line filter if concentration ≥20%	Wide range of concentrations are available; may see 3% as a continuous infusion; and up to 23.4% bolus in severe cases
Vascular access	Vesicant—central line may be required	Vesicant—central line may be required
Adverse effects	■ Dehydration ■ Acute kidney injury ■ Hypotension	■ Circulatory overload ■ Metabolic acidosis ■ CPM
Monitor	■ ICP ■ Renal function ■ Daily input/output ■ Serum electrolytes ■ Serum and urine osmolality	■ ICP ■ Daily input/output ■ Serum electrolytes ■ Urine osmolality

*Mannitol and hypertonic saline lower ICP by pulling fluid out of the cerebral cell and into the intravascular space.
CPM, central pontine myelinolysis; ICP, intracerebral pressure; IV, intravenous.

Table 9.7 Antidiabetics

NONINSULIN AGENTS (ORAL UNLESS OTHERWISE NOTED)		
THERAPEUTIC CLASS	GENERIC NAME	BRAND/TRADE NAME
Biguanide	metformin	Fortamet, Glucophage, Glumetza, Riomet
SGLT-2 inhibitor	canagliflozin	Invokana
	dapagliflozin	Farxiga
	empagliflozin	Jardiance
	ertugliflozin	Steglatro
GLP-1 receptor agonist	dulaglutide subQ	Trulicity
	exenatide subQ	Bydureon, Byetta
	liraglutide subQ	Victoza
	lixisenatide subQ	Adlyxin
	semaglutide	Ozempic (subQ), Rybelsus (oral)
DPP-4 inhibitor	alogliptin	Nesina
	linagliptin	Tradjenta
	saxagliptin	Onglyza
	sitagliptin	Januvia
Sulfonylurea	glimepiride	Amaryl
	glipizide	Glucotrol
	glyburide	Glynase

(continued)

Table 9.7 Antidiabetics (*continued*)

NONINSULIN AGENTS (ORAL UNLESS OTHERWISE NOTED) (*continued*)		
THERAPEUTIC CLASS	**GENERIC NAME**	**BRAND/TRADE NAME**
Thiazolidinedione	pioglitazone	Actos
Meglitinide	nateglinide	Starlix
	repaglinide	Prandin
Alpha-glucosidase Inhibitor	acarbose	Precose
	miglitol	Glyset
Amylinomimetic	pramlintide (subQ)	Symlin
INSULIN AGENTS (SUBQ UNLESS OTHERWISE NOTED)		
INSULIN TYPE	**GENERIC NAME**	**BRAND/TRADE NAME**
Rapid-acting	insulin aspart	Fiasp, NovoLOG
	insulin lispro	Admelog, HumaLOG
	insulin glulisine	Apidra
	inhaled insulin	Afrezza (inhaled)
Short-acting	insulin regular	HumuLIN R, NovoLIN R
Intermediate-acting	insulin NPH	HumuLIN N, NovoLIN N
Long-acting/basal	insulin detemir	Levemir
	insulin glargine	Basaglar, Lantus, Semglee, Toujeo
	insulin degludec	Tresiba

DPP-4, dipeptidyl peptidase 4; GLP-1, glucagon-like peptide-1; NPH, neutral protamine hagedorn; SGLT-2, sodium-glucose cotransporter-2; subQ, subcutaneous.

Table 9.8 Lipid Lowering Agents

THERAPEUTIC CLASS	GENERIC NAME	BRAND/TRADE NAME
Statin*	atorvastatin	Lipitor
	fluvastatin	Lescol
	lovastatin	Mevacor
	pitavastatin	Livalo
	pravastatin	Pravachol
	rosuvastatin	Crestor
	simvastatin	Zocor
Cholesterol absorption inhibitor	ezetimibe	Zetia
Fibric acid derivatives	fenofibrate	Lofibra, Tricor, Trilipix
	gemfibrozil	Lopid
OTHER (LESS COMMONLY USED CLASSES)		
THERAPEUTIC CLASS	**GENERIC NAME**	**BRAND/TRADE NAME**
ACL inhibitor	bempedoic acid	Nexletol
Bile acid sequestrant	cholestyramine	Questran
	colesevelam	Welchol
	colestipol	Colestid

(*continued*)

Table 9.8 Lipid Lowering Agents (*continued*)

THERAPEUTIC CLASS	GENERIC NAME	BRAND/TRADE NAME
Nicotinic acid	niacin	Niacor, Niaspan
Omega-3 fatty acids	omega-3-acid ethyl esters	Lovaza
	icosapent ethyl	Vascepa
PCSK9 inhibitor (subQ injection)	alirocumab	Praluent
	evolocumab	Repatha

Clinical Pearls: Statins are categorized as low, moderate, or high intensity based on degree of LDL-lowering and are the recommended lipid-lowering agents in the secondary prevention of ischemic stroke. They have insufficient data in the hemorrhagic stroke population; therefore, use is patient/provider specific.
ACL, adenosine triphosphate-citrate lyase; LDL, low-density lipoprotein; PCSK9, proprotein convertase subtilisin kexin type 9; subQ, subcutaneous.

Table 9.9 Antiepileptics

CATEGORY	GENERIC NAME (ROUTE OF ADMINISTRATION)	BRAND/TRADE NAME	CLINICAL PEARLS
Benzodiazepine	clonazepam (oral)	KlonoPIN	No recommendations exist for medication selection for treatment of seizure; however, phenytoin has been associated with poor outcomes in ICH and SAH Prophylactic anti-seizure medication isn't recommended for ischemic or hemorrhagic stroke; for SAH, it may be considered short term in the immediate post-hemorrhagic period
	diazepam (oral, rectal, nasal, IM, IV)	Diastat, Valium, Valtoco	
	lorazepam (oral, IM, IV)	Ativan	
	midazolam (oral, nasal, IM, IV)	Nayzilam, Versed	
Other	lacosamide (oral, IV)	Vimpat	
	levetiracetam (oral, IV)	Keppra	
	pentobarbital (IV)	Nembutal	
	phenobarbital (oral, IV)	Luminal	
	valproate (oral, IV)*	Depacon Depakene Depakote	

*Available as valproic acid, valproate sodium, and divalproex sodium salts.
ICH, intracerebral hemorrhage; IM, intramuscular; IV, intravenous; SAH, subarachnoid hemorrhage.

Table 9.10 Vasopressors and Inotropes

CATEGORY	GENERIC NAME	BRAND/TRADE NAME
Vasopressor	dopamine	Intropin
	epinephrine	Adrenalin
	norepinephrine	Levophed
	phenylephrine	Neo-Synephrine
	vasopressin	Vasostrict
Inotrope	dobutamine	Dobutrex
	isoproterenol	Isuprel
	milrinone	Primacor

It is day 4 for a 46-year-old man admitted with ischemic stroke and treated with intravenous (IV) thrombolytic in the ED. The patient's past medical history includes type 2 diabetes (diet controlled), hypertension (HTN), and hyperlipidemia. He quit smoking 10 years ago after his first baby was born. The National Institutes of Health Stroke Scale (NIHSS) today is 4 (right arm motor 2, sensory 1, and best language 1), blood pressure (BP) is 136/85, heart rate is 62, temperature is 36.8 °C (98.24 °F), blood sugar is 184, hemoglobin (Hgb) A1C is 8%, and total cholesterol is 143, with low-density lipoprotein (LDL) of 116. The plan is for the patient to be discharged to home tomorrow with his wife. He will get outpatient therapy.

1. Which of these medications would the nurse anticipate being added to the patient's discharge list?

   A. Lorazepam
   B. Atenolol
   C. Metformin
   D. Acetaminophen

2. The patient's provider knows that current recommendations are for a statin to be ordered after acute ischemic stroke if atherosclerotic origin is suspected and low-density lipoprotein (LDL) is above 100 mg/dL. Which of the following would have been ordered?

   A. Gemfibrozil
   B. Atorvastatin
   C. Niacin
   D. Cholestyramine

3. The patient admits having recently stopped taking his blood pressure (BP) medication at home after developing a dry cough. The patient had read on the internet that it was from that medication. Which BP medication is the patient referring to?

   A. Benazepril
   B. Losartan
   C. Nifedipine
   D. Pindolol

1. C) Metformin

Recommendations for secondary stroke prevention are to maintain hemoglobin (Hgb) A1C at ≤7%. He has failed diet control, and metformin is a commonly used antidiabetic medication. Lorazepam is used as an antiepileptic, which is not prescribed prophylactically. Atenolol is a beta blocker, which is not advisable with a heart rate of 62. Acetaminophen is an antipyretic/analgesic, neither of which is warranted.

2. B) Atorvastatin

Atorvastatin is a statin lipid-lowering agent. Gemfibrozil, niacin, and cholestyramine are not statins and will not be ordered.

3. A) Benazepril

Angiotensin-converting enzyme (ACE) inhibitors are the category of antihypertensives associated with development of a dry cough as a side effect. Benazepril is an ACE inhibitor and thus is associated with the development of a dry cough. Losartan, nifedipine, and pindolol are not ACE inhibitors and are not associated with a dry cough.

1. A patient tells their nurse that they have taken a baby aspirin every morning for years. How many milligrams of aspirin does the patient take?

    A. 25 mg
    B. 81 mg
    C. 162 mg
    D. 325 mg

2. Which of the following classifications does aspirin fall under?

    A. Analgesic
    B. Antiplatelet
    C. Antipyretic
    D. All of the above

3. Which antipyretic could be given to a febrile patient who is also on apixaban?

    A. Ibuprofen
    B. Naproxen
    C. Acetaminophen
    D. Aspirin

4. How many grams of acetaminophen should a patient not exceed per day?

    A. 1
    B. 2
    C. 3
    D. 4

5. Exceeding the daily limit of acetaminophen puts the patient at risk for which complication?

    A. Hepatoxicity
    B. Nephrotoxicity
    C. Neurotoxicity
    D. Stroke

6. Which of the following pain medications contain acetaminophen?

    A. Ultracet
    B. Vicodin
    C. Percocet
    D. All of the above

(See answers next page.) **161**

1. B) 81 mg
"Baby aspirin," commonly used in stroke prevention, refers to the 81-mg strength of aspirin, known as "low-dose" aspirin. 325 mg is considered "regular strength." 25 and 162 mg are not considered standard doses of aspirin.

2. D) All of the above
Aspirin has several pharmacological properties. It may be used for pain/inflammation, fever, and/or as an antithrombotic; therefore, it is classified as an analgesic, antiplatelet, and antipyretic.

3. C) Acetaminophen
There is an increased risk of bruising and bleeding with being on apixaban (Eliquis), which is an oral anticoagulant. As nonsteroidal anti-inflammatory drugs (NSAIDs)/aspirin also carry this risk, acetaminophen would be the preferred antipyretic in a patient on anticoagulation. Ischemic stroke patients often require oral anticoagulation and antipyretic therapy.

4. D) 4
The maximum recommended daily limit of acetaminophen is 4 g per day. Lower daily limits may be warranted if used for longer durations or in situations of heavy alcohol use, malnutrition, low body weight, advanced age, febrile illness, or liver disease.

5. A) Hepatoxicity
The use of more than 4 g of acetaminophen per day may lead to hepatotoxicity that can be life-threatening. Excess acetaminophen use is not associated with nephrotoxicity, neurotoxicity, nor stroke.

6. D) All of the above
Ultracet, Vicodin, and Percocet all contain acetaminophen (APAP): Ultracet contains tramadol + APAP, Vicodin contains hydrocodone + APAP, and Percocet contains oxycodone + APAP. This is important to be aware of in monitoring for daily cumulative doses of APAP, as too much can lead to adverse outcomes.

7. In the secondary prevention of ischemic stroke, statins are important for lowering which of the following?

   A. Blood glucose
   B. Blood pressure (BP)
   C. High-density lipoprotein (HDL) cholesterol
   D. Low-density lipoprotein (LDL) cholesterol

8. Nimodipine is used for what indication in the stroke population?

   A. Hypertension (HTN)
   B. Benign prostatic hyperplasia (BPH)
   C. Gastroesophageal reflux disease (GERD)
   D. Subarachnoid hemorrhage (SAH)

9. A patient states they are on a long-acting insulin at home but cannot remember the name. Which of the following could they be taking?

   A. Insulin lispro
   B. Insulin aspart
   C. Insulin neutral protamine hagedorn (NPH)
   D. Insulin detemir

10. Headache occurs in nearly 40% of patients starting which medication?

   A. Aggrenox
   B. Lisinopril
   C. Rivaroxaban
   D. Ticagrelor

7. D) Low-density lipoprotein (LDL) cholesterol
Statins effectively reduce LDL cholesterol levels and are routinely utilized in the secondary prevention of ischemic stroke that is atherosclerotic in etiology. They are categorized as low, moderate, or high intensity based on their degree of LDL lowering. Statins are not used to lower blood glucose, BP, nor HDL cholesterol.

8. D) Subarachnoid hemorrhage (SAH)
Nimodipine is an oral calcium channel blocker. This class of medication is typically used for the treatment of HTN. Nimodipine is unique in that it is only indicated for the improvement of neurological outcome in the aneurysmal SAH population (for a maximum duration of 21 days); however, it may also reduce blood pressure as a consequence of use. Nimodipine is not indicated for BPH or GERD.

9. D) Insulin detemir
Insulin detemir (Levemir) is the only long-acting insulin listed. Aspart and lispro insulins are classified as "rapid acting," and NPH insulin is "intermediate acting."

10. A) Aggrenox
Due to the dipyridamole content of Aggrenox, patients may experience a headache. Fortunately, tolerance usually develops. Lisinopril, rivaroxaban, and ticagrelor are not associated with increased incidence of headaches. It is important to know about the relationship between Aggrenox and headache, along with the fact that tolerance usually develops. It is an alternative antiplatelet for secondary stroke prevention.

BIBLIOGRAPHY

American Diabetes Association. (2021). Pharmacologic approaches to glycemic treatment: Standards of medical care in diabetes—2021. American Diabetes Association. *Diabetes Care, 44*(Suppl. 1), S111–S124. https://doi.org/10.2337/dc21-S009

Bryant, C., & Naik, N. (2019, May). Direct oral anticoagulants: Use in the setting of bariatric surgery and feeding tubes. Anticoagulation Forum Rapid Resource. https://acforum-excellence.org/Resource-Center/resource_files/-2020-05-14-124503.pdf

Clinical Resource, ACE Inhibitor Antihypertensive Dose Comparison. Pharmacist's Letter/Prescriber's Letter. (2016, November). https://pharmacist.therapeuticresearch.com/Content/Segments/PRL/2009/Aug/ACE-Inhibitor-Antihypertensive-Dose-Comparison-1719

Clinical Resource, Antiplatelets for Recurrent Ischemic Stroke. Pharmacist's Letter/Prescriber's Letter. (2020, October). https://pharmacist.therapeuticresearch.com/Content/Segments/PRL/2015/Sep/Antiplatelets-for-Recurrent-Ischemic-Stroke-8855

Clinical Resource, Comparison of Angiotensin Receptor Blockers (ARBs). Pharmacist's Letter/Prescriber's Letter. (2018, September). https://pharmacist.therapeuticresearch.com/Content/Segments/PRL/2010/Mar/Comparison-of-Angiotensin-Receptor-Blockers-2165

Clinical Resource, Non-Statin Lipid-Lowering Agents. Pharmacist's Letter/Prescriber's Letter. (2020, March). https://pharmacist.therapeuticresearch.com/Content/Segments/PRL/2015/Jul/Non-Statin-Lipid-Lowering-Agents-8617

Clinical Resource, Statin Dose Comparison. Pharmacist's Letter/Prescriber's Letter. (2018, April). https://pharmacist.therapeuticresearch.com/Content/Segments/PRL/2016/Jul/Statin-Dose-Comparison-9914

Connolly, E. S., Rabinstein, A. A., Carhuapoma, J. R., Derdeyn, C. P., Dion, J., Higashida, R. T., Hoh, B. L., Kirkness, C. J., Naidech, A. M., Ogilvy, C. S., Patel, A. B., Thompson, B. G., Vespa, P., the American Heart Association Stroke Council, the Council on Cardiovascular Radiology and Intervention, the Council on Cardiovascular Nursing, the Council on Cardiovascular Surgery and Anesthesia, & the Council on Clinical Cardiology. (2012). Guidelines for the management of aneurysmal subarachnoid hemorrhage: A guideline for healthcare professionals from the American Heart Association/American Stroke Association. *Stroke, 43*(6), 1711–1737. https://doi.org/10.1161/STR.0b013e3182587839

Gupta, R., & Elkind, M. S. V. (2021). Malignant cerebral hemispheric infarction with swelling and risk of herniation. *UpToDate.* https://www.uptodate.com/contents/malignant-cerebral-hemispheric-infarction-with-swelling-and-risk-of-herniation

Hemphill, J. C., Greenberg, S. M., Anderson, C. S., Becker, K., Bendok, B. R., Cushman, M., Fung, G. L., Goldstein, J. N., Macdonald, R. L., Mitchell, P. H., Scott, P. A., Selim, M. H., Woo, D., the American Heart Association Stroke Council, the Council on Cardiovascular and Stroke Nursing, & the Council on Clinical Cardiology. (2015). Guidelines for the management of spontaneous intracerebral hemorrhage: A guideline for healthcare professionals from the American Heart Association/American Stroke Association. *Stroke, 46*(7), 2032–2060. https://doi.org/10.1161/STR.0000000000000069

Johnston, S. C., Easton, J. D., Farrant, M., Barsan, W., Conwit, R. A., Elm, J. J., Kim, A. S., Lindblad, A. S., & Palesch, Y. Y. (2018). Clopidogrel and aspirin in acute ischemic stroke and high-risk TIA. *The New England Journal of Medicine, 379*, 215–225. https://doi.org/10.1056/NEJMoa1800410

Kernan, W. N., Ovbiagele, B., Black, H. R., Bravata, D. M., Chimowitz, M. I., Ezekowitz, M. D., Fang, M. C., Fisher, M., Furie, K. L., Heck, D. V., Johnston, S. C., Kasner, S. E.,

Kittner, S. J., Mitchell, P. H., Rich, M. W., Richardson, D., Schwamm, L. H., Wilson, J. A., the American Heart Association Stroke Council, the Council on Cardiovascular and Stroke Nursing, the Council on Clinical Cardiology, & the Council on Peripheral Vascular Disease. (2014). Guidelines for the prevention of stroke in patients with stroke and transient ischemic attack: A guideline for healthcare professionals from the American Heart Association/American Stroke Association. *Stroke, 45*(7), 2160–2236. https://doi.org/10.1161/STR.0000000000000024

Kim, A. S. (2020, April). Medical management for secondary stroke prevention. *Continuum, 26*(2), 435–456. https://doi.org/10.1212/CON.0000000000000849

Lexicomp Online. (2021). *UpToDate, Inc.* https://online.lexi.com

Manaker, S. (2021, April). Use of vasopressors and inotropes. *UpToDate.* https://www.uptodate.com/contents/use-of-vasopressors-and-inotropes

Parodi, G., & Storey, R. F. (2015). Dyspnoea management in acute coronary syndrome patients treated with ticagrelor. *The European Heart Journal – Acute CardioVascular Care, 4*(6), 555–560. https://doi.org/10.1177/2048872614554108

Peters, N. A., Farrell, L. B., & Smith, J. P. (2018). Hyperosmolar therapy for the treatment of cerebral edema. *U.S. Pharmacist, 43*(1), HS-8–HS-11. https://www.uspharmacist.com/article/hyperosmolar-therapy-for-the-treatment-of-cerebral-edema

Powers, W. J., Rabinstein, A. A., & Ackerson, T. (2019). Guidelines for the early management of patients with acute ischemic stroke: 2019 update to the 2018 guidelines for the early management of acute ischemic stroke: A guideline for healthcare professionals from the American Heart Association/American Stroke Association. *Stroke, 50*(12), e344–e418. https://doi.org/10.1161/STR.0000000000000211

Rodgers, M. L., Fox, E., Abdelhak, T., Franker, L. M., Johnson, B. J., Kirchner-Sullivan, C., Livesay, S. L., & Marden, F. A. (2021). Care of the patient with acute ischemic stroke (endovascular/intensive care unit-postinterventional therapy): Update to 2009 comprehensive nursing care scientific statement: A scientific statement from the American Heart Association. *Stroke, 52*(5), e198–e210. https://doi.org/10.1161/STR.0000000000000358

Schachter, S. C. (2021, April). Antiseizure medications: Mechanism of action, pharmacology, and adverse effects. *UpToDate.* https://www.uptodate.com/contents/antiseizure-medications-mechanism-of-action-pharmacology-and-adverse-effects

Wang, Y., Wang, Y., Zhao, X., Liu, L., Wang, D., Wang, C., Wang, C., Li, H., Meng, X., Cui, L., Jia, J., Dong, Q., Xu, A., Zeng, J., Li, Y., Wang, Z., Xia, H., & Johnston, S. C. (2013). Clopidogrel with aspirin in acute minor stroke or transient ischemic attack. *The New England Journal of Medicine, 369*(1), 11–19. https://doi.org/10.1056/NEJMoa1215340

Whelton, P. K., Carey, R. M., Aronow, W. S., Casey, D. E., Collins, K. J., Himmelfarb, C. D., DePalma, S. M., Gidding, S., Jamerson, K. A., Jones, D. W., MacLaughlin, E. J., Muntner, P., Ovbiagele, B., Smith, S. C., Spencer, C. C., Stafford, R. S., Taler, S. J., Thomas, R. J., Williams, K. A., Williamson, J. D., & Wright, J. T. (2018). 2017 ACC/AHA/AAPA/ABC/ACPM/AGS/APhA/ASH/ASPC/NMA/PCNA guideline for the prevention, detection, evaluation, and management of high blood pressure in adults: A report of the American College of Cardiology/American Heart Association Task Force on Clinical Practice Guidelines. *Hypertension, 71*(6), e13–e115. https://doi.org/10.1161/HYP.0000000000000065

Postacute Stroke Care

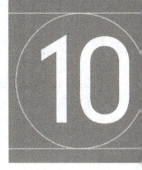

Over the past 20 years, significant progress has been made in the prehospital, hyperacute, and acute stroke levels of care, with improved outcomes as evidence. The postacute period may be seen as the next great frontier for stroke care as more evidence is emerging that it belongs in the stroke continuum of care. Models involving transitional and postdischarge support have demonstrated up to 50% reduction in readmission (Condon et al., 2016). A study reported by Prvu Bettger et al. (2015) showed that 44% of stroke patients were discharged home without any acute services, and of those under age 65, 65% were discharged home without any acute services. Since 2016, the Centers for Medicare & Medicaid Services (CMS) have mandated penalties for hospitals reporting an all-cause readmission rate that exceeds the national risk-adjusted readmission rate. In addition to reducing readmission rates, improvement efforts should also include preventing complications, maximizing recovery, reducing mortality, and preventing stroke and cardiovascular events. As more is being learned about how to improve stroke recovery, more is being expected of the healthcare team. Systems of care have the opportunity and responsibility to put processes and services in place to meet stroke patients' needs. Telemedicine has emerged as a practical and effective way for healthcare team members to interact with patients and families when in-person visits are not feasible.

POSTACUTE LEVELS OF STROKE CARE

Approximately 55% of stroke patients need additional inpatient care after their acute hospital stay in order to maximize recovery and return home. The American Stroke Association stroke rehabilitation guidelines recommend that stroke survivors who qualify for inpatient rehabilitation facility (IRF) care should receive treatment at this level of care (Winstein et al., 2016).

Table 10.1 includes the various levels of postacute inpatient and outpatient care for stroke survivors (American Academy of Physical Medicine and Rehabilitation [AAPMR], 2021).

Table 10.1 Postacute Levels of Stroke Care

Location	Patient Characteristics	Services Provided
IRF	■ Need for medical oversight ■ Able to do minimum of 3 hours of therapy daily 5 days/week ■ Expected plan for discharge is home ■ Average LOS is 2–3 weeks	■ Provider-led hospital level care (usually physiatrist) ■ Specialized nursing and social services ■ Physical, occupational, and speech therapy
SNF	■ Need for skilled nursing care ■ Able to do less than 3 hours of therapy up to 5 days/week ■ Expected plan is improved function ■ Average LOS is 32.5 days	■ Skilled nursing on site ■ Provider-led plan of care ■ Physical, occupational, and speech therapy as needed ■ Referred to as "subacute rehab" if therapy provided

(continued)

Table 10.1 Postacute Levels of Stroke Care (*continued*)

Location	Patient Characteristics	Services Provided
LTACH	▪ Multiple medical conditions ▪ Need for hospital-level care for ≥25 days	▪ Specialized medical and nursing care ▪ Extended rehab services
Nursing home	▪ No need for skilled nursing care	▪ Long-term care for patients who cannot live independently ▪ Referred to as "custodial care" if no therapy provided
Outpatient clinic	▪ No need for inpatient care	▪ Specialized medical review and therapy services
Home health agency	▪ Homebound except for medical appointments	▪ Physical, occupational, and speech therapy as needed ▪ Home health aide as needed ▪ Skilled nursing ▪ Social services ▪ Transition of care to primary provider
Day rehabilitation program	▪ Transition from inpatient rehabilitation to home; sleep and eat 2 meals at home; spend day in clustered therapy sessions	▪ Physical, occupational, and speech therapy ▪ Recreational therapy ▪ Vocational rehabilitation
Hospice care	▪ Decision to or need to prioritize comfort and support for end of life	▪ Specialized nursing and social services ▪ Health aides

IRF, inpatient rehabilitation facility; LOS, length of stay; LTACH, long-term acute care hospital; SNF, skilled nursing facility.

Source: Adeoye, O., Nyström, K. V., Yavagal, D. R., Luciano, J., Nogueira, R. G., Zorowitz, R. D., Khalessi, A. A., Bushnell, C., Barsan, W. G., Panagos, P., Alberts, M. J., Tiner, A. C., Schwamm, L. H., & Jauch, E. C. (2019). Recommendations for the establishment of stroke systems of care: A 2019 update. *Stroke, 50*(7), e187–e210. https://doi.org/10.1161/STR.0000000000000173. Copyright 2019 American Heart Association, Inc.

CLINICAL PEARL

Although rehabilitation nurse certification is not stroke specific, research has shown that the presence of Certified Rehabilitation Registered Nurses (CRRNs) in inpatient rehabilitation facilities reduces length of stay (LOS) by 6% (Nelson et al., 2007). This is additional proof that nurses with additional certifications provide a higher quality of care, which results in better outcomes for patients.

FOLLOW-UP OPTIONS

Follow-up no longer refers to only in-person clinic or office visits. Prior to 2020, telemedicine was emerging as an excellent option for those stroke patients who were unable to get transportation to appointments or for whom transportation was difficult, and the COVID-19 pandemic has only made that demand greater.

- Telemedicine: utilization of telephone or two-way audio-video technology to connect with the patient/family in their home or facility.
  - Two-way audio-video technology involves use of computer, tablet, or smartphone and facilitates face-to-face assessment and discussion; also provides ability to view home setup.
  - Telephone follow-up has been used by nurses for years to check on patients, provide education, and capture outcomes and patient satisfaction data; has been used for follow-up by providers during the COVID-19 pandemic for patients who lack technology to support audio-video connection.
- In-person clinic or office visit: **still considered to be the gold standard for follow-up as it allows for hands-on examination**; a significant percentage of stroke survivors find it prohibitive to attend in-person appointments **due to mobility or transportation concerns**; multiple comorbid conditions also necessitate other specialty appointments.

CLINICAL PEARL

Primary care clinicians provide the majority of poststroke care. Unfortunately the vast amount of evidence for clinical care is dispersed across multiple publications and guidelines. The American Heart Association/American Stroke Association's scientific statement *Primary Care of Adult Patients After Stroke* is a summary of the literature to guide providers in best practice for their stroke patients (Kernan et al., 2021).

▶ PRIMARY CARE GOALS

The first poststroke visit should occur soon after discharge, within 1 to 3 weeks, in order to reduce readmissions and address gaps in care. There are optimally five goals addressed with each visit (Kernan et al., 2021).

1. To provide patient-centered care
   a. Alleviation of pain, fear, and anxiety.
   b. Emphasizes patient autonomy and values/preferences.
2. To prevent recurrent stroke
   a. Review what caused the stroke and if any diagnostic tests were deferred until after discharge.
   b. Review and manage risk factors—some may have been present prestroke that the patient had deferred treatment for.
   c. Provide education to patient and family members.
3. To maximize function
   a. Assess what the patient could do prior to the stroke and what their current goals are.
   b. Assess ability to perform activities of daily living, communication ability, and functional mobility.
   c. Ensure continued therapy services.
4. To prevent late complications
   a. Close communication and monitoring for compliance might include an advanced practice clinician and/or case manager.
5. To optimize quality of life
   a. Life-changing effects such as depression, loss of income, and social isolation should be addressed.
   b. Link patient/family to community resources such as support groups and exercise programs.

PREVENTING READMISSIONS

All-cause readmissions are tracked by the CMS, with financial penalties to organizations that exceed the national average.

- All-cause readmissions include scheduled procedures such as carotid endarterectomy and aneurysm obliteration done for secondary stroke prevention.
- Stroke experts have recommended that stroke readmissions be calculated as cause specific to facilitate pattern detection and strategic planning to prevent readmissions; it would also delineate which were planned.
- Thirty days from discharge from the acute hospital stay is the time frame for reportable stroke readmissions.
- Readmission incidence:
  - Intracerebral hemorrhage (ICH): 13.7%
  - Acute ischemic stroke (AIS): 12.4%
  - Subarachnoid hemorrhage (SAH): 11.4%
- Causes of unplanned readmissions:
  - Recurrent stroke: 33%
  - Infections (septicemia, pneumonia, and urinary tract infection [UTI]): 14.5%
  - Cardiopulmonary disease: 9.1%
  - Diabetes: 2.2%

CLINICAL PEARL

Overall stroke readmission rates have been reported to have declined by 3.3% recently; however, the readmission rate for recurrent stroke specifically has gone up. Prevention strategies for recurrent stroke are still immensely needed (Bambhroliya et al., 2018).

- Readmission prevention strategies:
  - Readmission predictor tools have been created by many institutions, but nothing standardized has been established.
  - Focused assessment of temperature, pulmonary status, white blood cell count, urinalysis close to discharge to facilitate early detection/treatment of infection.
  - Early follow-up by the advanced practice provider (APP), nurse, or pharmacist to review medications, current neuro status to compare to discharge status, knowledge of signs of recurrent stroke, and follow-up appointments/therapy.
  - Focused stroke education for nurses/providers in inpatient rehabilitation facilities, skilled nursing facilities (SNFs), long-term acute care (LTAC) facilities, as well as primary care offices and cardiology offices.

PREVENTING COMPLICATIONS

- Shoulder pain
  - Shoulder pain occurs in up to 75% of stroke patients with upper extremity paresis. Probable causes include shoulder subluxation due to the weight of the paretic arm and improper positioning or support of the limb, traction on the arm during transfers and repositioning, and spasticity of the shoulder muscles.

- Treatment involves progressive range-of-motion (ROM) exercises, electrical stimulation, heat, anti-inflammatory agents, and analgesics.
- Nursing considerations:
  - Ensure proper handling during transfers, ambulation, and repositioning in bed.
  - Provide careful positioning of the affected limb at rest—either in a chair or in bed.
  - Use of sling during ambulation.
- Incontinence and constipation
  - Urinary and fecal incontinence are common but usually resolve within 2 to 4 weeks.
  - Constipation becomes more common after first 2 weeks.
    - Inactivity, decreased fluid intake, and depression are causes.
  - Nursing considerations:
    - Establish timed voiding and bowel training programs.
    - Encourage activity to facilitate bowel motility.
    - Ensure adequate hydration and a diet high in fiber.
    - Stool softeners and laxatives may be needed, at least temporarily.
- Depression
  - Depression is common after stroke, with an incidence rate of approximately 33% (Tamburri et al., 2020).
  - Caused by the psychological impact of loss of function/independence and/or is due to biological impact of alteration of brain neurotransmitter function.
  - Treatment involves antidepressants and psychotherapy.
  - A variety of screening tools exist, but an optimal tool or time for screening has not yet been determined.
    - The most highly regarded are the Center for Epidemiological Studies Depression Scale (CES-D), the Hamilton Depression Rating Scale (HDRS), and the nine-item Patient Health Questionnaire (PHQ-9), which has recently been endorsed by the American Heart Association/American Stroke Association (Tamburri et al., 2020).
  - Nursing considerations:
    - Notify provider if the following are noted: apathy, crying, or overt sadness; constant fatigue; sleep disturbance; appetite change; or suicidal thoughts.

CLINICAL PEARL

Evidence has shown that patients treated with antidepressants even without depressive symptoms had better functional recovery. For several years, many providers started all their stroke patients on antidepressants during the acute hospital stay to ensure an adequate blood level during the early rehabilitation phase. However, the side effects and drug interactions with these medications have led to recommendations that treatment be instituted only when symptoms are noted. Therefore, close monitoring is essential.

- Falls
  - Forty percent of stroke patients experience falls during the early rehabilitative phase; 22% sustain injuries as a result.
  - Deficits that increase risk of falls are paralysis, paresthesias, communication disorders, hemineglect, hemianopia, and cognitive impairment.
  - Nursing considerations:
    - Call bells or a mechanism for patient to summon help should be within reach on the unaffected side.

- Ensure glasses, proper lighting, and nonskid footwear are in place when ambulating.
- Environmental adaptations such as handrails, grab bars, nonslip mats, raised toilet seats, limited use of throw rugs, elimination of clutter, and avoiding overexertion should be implemented.
    - It may be helpful to instruct patients and family members how to get up after a fall because injury during the attempt to get up is common, as is the danger of being stuck out of reach of the phone or bell for extended periods of time.
- Malnutrition
    - At 2 to 3 weeks after stroke, malnutrition is reported in 50% of severe stroke patients.
    - Nursing considerations:
        - Weight loss greater than 3 kg indicates need for close review of nutritional status.
        - If imbalance is suspected, monitor urinary output for color as well as amount in contrast to oral fluid intake.
        - Collaboration with a speech–language pathologist (SLP) and a dietician is essential to determine the cause of malnutrition.
    - Treatment involves supplemental feedings and fluid intake.
- Osteoporosis
    - Bone mineral density in the paretic lower limb can decrease by 10% within the first year if nonambulatory, compared to a 3% reduction if ambulatory (Winstein et al., 2016).
    - Nursing considerations:
        - Support for and facilitation of ambulation will be beneficial.
        - Dietary and supplemental calcium and vitamin D should be encouraged.
- Spasticity
    - It occurs in up to 65% of stroke patients.
    - Treatment involves stretching, splinting, and medications.
        - Botulinum toxin injection into the spastic muscle has proven effective in improving ROM and preventing contractures when used for focal spasticity.
        - Oral baclofen, benzodiazepines, and tizanidine have been used for generalized spasticity, but their usefulness is limited secondary to sedative effects.
        - Intrathecal baclofen can be administered with an implanted pump.
    - Nursing considerations:
        - Provide/encourage ROM exercises throughout the day; follow the therapist's recommendations. Nurses can/should facilitate exercises being done, even when therapists are not present.
        - Understand proper placement of splints and ensure they are used according to therapist's recommendations.
        - Monitor for somnolence and notify care team.

FAMILY AND CAREGIVER SUPPORT

- Family/caregiver stress and inability to continue to provide care are the leading causes of institutionalization of stroke patients.
- There is an increased risk of depression, social isolation, health deterioration, and mortality for caregivers.
    - There is a 52% incidence of depression and a 63% higher mortality risk in caregivers compared to others their age who are not caregivers (Steiner et al., 2008).

- Nursing considerations:
  - An assessment of family/caregiver's needs and concerns should be done on an ongoing basis.
    - ○ Strength of the caregiver/stroke survivor relationship.
    - ○ Caregiver's understanding/willingness to provide care.
    - ○ Caregiver's capacity to provide care: preexisting health conditions of their own, time availability, financial resources.
  - Assessment tools are available for use throughout the rehabilitation process (Miller et al., 2010).
    - ○ A list of community resources and websites should be provided.

● REHABILITATION TREATMENTS

Regardless of the level of poststroke rehabilitation, there are two distinct purposes to be accomplished through the use of devices and therapies:
- Facilitating neuroplasticity: With research having demonstrated that functions previously located in the area of infarct can be taken over by adjacent areas of the brain, repetitive practice helps to facilitate rewiring of the brain circuits.
- Compensatory training: Repetitive practice of new strategies and techniques to accomplish tasks and functions for the remaining disabilities, for instance, how to dress using one arm or use of assistive devices if language has been affected.

▶ DEVICES

- Functional electrical stimulation therapy
  - Electrodes placed on an affected limb can cause movement of the limb; repetition can result in some degree of functional improvement.
- Dynamic splinting
  - Used for wrist and hand to mechanically assist in straightening.
- Partial body weight–supported treadmill training (BWSTT)
  - Uses a harness to reduce weight bearing while practice walking.
- Robotic techniques
  - Sophisticated exercise machines that guide the patient through repetitive movements.

▶ THERAPIES

- Constraint-induced movement therapy (CIMT)
  - The unaffected arm is placed in a restrictive mitt to encourage use of the weak upper limb; classic therapy occurs for 6 hours, 5 days per week for a 2-week period.
- Botulinum toxin
  - See "Spasticity" section in this chapter.
- Brain stimulation
  - Repetitive stimulation over the area of infarction to enhance the brain's ability to rewire itself.
  - Transcranial magnetic stimulation (TMS) and transcranial direct current stimulation (TDCS), as well as deep brain stimulation (DBS), have been used.

- Virtual reality (VR)
  - Computerized artificial environment used to practice movements, to improve arm and leg mobility and strength, and to foster better reaction time and decision-making.
  - Advantages include increased engagement and immediate feedback to the patient.
  - "Wii-hab" or "Wii-habilitation": Nintendo Wii and Kinect have become widely used in physical rehabilitation for a variety of populations.
- Mental practice
  - Involves imagining movement of the affected limb, usually the arm, with the aid of an audio recording to facilitate focus.
  - Effective as an adjunct therapy to CIMT.
- Mirror therapy
  - Use of a mirror to create the appearance of the affected arm moving normally in a symmetric, two-armed activity; the patient is actually seeing the unaffected arm in the mirror.
- Cognitive therapy
  - There are two general treatment approaches:
    - Retraining impaired cognitive skills that are task specific
    - Training strategies to compensate for impaired skills
  - Cognitive therapy is performed by a variety of healthcare disciplines—communication among team members is imperative to avoid omission or duplication of services.

CLINICAL PEARL

Motor, cognitive, and sensory rehab have been greatly advanced by VR technologies. This is thought to be due to the ability to simulate the real world with an interactive environment. Several studies have confirmed that VR fosters the reactivation and improvement of various cortical functions and optimizes sensory cortex function (Maggio et al., 2019).

EMERGING STRATEGIES AND RESEARCH IN STROKE REHABILITATION

The National Institute of Neurological Disorders and Stroke (NINDS) is a subsidiary of the National Institutes of Health (NIH). The NIH has been a leader in advancing research in stroke care, recovery, and rehabilitation. Below are some examples of how technology is being studied to impact stroke rehabilitation.

- Telerehabilitation is a home-based telehealth system designed to improve motor recovery and patient education after stroke.
- Transcranial Direct Current Stimulation for Post-Stroke Motor Recovery: A Phase II Study (TRANSPORT 2) aims to find out if brain stimulation at different dosage levels combined with an efficacy-proven rehabilitation therapy can improve arm function.
- The Locomotor Experience Applied Post-Stroke (LEAPS) trial found that people who had a stroke and had physical therapy at home improved their ability to walk just as well as those who were treated with a locomotor training program using treadmill walking with body weight support followed by walking practice. Study investigators also found that patients continued to improve up to 1 year after stroke.

- The multi-site I-ACQUIRE trial in infants with perinatal arterial stroke will determine the effectiveness of intensive infant rehabilitation to increase upper extremity skills.
- Sleep-SMART (Sleep for Stroke Management and Recovery Trial) will determine whether treatment of sleep-disordered breathing with positive airway pressure after AIS or high-risk transient ischemic attack prevents recurrent stroke, and whether treatment of sleep-disordered breathing shortly after AIS improves stroke outcomes at 3 months (NINDS, 2020).

CLINICAL PEARL

Research trials in stroke rehabilitation have become the fastest growing area of therapeutic research for the NIH. And as technology advances, we can anticipate more innovative methods and devices that will guide new therapeutic treatments and improve on existing ones (NINDS, 2020).

CASE STUDY

Mrs. Thomas is a 67-year-old woman who is nearing discharge after a hospital stay for subarachnoid hemorrhage (SAH). Her current National Institutes of Health Stroke Scale (NIHSS) score is 8 resulting from language difficulty, left arm and leg weakness, and sensory deficit. The aneurysm that ruptured and caused her to bleed had been coiled successfully on day 3, and she has not experienced any seizures in the 12 days since admission. Incidentally, a second smaller aneurysm was found, and a plan for its obliteration is set for 4 weeks from now. Prior to her stroke, she lived independently with her 69-year-old partner who has emphysema and had a hip replacement 1 month ago. Her past medical history includes coronary artery disease for which she takes clopidogrel and diltiazem. No new diagnoses have been made during her hospital stay. She is to follow up with her neurosurgeon and neurologist in 30 days.

1. Which of the following discharge destinations would be most appropriate?

    A. Home with outpatient therapy
    B. Skilled nursing facility (SNF)
    C. Inpatient rehabilitation facility (IRF)
    D. Day rehabilitation program

2. How will an inpatient rehabilitation hospital stay impact her planned admission for aneurysm obliteration in 4 weeks?

    A. It will likely necessitate postponing the obliteration due to average length of stay (LOS) in rehab of 3 to 4 weeks
    B. The obliteration will have to be postponed because it cannot be done within 30 days of discharge from the hospital
    C. The obliteration will have to be moved up because it can only be done while an inpatient in either an acute hospital or an acute rehabilitation facility
    D. It should not impact her obliteration admission due to average LOS in rehab of 2 to 3 weeks

3. What nursing considerations would be most important to include in her plan of care?

    A. Detailed instructions on how to not fall
    B. Scheduled bolus feedings via percutaneous endoscopic gastrostomy (PEG) tube
    C. Call bell within reach on unaffected side
    D. Use of arm immobilizer while in bed

4. Which of the following represents the greatest barrier to two-way audio-video follow-up?

    A. Living in a rural setting with poor internet access
    B. Partner's recent surgery
    C. Patient will not be able to drive
    D. Patient may have residual language difficulty

(See answers next page.)

1. C) Inpatient rehabilitation facility (IRF)

Her National Institutes of Health Stroke Score (NIHSS) indicates disabilities that require multiple therapies. She was independent prior to her stroke, and her partner can be anticipated to be helpful by the time she is ready for discharge to home from rehab. Her partner likely cannot drive her to outpatient therapy appointments or day rehab sessions due to a recent hip surgery. An SNF is not necessary since she will have support at home and good potential for progress in rehabilitation.

2. D) It should not impact her obliteration admission due to average LOS in rehab of 2 to 3 weeks

With average LOS of 2 to 3 weeks, it should not impact her planned procedure. There is no rule that the procedure cannot be done within 30 days of discharge or that it can only be done on inpatients.

3. C) Call bell within reach on unaffected side

Keeping the call bell within reach on the unaffected side has been proven to prevent falls, one major poststroke complication. Instructions for how to not fall may be helpful but is not as important as keeping the call bell within reach. This patient did not have a PEG tube. Arm immobilizers are used during mobilization, not while on bedrest.

4. A) Living in a rural setting with poor internet access

Two-way audio-video follow-up requires dependable internet access. Two-way audio-video follow-up negates concerns regarding driving, as it provides connection between home and provider. As long as the partner can communicate or help the patient communicate, two-way audio-video follow-up is possible.

1. What is the leading cause of unplanned readmissions to acute care?

   A. Noncompliance with medications resulting in complications
   B. Recurrent stroke
   C. New-onset seizure disorder
   D. Aspiration pneumonia

2. A 75-year-old hemiparetic patient demonstrates the ability to tolerate 1 to 1.5 hours of therapy a day. The patient can eat with assistance and has a daughter who lives an hour away. Which discharge disposition is anticipated?

   A. Inpatient rehabilitation facility (IRF)
   B. Skilled nursing facility (SNF)
   C. Long-term acute care (LTAC) facility
   D. Home

3. Botulinum toxin injection has proven effective poststroke for which condition?

   A. Urinary incontinence
   B. Focal spasticity
   C. Facial palsy
   D. Balance deficit

4. Subacute rehabilitation is a term used for which level of postacute care?

   A. Inpatient rehabilitation facility (IRF)
   B. Skilled nursing facility (SNF)
   C. Long-term acute care hospital (LTACH)
   D. Home health care agency (HHCA)

5. Which of the following is most common during the first 6 months after discharge from the hospital or rehabilitation facility?

   A. Swallowing difficulties
   B. Urinary tract infection (UTI)
   C. Falling
   D. Shoulder subluxation

1. B) Recurrent stroke

Recurrent stroke accounts for 33% of unplanned stroke readmissions, higher than noncompliance with medication, aspiration pneumonia, or complications resulting from noncompliance with medications.

2. B) Skilled nursing facility (SNF)

The criteria for an inpatient acute rehabilitation stay are the ability to tolerate 3 hours of therapy a day. Because this patient could only tolerate 1 to 1.5 hours and their daughter is an hour away, an IRF is not advised. This patient does not have acute care needs to warrant an LTAC facility and is not independent enough for home discharge.

3. B) Focal spasticity

Botulinum toxin, a neurotoxin that blocks the chemicals that make muscles tight, has been proven effective poststroke for treatment of spasticity. This therapy intends to loosen the muscles enough to facilitate physical therapy and recovery of function. It is not indicated for urinary incontinence, facial palsy, or balance deficit and will not be effective in treating these conditions.

4. B) Skilled nursing facility (SNF)

SNFs have also been referred to as subacute rehabilitation facilities because they provide therapy services for patients who cannot tolerate acute rehabilitation–level therapies.

5. C) Falling

Up to 70% of individuals with a stroke experience a fall during the first 6 months after discharge from a hospital or rehabilitation facility. Shoulder subluxation occurs in up to 22% of patients, UTI occurs in 10% of patients postdischarge, and dysphagia occurs in up to 30% of stroke patients.

6. An 87-year-old inpatient rehabilitation patient has just told their rehab nurse that they are stronger now and insist on going home. Today is day 11, and the patient's progress has been slow. An additional week has been strongly recommended by the physiatrist as the patient's balance is bad, coupled with a reluctance to use a walker. What is the best nursing action?

   A. Double therapy times for 2 days, then discharge home in the evening
   B. Increase dose of antidepressant
   C. Ask the patient's niece next door to check on them daily
   D. Confirm the son's offer to move in with them for 6 months

7. It is day 9 for an acute ischemic stroke patient. Their history of renal failure requires dialysis, and labile hypertension has complicated and extended their hospital stay. The patient is able to participate in some therapy services but still requires tube feed support. Discharge is planned for tomorrow. What is the most likely discharge disposition?

   A. Inpatient hospice facility
   B. Long-term acute care hospital (LTACH)
   C. Home with full-time homecare
   D. Skilled nursing facility (SNF)

8. For Mr. White, a 74-year-old ischemic stroke patient, to qualify for home healthcare, what condition must be present?

   A. He must have supplemental insurance that covers home healthcare
   B. He must be homebound
   C. He must require at least two therapies and one nursing care need
   D. He must be able to answer the door when the staff arrive

9. A patient receives cognitive therapy during their acute rehabilitation stay. Which care team member would provide this therapy?

   A. Neuropsychologist
   B. Occupational therapist
   C. Speech–language pathologist
   D. All of the above

10. Poststroke depression is attributable to which of the following causes?

   A. Organic, related to the neuronal damage of the stroke
   B. Premorbid, related to having risk factors for depression prior to stroke
   C. Reactive, related to the loss of prestroke independence
   D. All of the above

6. D) Confirm the son's offer to move in with them for 6 months

An important consideration for readiness for discharge from acute rehabilitation is readiness/willingness of a caregiver to provide support, for example, the patient's son's ability to move in with the patient. Doubling therapy sessions for an 87-year-old is not feasible. Increasing the dose of antidepressant is possible, but it is not as helpful as lining up help at home and does not directly address the patient's needs. Asking someone to check in daily does not provide adequate care to meet this patient's needs.

7. B) Long-term acute care hospital (LTACH)

Patients with complex medical needs requiring acute care stays of at least 25 days are discharged to LTACHs. Inpatient hospice is not appropriate as there is no life-limiting condition present. Discharge to neither a home with homecare nor an SNF is adequate with the patient's needs for parenteral nutrition and tight blood pressure control.

8. B) He must be homebound

For Medicare patients to qualify for home healthcare, they must be certified as homebound by a physician. Supplemental insurance will be helpful but not necessary. There is no requirement for number of therapies or nursing care needs or for him to be able to answer the door.

9. D) All of the above

A neuropsychologist, occupational therapist, and speech–language pathologist all provide different aspects of cognitive therapy. A strong rehabilitation care team employs all three types of professionals.

10. D) All of the above

Poststroke depression can occur because of the physical damage of the stroke or a result of the person's reaction to the effect of the stroke. It is also more likely with people who had a history of risk factors for stroke.

11. A skilled nursing facility nurse is an expert in managing fecal incontinence and constipation in poststroke patients. Why do so many of these patients have this trouble?

   A. Decreased mobilization and limited access to toilet cause many to become constipated
   B. Frequent therapy daily sessions interrupt their bathroom schedule, which frustrates them
   C. Spasticity of the smooth muscles of the bowel is the result of polypharmacy
   D. Bowel motility is decreased by tube feedings

12. Which of the following is NOT a reason for healthcare professionals to strive to prevent stroke readmissions?

   A. The Centers for Medicare & Medicaid Services' (CMS's) financial penalty to institutions for exceeding national average of stroke readmissions
   B. Providers are penalized for more than 30 stroke readmissions annually
   C. Readmissions represent complications or recurrent stroke, which are bad for patients
   D. Readmitted stroke patients are less satisfied with their care

13. Which is true of custodial care?

   A. Refers to guardianship cases when there are no family members
   B. Refers to the level of care in a nursing home without therapy services
   C. Synonymous to home hospice care
   D. Refers to care of patients in nursing homes who have run out of money

14. After mobilizing a patient from the bed to the chair, which of the following actions should occur?

   A. Elevate their affected arm above their shoulder to prevent dependent edema
   B. Elevate their affected leg above their hip to prevent dependent edema
   C. Elevate their affected arm on a pillow to prevent shoulder subluxation
   D. Both A and B

15. A patient has exhibited signs of spasticity of their affected arm, and the provider has ordered treatment for them. Which of the following will be added to their plan of care?

   A. Monitor for tachycardia
   B. Ensure bedrest during splinting sessions
   C. Monitor for somnolence
   D. Patient education to not use the splinted limb

11. A) Decreased mobilization and limited access to toilet causes many to become constipated

Fecal incontinence and constipation often occur because of decreased mobilization and limited access to a toilet. Bowel motility is stimulated by physical activity. Many patients will suppress the urge to move their bowels if their only option is a bedpan or bedside commode. Therapy sessions in a nursing home are not frequent or lengthy, as in inpatient rehabilitation, so it should not impact their bathroom schedule. Polypharmacy and tube feedings are more likely to result in diarrhea than constipation.

12. B) Providers are penalized for more than 30 stroke readmissions annually

There is no penalty specific to providers who have readmitted stroke patients; however, there is a penalty for institutions that exceed the national average. It is true that readmissions represent complications or recurrent stroke, which are negative patient outcomes, and readmitted stroke patients tend to be less satisfied with their care.

13. B) Refers to the level of care in a nursing home without therapy services

Custodial care is a term used to differentiate a nursing home from skilled nursing facility care in which skilled services are provided. Most facilities provide therapy as ordered, but if a patient cannot tolerate it, or hasn't progressed with therapy, their care is deemed to be custodial care. It is not associated with guardianship, hospice, or indigent care.

14. C) Elevate their affected arm on a pillow to prevent shoulder subluxation

Shoulder subluxation is a common and painful complication of poor positioning and support of the affected arm. Proper positioning with both the affected arm and leg is important to prevent dependent edema, but elevation of the arm above the shoulder and the leg above the hip is improper.

15. C) Monitor for somnolence

If oral medications such as benzodiazepines are used, somnolence is a likely result and may be a safety risk as well as inhibit therapy. There is no need for monitoring for tachycardia, bedrest, or limited use of the limb.

16. Which of the following therapies involves restricting use of the unaffected arm?

    A. Constraint-induced movement therapy (CIMT)
    B. Mental imaging movement therapy
    C. Leg restraint incentive therapy
    D. Dynamic splinting therapy

17. Which of the following statements is true?

    A. Telemedicine technology is useful for follow-up visits with a provider, but evidence has shown it cannot be utilized for therapies
    B. Stroke recovery research has been hindered by lack of interest and apathy on the part of stroke survivors
    C. The sole purpose of stroke rehabilitation services is to teach patients how to work around their deficits
    D. Stroke recovery has been enhanced significantly with the addition of technology such as virtual reality

18. Which of the following is NOT a reason for nurses to facilitate ambulation during the postacute phase?

    A. Prevention of osteoporosis
    B. Prevention of dysphagia
    C. Prevention of pneumonia
    D. Prevention of muscle atrophy

19. Which of the following is NOT true of readmission prevention strategies?

    A. Early follow-up by members of the healthcare team is beneficial
    B. Evidence-based readmission predictor tools are available and proven to reduce readmission
    C. Education for primary care providers is beneficial
    D. Monitoring for signs of infection prior to discharge may facilitate treatment and prevent readmission

20. During a patient's 30-day follow-up visit via two-way audio-video connection, the nurse notices that the patient's partner is tearful and is barely engaged in the conversation. What would be the best nursing action?

    A. Ask to meet with the patient's partner
    B. Note the partner's behavior and sympathize that it would be tough to be a caregiver
    C. Ask if the partner is feeling overwhelmed by the patient's needs and loss of independence
    D. Speak with the provider about ordering her antidepressant

(See answers next page.)

16. A) Constraint-induced movement therapy (CIMT)
By immobilizing the unaffected arm, the patient is incentivized to use their affected arm. The other choices do not involve restriction of arm movement.

17. D) Stroke recovery has been enhanced significantly with the addition of technology such as virtual reality
The marriage of technology and therapies has shown to improve outcomes. Studies are currently underway to determine if telerehabilitation is feasible. There is no evidence that stroke survivors don't care about research. Stroke rehabilitation has a dual purpose—to facilitate neuroplasticity and for compensatory training.

18. B) Prevention of dysphagia
There is no evidence that ambulation prevents dysphagia, but it does help to prevent osteoporosis, atelectasis and pneumonia, and muscle atrophy.

19. B) Evidence-based readmission predictor tools are available and proven to reduce readmission
Predictor tools have been developed and utilized, but research is pending as to their efficacy. Early follow-up by members of the healthcare team, education for primary care providers, and monitoring for signs of infection prior to discharge all have many benefits, which can help to mitigate patient readmission.

20. A) Ask to meet with the patient's partner
Checking in with the partner later will give the opportunity to communicate apart from the patient. Sympathy is important, but not as useful as speaking with the partner. Pointing out the enormity of their life changes is not beneficial for the patient or their partner. Until more information is known, medications are premature and not indicated.

REFERENCES

Adeoye, O., Nyström, K. V., Yavagal, D. R., Luciano, J., Nogueira, R. G., Zorowitz, R. D., Khalessi, A. A., Bushnell, C., Barsan, W. G., Panagos, P., Alberts, M. J., Tiner, A. C., Schwamm, L. H., & Jauch, E. C. (2019). Recommendations for the establishment of stroke systems of care: A 2019 update. *Stroke, 50*(7), e187–e210. https://doi.org/10.1161/STR.0000000000000173

American Academy of Physical Medicine and Rehabilitation. (2021). *The post-acute continuum for stroke care.* Author. https://www.aapmr.org/docs/default-source/career-center/aapmr-stroke-brochure-4-28-printhighres.pdf?sfvrsn=0

Bambhroliya, A. B., Donnelly, J. P., Thomas, E. J., Tyson, J. E., Miller, C. C., McCullough, L. D., Savitz, S. I., & Vahidy, F. S. (2018). Estimates and temporal trend for US nationwide 30-day hospital readmission among patients with ischemic and hemorrhage stroke. *JAMA Network Open, 1*(4), e181190. https://doi.org/10.1001/jamanetworkopen.2018.1190

Condon, C., Lycan, S., Duncan, P., & Bushnell, C. (2016). Reducing readmissions after stroke with a structured nurse practitioner/registered nurse transitional stroke program. *Stroke, 47*(6), 1599–1604. https://doi.org/10.1161/STROKEAHA.115.012524

Kernan, W. N., Viera, A. J., Billinger, S. A., Bravata, D. M., Stark, S. L., Kasner, S. E., Kuritzky, L., Towfighi, A., the American Heart Association Stroke Council, the Council on Arteriosclerosis, Thrombosis and Vascular Biology, the Council on Cardiovascular Radiology and Intervention, & the Council on Peripheral Vascular Disease. (2021). Primary care of adult patients after stroke: A scientific statement from the American Heart Assocation/American Stroke Association. *Stroke, 52*(9), e1–e14. https://doi.org/10.1161/STR.0000000000000382

Maggio, M. G., Latella, D., Maresca, G., Sciarrone, F., Manuli, A., Naro, A., De Luca, R., & Calabrò, R. S. (2019). Virtual reality and cognitive rehabilitation in people with stroke: An overview. *Journal of Neuroscience Nursing, 51*(2), 101–105. https://doi.org/10.1097/JNN.0000000000000423

Miller, E. L., Murray, L., Richards, L., Zorowitz, R. D., Bakas, T., Clark, P., Billinger, S. A., & the American Heart Association Council on Cardiovascular Nursing and the Stroke Council. (2010). Comprehensive overview of nursing and interdisciplinary rehabilitation care of the stroke patient: A scientific statement from the American Heart Association. *Stroke, 41*(10), 2402–2448. https://doi.org/10.1161/STR.0b013e3181e7512b

National Institute of Neurological Disorders and Stroke. (2020). Post-stroke rehabilitation fact sheet. https://www.ninds.nih.gov/Disorders/Patient-Caregiver-Education/Fact-Sheets/Post-Stroke-Rehabilitation-Fact-Sheet

Nelson, A., Powell-Cope, G., Palacios, P., Luther, S. L., Black, T., Hillman, T., Christiansen, B., Nathenson, P., & Gross, J. C. (2007). Nurse staffing and patient outcomes in inpatient rehabilitation settings. *Rehabilitation Nursing, 32*(5), 179–202. https://doi.org/10.1002/j.2048-7940.2007.tb00173.x

Prvu Bettger, J., McCoy, L., Smith, E. E., Fonarrow, G. C., Schwamm, L. H., & Petersen, E. D. (2015). Contemporary trends and predictors of postacute service use and routine discharge home after stroke. *Journal of the American Heart Association, 4*(2), e001038. https://doi.org/10.1161/JAHA.114.001038

Schwamm, L. H., Chumbler, N., Brown, E., Fonarow, G. C., Berube, D., Nystrom, K., Suter, R., Zavala, M., Polsky, D., Radhakrishnan, K., Lacktman, N., Horton, K., Malcarney, M.-B., Halamka, J., Tiner, A. C., & the American Heart Association Advocacy Coordinating Committee. (2017). Recommendations for the implementation of telehealth in cardiovascular and stroke care: A policy statement from the

American Heart Association. *Circulation, 135*(7), e24–e44. https://doi.org/10.1161/CIR.0000000000000475

Steiner, V., Pierce, L., Drahuschak, S., Nofziger, E., Buchman, D., & Szirony, T. (2008). Emotional support, physical help, and health of caregivers of stroke survivors. *Journal of Neuroscience Nursing, 40*(1), 48–54. https://doi.org/10.1097/01376517-200802000-00008

Tamburri, L. M., Hollender, K. D., & Orzano, D. (2020). Protecting patient safety and preventing modifiable complications after acute ischemic stroke. *Critical Care Nurse, 40*(1), 56–65. https://doi.org/10.4037/ccn2020859

Towfighi, A., Ovbiagele, B., El Husseini, N., Hackett, M. L., Jorge, R. E., Kissela, B. M., Mitchell, P. H., Skolarus, L. E., Whooley, M. A., Williams, L. S., the American Heart Association Stroke Council, the Council on Cardiovascular and Stroke Nursing, & the Council on Quality of Care and Outcomes Research. (2016). Poststroke depression: A scientific statement for healthcare professionals from the American Heart Association/American Stroke Association. *Stroke, 48*(2), e30–e43. https://doi.org/10.1161/STR.0000000000000113

Winstein, C. J., Stein, J., Arena, R., Bates, B., Cherney, L. R., Cramer, S. C., Deruyter, F., Eng, J. J., Fisher, B., Harvey, R. L., Lang, C. E., MacKay-Lyons, M., Ottenbacher, K. J., Pugh, S., Reeves, M. J., Richards, L. G., Stiers, W., Zorowitz, R. D., the American Heart Association Stroke Council, the Council on Cardiovascular and Stroke Nursing, the Council on Clinical Cardiology, & the Council on Quality of Care and Outcomes Research. (2016). Guidelines for adult stroke rehabilitation and recovery: A guideline for healthcare professionals from the American Heart Association/American Stroke Association. *Stroke, 47*(6), e98–e169. https://doi.org/10.1161/STR.0000000000000098

Primary and Secondary Preventive Care

Of the 795,000 people annually in the United States who have had strokes, approximately 610,000 of these are first events. The annual incidence is unchanged since 2014, but the incidence among various age groups has changed: down 28% in age >65 years, and up 44% in ages 25 to 44 years. Experts have theorized that the drop in older adults is the result of better blood pressure (BP), cholesterol, and diabetes management. The rise in younger adults is thought to be the result of risk factors occurring in childhood such as type 2 diabetes, obesity, and inactivity. Stroke primary prevention education is critical—for all ages.

Experts anticipate that the cost of stroke care will be $56 billion by 2030, with the loss of productivity and quality of life being much more than just dollars. For many patients, their stroke hospital stay is their first comprehensive health assessment in some time and represents the healthcare team's one opportunity to promote secondary prevention.

This chapter will provide an overview of the risk factor management recommendations for primary and secondary prevention for both a transient ischemic attack (TIA) and stroke, as the physiological mechanisms for both are the same.

PREVENTION PRIMER

- Primordial prevention
  - Interventions to prevent risk factors from developing in the first place, a key part of population health initiatives.
    - Examples of primordial prevention strategies: school initiatives to keep students active, limiting calories in meals served, and elimination of fast foods and vending machines from cafeterias.
    - In this book, primordial prevention strategies will be included in the primary prevention strategies.
- Primary prevention
  - Interventions designed to modify risk factors once present with the goal of preventing an initial stroke event.
    - With over 76% of strokes annually being first events, and 90% of all strokes being attributable to five risk factors, it seems essential and doable to develop effective primary prevention strategies.
- Secondary prevention
  - Interventions to modify risk factors after an initial stroke or TIA with the goal of preventing a subsequent event.
    - The risk for stroke recurrence is ~8% during the first year post ischemic stroke, then falls to ~2%, which is still approximately four times higher than the risk of a first stroke (Kernan et al., 2021).
- Tertiary prevention
  - Efforts to soften the impact of an ongoing illness or injury that has lasting effects by helping to manage long-term, complex health problems to improve as much as possible a person's ability to function, quality of life, and life expectancy.

RISK FACTORS

▶ NONMODIFIABLE RISK FACTORS

Individuals with one or more of the following risk factors should also be advised to pay close attention to their modifiable risk factors:

- Age
  - Risk doubles with each decade after age 55.
  - Recent studies have shown that the incidence of stroke is rising among young adults.
  - A 44% increase in hospitalizations for stroke has occurred in those aged 24 to 44 years, attributed to the rise in type 2 diabetes, hypercholesterolemia, and obesity in children and young adults.
  - A 29% decrease was seen in those aged 65 to 84 years, attributed to better control of risk factors like hypertension (HTN), cholesterol, and diabetes (Béjot et al., 2016).
- Gender
  - Annually, ~55,000 more females than males have a stroke.
  - Incidence rates are substantially lower in females than males in younger and middle-aged groups, but that changes after age 55 when the incidence rates in females are approximately equal to or even higher than those in males (Virani et al., 2021).
- Low birth weight
  - Risk is more than double for babies with a birth weight below 2,500 g (5 lb., 8 oz).
- Race/ethnicity
  - Black people have the highest incidence of stroke in the United States and a higher death rate from stroke than any other racial group.
  - Over two-thirds of Black populations have at least one risk factor for stroke, with high BP being most common.
  - Black and Hispanic females ≥70 years of age had higher risk of stroke compared with White females; this increased risk was not present with elderly Black or Hispanic males compared with White males.
  - Hispanic, non-Hispanic White, Pacific Islander, and Native American populations have similar incidence of stroke.
  - Fifty percent of Hispanic men and 40% of Hispanic women have heart disease, HTN, and diabetes.
  - Stroke incidence in Hispanic people is expected to rise by 29% (Virani et al., 2021).
- Genetics
  - Coagulopathies and intracranial aneurysms have been shown to have familial tendencies; Marfan syndrome, sickle cell disease, and Fabry disease are associated with increased stroke risk.
  - Parental ischemic stroke by the age of 65 years was associated with a threefold increase in ischemic stroke risk in offspring (Benjamin et al., 2018).
  - Variants in the *HDAC9* gene, as well as chromosome 9p21, have been associated with large-artery stroke.
  - A variant on chromosome 16q24.2 has been associated with small vessel stroke.
  - Variants on chromosomes 205, PMF1, and SLC25A44, and the APOE gene have been linked to intracranial hemorrhage (ICH).

● CLINICAL PEARL

It is important to improve stroke awareness and provide education to primary care providers (PCPs) and gynecologists regarding women at younger ages due to the risks of stroke associated with pregnancy, gestational HTN, and hormonal contraception; and the onset of stroke risk factors such as obesity, HTN, and diabetes at younger ages.

▶ MODIFIABLE RISK FACTORS

Five risk factors account for up to 90% of ischemic and hemorrhagic strokes: HTN, poor diet, physical inactivity, smoking, and abdominal obesity (Kleindorfer et al., 2021).

Table 11.1 lists the most commonly cited vascular and lifestyle risk factors for ischemic and hemorrhagic stroke along with primary and secondary prevention recommendations. The first five (highlighted) have been associated with 90% of strokes.

Table 11.1 Primary and Secondary Prevention

Risk Factor	Primary Prevention	Secondary Prevention
Hypertension a. Borderline: 120–129/80 mmHg b. Stage 1: 130–139/80–89 mmHg c. Stage 2: ≥140/90 mmHg	a. Lifestyle changes: weight loss; healthy, low sodium diet; physical activity b. Medication, lifestyle changes; target <130/80 mmHg c. Same as b	Medications: thiazide diuretic, ACE I, ARB—in addition to lifestyle changes with goal of office follow-up BP <130/80 mmHg
Smoking	Behavioral modification and/or medication for cessation	Same as primary prevention
Physical inactivity	Moderate- to vigorous-intensity physical activity at least 40 min/d, 3 to 4 d/wk	Moderate physical activity at least 10 min/d, 4 d/wk or Vigorous physical activity at least 20 min/d, twice a week Addition of exercise class and counseling may be beneficial
Unhealthy diet	DASH-style diet or Mediterranean diet supplemented with nuts; reduced sodium	Mediterranean diet; reduced sodium
High BMI ■ Overweight: BMI 25–29 kg/m² ■ Obese: BMI 30–39 kg/m² ■ Morbid obesity: > 40 kg/m²	Weight reduction with goal of BMI <25 kg/m²	Referral to behavioral lifestyle modification program for weight reduction with goal of BMI <25 kg/m²
■ **Diabetes**	Glucose-lowering medications to maintain Hgb A1C <7.0%; tight BP control; statin therapy	Glucose-lowering medications to maintain Hgb A1C <7.0%; nutritional therapy; diabetes self-management education

(continued)

Table 11.1 Primary and Secondary Prevention (*continued*)

Risk Factor	Primary Prevention	Secondary Prevention
Hyperlipidemia	■ LDL <160 mg/dL: statin; lifestyle changes ■ Family history of cardiovascular disease and LDL <160 mg/dL: statin; lifestyle changes	■ LDL <100 mg/dL: statin; lifestyle changes ■ LDL <70 mg/dL and atherosclerotic disease: statin plus ezetimibe
Atrial fibrillation (Afib) a. Valvular Afib with CHA_2DS_2-VASc score of ≥2 b. Nonvalvular Afib with CHA_2DS_2-VASc score of ≥2 c. Nonvalvular Afib with CHA_2DS_2-VASc score of 0 or 1	a. Warfarin with a target INR of 2.0 to 3.0 b. Oral anticoagulants: Warfarin (INR, 2.0 to 3.0) Dabigatran Apixaban Rivaroxaban ■ Closure of the left atrial appendage if intolerant of anticoagulants c. No antithrombotics	a. Warfarin with a target INR of 3.0 b. Oral anticoagulants: Warfarin (INR, 2.0 to 3.0) Dabigatran Apixaban Rivaroxaban ■ Closure of the left atrial appendage if intolerant of anticoagulants c. Oral anticoagulants: Warfarin (INR, 2.0 to 3.0) Dabigatran Apixaban Rivaroxaban ■ Closure of the left atrial appendage if intolerant of anticoagulants
Carotid artery stenosis Asymptomatic: a. <70% stenosis b. >70% stenosis	a. Aspirin and statin; lifestyle changes b. Carotid endarterectomy or stent	
Symptomatic: Extracranial: a. ≥50% stenosis ipsilateral to stroke Intracranial: a. >50–69% stenosis ipsilateral to stroke b. ≥70% stenosis ipsilateral to stroke		a. Carotid endarterectomy within 2 weeks; antiplatelet, lipid-lowering, and hypertension therapies b. Aspirin 325 mg/d c. Aspirin 325 mg/d; SBP <140 mmHg; statin; moderate physical activity

Note: Highlighted fields indicate the five risk factors that account for 90% of strokes.

ACE I, angiotensin converting enzyme inhibitor; Afib, atrial fibrillation; ARB, angiotensin receptor blocker; BMI, body mass index; BP, blood pressure; DASH, dietary approaches to stop hypertension; Hgb, hemoglobin; INR, international normalized ratio; LDL, low-density lipoprotein; SBP, systolic blood pressure.

Sources: Data from Arnett, D. K., Blumenthal, R. S., Albert, M. A., Buroker, A. B., Goldberger, Z. D., Hahn, E. J., Himmelfarb, C. D., Khera, A., Lloyd-Jones, D., McEvoy, J. W., Michos, E. D., Miedema, M. D., Muñoz, D., Smith, S. C., Virani, S. S., Williams, K. A., Yeboah, J., & Ziaeian, B. (2019). 2019 ACC/AHA guideline on the primary prevention of cardiovascular disease: A report of the American College of Cardiology/American Heart Association Task Force on Clinical Practice Guidelines. *Journal of the American College of Cardiology, 74*(10), e177–e232. https://doi.org/10.1016/j.jacc.2019.03.010; Kleindorfer, D. O., Towfighi, A., Chaturvedi, S., Cockroft, K. M., Gutierrez, J., Lombardi-Hill, D., Kamel, H., Kernan, W. N., Kittner, S. J., Leira, E. C., Lennon, O., Meschia, J. F., Nguyen, T. N., Pollak, P. M., Santangeli, P., Sharrief, A. Z., Smith, S. C., Turan, T. N., & Williams, L. S. (2021). 2021 guideline for the prevention of stroke in patients with stroke and transient ischemic attack: A guideline from the American Heart Association/American Stroke Association. *Stroke, 52*(7), e364–e467. https://doi.org/10.1161/STR.0000000000000375; Meschia, J. F., Bushnell, C., Boden-Albala, B., Braun, L. T., Bravata, D. M., Chaturvedi, S., Creager, M. A., Eckel, R. H., Elkind, M. S. V., Fornage, M., Goldstein, L. B., Greenberg, S. M., Horvath, S. E., Iadecola, C., Jauch, E. C., Moore, W. S., & Wilson, J. A. (2014). Guidelines for the primary prevention of stroke: A statement for healthcare professionals from the American Heart Association/American Stroke Association. *Stroke, 45*(12), 3754–3832. https://doi.org/10.1161/STR.0000000000000046.

CLINICAL PEARL

Uncontrolled HTN is the most common cause of both ischemic and hemorrhagic stroke. Each 10-mmHg increase in systolic BP is associated with a 24% increase in stroke risk (Benjamin et al., 2018).

Strokes are more than four times more common among people with elevated BP at age 30 and nearly six times more common for such people by age 40 (Gerber et al., 2021).

ADDITIONAL MODIFIABLE RISK FACTORS

- Sleep-disordered breathing
  - Loud snoring and sleep apnea are associated with increased carotid atherosclerosis, cardiomyopathy, atrial fibrillation (Afib), and HTN.
    - Recommendation is to maintain healthy weight to reduce risk of snoring and to treat sleep apnea.
- Hormone therapy
  - Postmenopausal hormone therapy with estrogen and/or progestin increases stroke risk.
  - High-dose estrogen patches increase stroke risk at any age.
    - Recommendation is to use alternate therapies to control menopausal symptoms and to avoid high-dose patches for birth control.
- Migraine with aura
  - Young women with migraines who also smoke and take oral contraception have nine-fold increased risk of stroke.
    - Recommendation is to avoid triggers and take medication to control migraines; do not smoke; and use an alternate form of contraception.
- Alcohol consumption
  - Heavy alcohol use (more than 21 drinks per week) is associated with HTN, hypercoagulability, reduced cerebral blood flow, and Afib.
    - Recommendation is two drinks or less per day for men and one drink or less per day for women.
- Drug abuse
  - Cocaine, amphetamines, and heroin are linked to HTN, cerebral vasospasm, vasculitis, infectious endocarditis, increased blood viscosity, and ICH.
    - Recommendation is to avoid use of these drugs.
- Hypercoagulability
  - Condition that increases likelihood of clot formation.
    - Recommendation is to screen stroke patients under age 50 with no other etiology identified; if present, treatment with anticoagulation may be initiated.
- Inflammation
  - Chronic conditions, such as rheumatoid arthritis and lupus, have been associated with initiation, growth, and destabilization of atherosclerotic plaque.
    - Recommendation is to avoid triggers and take medications to control these chronic conditions.

PROCEDURES FOR PREVENTION

▶ CAROTID ENDARTERECTOMY

- First performed in 1953
- Indicated for symptomatic carotid stenosis with greater than 60% loss of lumen or asymptomatic high-grade carotid stenosis with greater than 70% loss of lumen
- Recommended over stenting for people >70 years of age
- Benefit is highest if done during the initial 2 weeks after the TIA or mild stroke for neurologically stable patients

▶ CAROTID ARTERY STENTING

- Approved by the U.S. Food and Drug Administration (FDA) in 2004.
- Indicated for symptomatic, high-risk patients with greater than 70% stenosis; not recommended over age 70.
- Benefits are that there is no need for anesthesia, no surgical incision, and shorter hospital stays.

▶ LEFT ATRIAL APPENDAGE OCCLUSION

- For patients with Afib to prevent pooling of blood.
- Endovascular placement.
- Clinical utility likely will be in patients at high risk for stroke who are poor candidates for medical management with anticoagulants.

▶ CARDIOVERSION

- Indicated for symptomatic Afib, acute dyspnea, or heart failure symptoms
- Only with new onset of Afib with no evidence of clot present in heart on transesophageal echocardiography (TEE)
- Not indicated in the acute phase of stroke management

CLINICAL PEARL

Older people are more prone to Afib because the myocardium tends to stretch with age and with long-standing HTN. With stretching, the electrical conduction of the impulse between the sinoatrial (SA) node and the atrioventricular (AV) node is interrupted, and Afib is the result.

▶ PATENT FORAMEN OVALE CLOSURE

- Patent foramen ovale (PFO) is present in up to 25% of the adult population.
- PFO was detected in cryptogenic stroke more often in younger patients: 43.9% (vs. 28.3% in older patients).
- Recommended if deep vein thrombosis (DVT) is also present; otherwise, antithrombotic is the only recommendation.
- Devices available for surgical and endovascular approach.

▶ ANEURYSM OBLITERATION

- Designed to isolate the aneurysm, or reduce the arterial pressure within it, in order to promote its thrombosis.
- Intervention should be done within the first 72 hours, if possible.
  - Risk of rebleed is highest within first 24 hours.
- Although clipping provides better results in terms of decreased mortality rate, rebleeding, and retreatments, endovascular coiling has better results related to postoperative complications, favorable outcomes (modified Rankin Scale [mRS] scores ranging 0 to 2), and rehabilitation (Ahmed et al., 2019).
- Patients who receive either intervention should have follow-up vascular imaging (time frame to be individualized) with strong consideration of retreatment if there is remnant growth.

CLIPPING

- First performed in 1937
- Involves opening the skull and manipulating brain tissue to access the aneurysm, increasing risk of complications (i.e., infection and secondary injury)

ENDOVASCULAR COILING

- First performed in 1991; earlier technique of balloon occlusion was done in the 1980s but had very high complication rates
- Involves large-artery access (usually femoral), with threading of the catheter up to the brain, similar to the process described in ischemic stroke mechanical intervention
- Less invasive than craniotomy for clipping; shorter recovery time and shorter length of stay (LOS) than craniotomy

ENDOVASCULAR FLOW DIVERSION

- First performed in the 1990s
- Indicated for all aneurysms, but particularly suited for complex and wide-necked aneurysms
- Flexible self-expanding cylindrical construct composed of braided strands of cobalt, chromium, and platinum; positioned in the parent artery across the aneurysm neck

▶ARTERIOVENOUS MALFORMATION OBLITERATION

- The following procedures are designed to remove or isolate the arteriovenous malformation (AVM).
- Combination therapy involving embolization followed by surgery or radiation therapy provides the greatest success.

SURGICAL REMOVAL

- Involves craniotomy approach and surgical excision of the lesion
- Indicated for medically stable patients with small, uncomplicated lesions

ENDOVASCULAR EMBOLIZATION

- Involves a large-artery approach and use of particulate or embolizing agents
- Often used to stabilize or reduce the lesion size prior to surgery to reduce the incidence of intraoperative bleeding
- Most successful when combination therapy is used and embolization is followed by surgery or radiation therapy

FOCUSED RADIATION

- Indicated for those patients for whom surgery or the endovascular approach is not feasible
  - Examples are lesions in the thalamus, basal ganglia, and brainstem
- Involves use of gamma knife, linear accelerators, or proton beam radiation
- Often utilized after surgery or endovascular embolization to eliminate any remaining lesion
- Not indicated for large AVMs unless a staged approach using multiple treatments is possible

⬤ CLINICAL PEARL

The first operative microscope was used in 1960, so early neurosurgeons performed aneurysm clippings without the benefit of the microscope.

⬤ OPPORTUNITIES FOR PREVENTIVE HEALTH SERVICES

Numerous first-time stroke risk-assessment tools have been utilized, but experts agree that an ideal, comprehensive tool does not yet exist. These risk assessment tools seek to identify people at elevated risk who might be unaware of their risk, to assess risk in the presence of >1 condition, to measure an individual's risk that can be tracked and lowered by appropriate modifications, and to guide appropriate use of further diagnostic testing.

- Framingham Stroke Risk Profile is one of the most widely used
  - Analyzes risk factors and provides a gender-specific, 10-year cumulative stroke risk.

- The American Heart Association (AHA)/American College of Cardiology (ACC) Cardiovascular (CV) Risk Calculator (https://static.heart.org/riskcalc/app/index.html#!/baseline-risk)
  - Identifies individuals who could benefit from therapeutic interventions as well as those who may not be treated on the basis of any single risk factor.
- ED
  - Visits to the ED are increasing due to several factors: increased number of people without insurance, lack of PCPs, decreased availability of medical specialists, and inadequate preventive and chronic care management.
  - The ED represents the opportunity to screen and initiate treatment for patients with HTN, diabetes, Afib, and other risk factors such as smoking and alcohol and drug abuse.
- Primary care and specialty practices
  - Strategies aimed at provider practice to improve adherence with guideline recommendations include physician education, audit and feedback of practice patterns, and physician and patient profiling.
    - PCPs and specialty providers such as cardiology and endocrinology providers represent the opportunity to manage risk factors, thus preventing 90% of strokes.
  - Strategies aimed at systems have been more effective; these include computer-based clinical reminders, use of electronic medical records, support personnel to implement preventive health protocols, and separate clinics devoted to screening and preventive services.
- Community education
  - Provision of education regarding stroke risk factors, symptom recognition, and calling 911 represent true primordial prevention.
  - Community health fairs and lectures to community groups such as churches, social groups, clubs, and so on.
  - Resources and materials for use are available:
    - Stroke.org
    - Stroke.nih.gov
    - Strokefocus.net
    - Strokeawareness.com
    - Strokerecoveryfoundation.org
  - FAST versus BE FAST
    - FAST stands for face, arm, speech, time and was first introduced in the United Kingdom in 1996 to facilitate greater stroke symptom recognition.
    - BE FAST stands for balance, eyesight, face, arm, speech, time and has been shown to improve accuracy of stroke symptom recognition to 95%.
    - Researchers at the University of Texas Health Center have recently developed a Spanish version, RAPIDO (Kozak, 2021). It stands for rostro caido, alteración del equilibrio, pérdida de fuerza, impedimento visual, dificultad para hablar, obtenga ayuda rapido. Translated into English, it is: fallen/drooped face, change in balance, loss of strength, eyesight issues, speech difficulty, get help quickly.

CLINICAL PEARL

Focusing community education on children can be a smart strategy. Adults are interested in children's health and well-being and often don't pay attention to their own. By having interactive games and activity books, the parents receive information along with their children. It is useful to include statistics about children and young adult stroke incidence, risk factors, recognition of symptoms, and the importance of calling 911.

TARGET POPULATIONS

- Black and Hispanic populations
  - Access to care has been identified as a barrier for both groups.
    - Lower socioeconomic status and fewer community resources exist.
  - Lack of knowledge about stroke symptoms and risk factors.
    - 58% of Hispanic adults and 64% of Black adults knew the signs of stroke compared to 71% of White adults.
  - Now that there is recognition of this disparity, concerted efforts are underway to address provider shortages, provide culturally focused risk factor education, and improve use of emergency medical services, which expedites ED care.
- The Stroke Belt
  - Located in the southeastern United States, people living in the following states have the highest mortality rate from stroke: Alabama, Arkansas, Georgia, Indiana, Kentucky, Louisiana, Mississippi, North Carolina, South Carolina, Tennessee, and Virginia.
  - Twenty years of research has determined the cause to be a combination of higher risk-factor burden (HTN, diabetes, and smoking), race, lower socioeconomic status, and limited access to care (Howard & Howard, 2020).
    - The disparity has lessened over the past 10 years due to focused improvements in care access and prevention support.
- Children
  - Incidence is reported as 4.6 to 6.4/100,000 (Benjamin et al., 2018).
    - Boys have slighter higher incidence than girls.
    - Black children have a two-fold higher incidence than White children.
  - Half of all childhood strokes are hemorrhagic, with the most common cause being aneurysm or AVM rupture.
  - Most common cause of arterial ischemic stroke (AIS) is cerebral arteriopathy and sickle cell disease.
  - Risk factors, such as hyperlipidemia, obesity, and type 2 diabetes, have been increasing in adolescents since 1995.
    - Although incidence is not high, the presence of risk factors in childhood is accountable for the rise in stroke among young adults.
  - Management of activity levels, diet, and weight are essential in controlling modifiable risk factors.
  - Schools, after-school programs, summer camps, churches, scout troops, and team activities offer an opportunity to teach children about stroke.
  - Encourage children to become "stroke detectives."
    - Teach them the FAST, BE FAST, or RAPIDO acronyms and the importance of calling 911.
    - Stroke Hero Toolkit (American Stroke Association [ASA] & AHA, 2020) is an excellent resource.
    - Make a game of healthy lifestyle choices: choosing healthy foods and engaging in family-friendly physical activity.
    - Make them MyPlate Champions—resources available at www.myplate.gov/life -stages/kids.
    - Make BE FAST/RAPIDO bookmarks, doorhangers, and posters; offer coloring activities, crossword puzzles, and word searches.
    - Encourage children to share their knowledge with others by providing them with pocket cards that have BE FAST/RAPIDO on one side and risk factors on the other.

⬤ MEASURING IMPACT

Some progress has been made in secondary prevention, as evidenced by the vastly improved outcomes seen in the Get With the Guidelines (GWTG) Stroke database. This database, started in 2003, now has over 2,000 hospitals participating and more than 5 million patient records. There has been significant reduction in mortality rates and improved functional outcomes as a result of quality measures compliance, but stroke recurrence hasn't shown significant reduction.

It continues to be challenging to measure primary prevention effectiveness. The ASA has provided formal recommendations that put the responsibility for primary prevention strategies and tracking on Stroke Systems of Care (Adeoye et al., 2019).

- Support for community and providers in initiating prevention strategies
- Support for community education to increase stroke awareness
- Monitoring the effectiveness of these efforts by tracking:
  - Rate of behavioral responses to warning signs (calling 911)
  - Rate of stroke incidence
  - Percentage of those who arrive within the treatment window

J.B. is a nurse practitioner in a primary care office, seeing patients for healthy checkups and treating minor injuries or illnesses. J.B. loves the variety of cases this position offers and feels like the work is important. He also enjoys participating in community health fairs and providing lectures at local senior centers. This morning he saw Mr. Bell, a 52-year-old Black man, for management of his diabetes; his hemoglobin (Hgb) A1C had risen to 9%, so J.B. prescribed insulin and set Mr. Bell up for a session with the diabetic educator. His blood pressure (BP) was 166/86, and Mr. Bell declined any change in his antihypertensive medications.

After Mr. Bell, J.B. saw Mrs. Cook, a 77-year-old White woman, for stroke follow-up after discharge from the hospital. He noted her new medical regimen of apixaban for newly diagnosed atrial fibrillation and a change to lisinopril for her hypertension management. However, her BP recordings from home indicate that her BP is still too high, ranging from 158/80 to 176/88. J.B. commends her for checking her BP and explains that he would like to increase the dose of lisinopril and that she should keep checking it at home and notify him if it drops below 130/70 or stays above 150/80.

1. What type of prevention does J.B. engage in when lecturing at the local senior center?

   A. Primary
   B. Primordial
   C. Secondary
   D. Tertiary

2. What type of prevention does J.B. engage in when treating Mr. Bell's high hemoglobin (Hgb) A1C?

   A. Primary
   B. Primordial
   C. Secondary
   D. Tertiary

3. What type of prevention does J.B. engage in when adjusting Mrs. Cook's lisinopril dose in her follow-up appointment?

   A. Primary
   B. Primordial
   C. Secondary
   D. Tertiary

4. How many risk factors did Mr. Bell and Mrs. Cook each present with, respectively?

   A. 0 and 4
   B. 3 and 2
   C. 2 and 2
   D. 3 and 4

1. B) Primordial
Primordial prevention refers to efforts to prevent a disease from developing. Primary prevention refers to efforts to stop an event such as stroke or transient ischemic attack (TIA) once risk factors like hypertension (HTN), diabetes, and so on, exist. Secondary prevention refers to efforts to prevent a second major event by managing risk factors. Tertiary prevention refers to efforts to soften the impact of an ongoing illness or injury that has lasting effects by helping to manage long-term, complex health problems to improve as much as possible a person's ability to function, quality of life, and life expectancy.

2. A) Primary
Primary prevention involves modifying risk factors, like a high Hgb A1C, to prevent stroke or other major event from occurring. Secondary prevention refers to prevention of a second major event by managing risk factors. Tertiary prevention refers to efforts to soften the impact of an ongoing illness or injury that has lasting effects by helping to manage long-term, complex health problems. Primordial prevention focuses on preventing the disease from developing.

3. C) Secondary
Secondary prevention involves modifying risk factors, like hypertension control, after an initial stroke or transient ischemic attack (TIA) to prevent subsequent event. Primordial prevention focuses on preventing the disease from developing. Primary prevention focuses on modifying risk factors to prevent stroke or TIA. Tertiary prevention will soften the impact of an ongoing illness or injury with lasting effects by helping to manage long-term, complex health problems.

4. D) 3 and 4
Mr. Bell's risk factors are as follows: race, uncontrolled diabetes, and uncontrolled hypertension. Mrs. Cook's risk factors are as follows: age, gender, atrial fibrillation, and uncontrolled hypertension.

1. A primary care provider (PCP) who initiates a statin medication for a patient whose medical history includes type 2 diabetes and hypertension would be providing what type of stroke care?

   A. Secondary prevention
   B. Tertiary prevention
   C. Primary prevention
   D. Primordial prevention

2. A 78-year-old transient ischemic attack (TIA) patient has been recommended carotid endarterectomy (CEA) for the left carotid artery stenosis of 80%. They are reluctant because they never had a TIA before and do not like the idea of surgery on the neck. The nurse's best response would be:

   A. To listen and validate the patient's concerns and reassure them that the surgeon is the best at the hospital
   B. To listen and then provide education that research supports this intervention for patients with higher than 70% stenosis and risk factors for stroke (the recent TIA)
   C. To calculate the patient's ABCD2 (age [>60], blood pressure, clinical features of TIA, duration, and diabetes) score and notify the patient that the score is only 5
   D. To reassure the patient that the neck incision is nearly invisible within 5 years

3. For community members with a family history of atrial fibrillation, what advice should be included regarding self-assessment?

   A. The value of purchasing a blood pressure (BP) cuff to monitor for hypotension
   B. YouTube instructions for monitoring for palpitations and dyspnea
   C. Deep breathing strategies to regulate heart rhythm
   D. Demonstration of radial pulse assessment for rate and rhythm regularity

4. A stroke patient is angry with himself because he has smoked for over 30 years and feels like he is doomed. What is the nurse's best response?

   A. Switching to vaping will be less bothersome to his family
   B. Smoking cessation may not help him anymore, but he has a responsibility to those around him
   C. Smoking cessation can result in rapid reduction in stroke risk
   D. Switching to filtered cigarettes reduces the risk of stroke by 50%

5. The INTERSTROKE study found that five risk factors accounted for the majority of stroke, both ischemic and hemorrhagic. Which one is NOT one of the five?

   A. Carotid stenosis
   B. Smoking
   C. Obesity
   D. Physical inactivity

1. C) Primary prevention

Primary prevention seeks to prevent the onset of specific diseases via risk reduction, that is, by altering behaviors that can lead to disease. Primary prevention refers to control of risk factors that already exist in specific populations: people who smoke, people with diabetes, people with hypertension, and so on. Primordial prevention refers to strategies designed to decrease the development of disease risk factors: efforts to decrease the development of obesity, increase exercise, and provide a well-balanced diet. Primordial prevention encompasses the entire population and is not limited to individuals with recognized risk factors. Secondary prevention refers to measures taken to limit risk of another event, such as stroke or transient ischemic attack (TIA). Tertiary prevention refers to efforts to soften the impact of an ongoing illness or injury that has lasting effects by helping to manage long-term, complex health problems to improve as much as possible a person's ability to function, quality of life, and life expectancy.

2. B) To listen and then provide education that research supports this intervention for patients with higher than 70% stenosis and risk factors for stroke (the recent TIA)

The American Heart Association/American Stroke Association guidelines recommend CEA for TIA and stroke patients with ipsilateral (same side as their TIA or stroke symptoms) carotid stenosis of 70% to 99% and for patients older than 70 years. Patients younger than age 70 would also have the option of carotid artery stent (CAS). There is little value in telling a patient that their surgeon is the best at that hospital. An ABCD2 score of 5 is a high–moderate score and indicates higher risk of subsequent stroke, which would do nothing to address the patient's concerns. There is no guarantee that the incision will be nearly invisible.

3. D) Demonstration of radial pulse assessment for rate and rhythm regularity

Knowledge of how to monitor heart rate and rhythm would be the most helpful for someone with a family history of atrial fibrillation, advancing age, but without documented dysrhythmia. Hypotension may or may not result from atrial fibrillation, so a BP cuff is not the most helpful self-assessment tool. While YouTube has some valuable educational material, it would only be an adjunct to personal demonstration of radial pulse assessment. Deep breathing strategies have been shown to impact heart rate/rhythm; it would be used as a secondary tool for managing rate/rhythm, not the first-line method for self-assessment in someone with no personal history of atrial fibrillation.

4. C) Smoking cessation can result in rapid reduction in stroke risk

The American Heart Association/American Stroke Association guidelines indicate that "smoking cessation is associated with a rapid reduction in risk of stroke and other cardiovascular events to a level that approaches but does not reach that of those who never smoked" (Goldstein et al., 2011, p. 528), so it is still beneficial for persons to stop smoking even with a long history. There is evidence that quitting will benefit him, so it is incorrect to say otherwise. There is no evidence of vaping or filtered cigarettes reducing stroke risk.

5. A) Carotid stenosis

The INTERSTROKE study demonstrated that the following five risk factors accounted for 90% of strokes: hypertension, current smoking, abdominal obesity, high-fat diet, and physical inactivity.

6. Overall stroke incidence has remained steady at 800,000 new and recurrent strokes per year, despite the 44% increase in stroke among people aged 24 to 44 years. Which age group has shown a 29% decrease in stroke incidence?

    A. Ages 65 to 84 years
    B. Ages 50 to 64 years
    C. Ages 12 to 18 years
    D. Ages 85 to 98 years

7. Which of the following is a modifiable risk factor for stroke?

    A. Low birth weight
    B. Gender
    C. Migraine with aura
    D. Race/ethnicity

8. Which racial group has similar stroke incidence to White Americans?

    A. Hispanic/Latinx Americans
    B. Native Americans
    C. Pacific Islanders
    D. All of the above

9. Primary prevention of stroke recommendations for physical activity are which of the following?

    A. Vigorous aerobic activity for 30 minutes, twice a day, three times a week
    B. Moderate aerobic activity for a minimum of 60 min/d, twice a week
    C. Moderate to vigorous aerobic activity for a minimum of 40 min/d, three to four times a week
    D. Moderate to vigorous aerobic activity daily for a minimum of 45 min/d

10. In preparing a patient for discharge to home from the acute rehabilitation hospital, the nurse senses reluctance from the patient's partner. The partner says that all of the information they have been getting is overwhelming, and they are terrified that the patient will have another stroke. What is the nurse's best response?

    A. Review the resource guide with the partner to ensure that they know the signs of stroke
    B. Inform the partner that their concerns have been communicated to the care team and ensure that a community resource guide will provided
    C. Review the plan of care, reassuring the partner that the patient's risk factors have been addressed, and impress the importance of follow-up
    D. None of the above

11. In planning community education about stroke, identify what information would help develop the best strategy for hospital stroke teams.

    A. The number of healthcare providers interested in participating
    B. The time frame for sufficient stroke flyers to be produced
    C. Regional demographic information: race, age, and socioeconomic status
    D. The number of stroke survivors in the region

(See answers next page.)

6. A) Ages 65 to 84 years

There has been a decrease of 29% among ages 65 to 84.

7. C) Migraine with aura

Migraine with aura can be modified by avoiding triggers and maintaining compliance with medications. Low birth weight, gender, and race/ethnicity cannot be modified.

8. D) All of the above

Hispanic/Latino Americans, Pacific Islanders, and Native Americans have similar stroke incidence to Non-Hispanic White Americans. Black Americans have the highest incidence.

9. C) Moderate to vigorous aerobic activity for a minimum of 40 min/d, three to four times a week

The recommendations are for moderate to vigorous activity 40 min/d, three to four times a week.

10. C) Review the plan of care, reassuring the partner that the patient's risk factors have been addressed, and impress the importance of follow-up

Support for the caregiver is critical in prevention of recurrent stroke and readmission. Simply ensuring knowledge of the signs of stroke is inadequate for this situation, as it does not address the partner's concerns directly. Although it is valuable to inform the partner that their concerns have been communicated to the care team and that a resource guide will be provided, it is not as comprehensive a solution as reviewing the plan of care, reassuring the partner, and making sure a follow-up occurs.

11. C) Regional demographic information: race, age, and socioeconomic status

To develop an effective and efficient education plan for the community, it would be helpful to determine the demographic makeup so that the focus can be on the highest need areas. Although it is helpful to know about the number of healthcare providers who would like to participate, the time frame for stroke flyers to be produced, and the amount of stroke survivors in the area, they do not provide as much actionable value as demographic information of the community.

12. In what circumstance would a nurse expect a right-sided carotid artery stenosis to be treated with a stent rather than an endarterectomy?

   A. When the degree of stenosis is less than 50% and the patient is over age 80 years
   B. When the procedure needs to be performed within 2 weeks
   C. When the degree of stenosis is higher than 70% and there are anatomic or medical conditions present that increase risk of surgery
   D. When the provider who performs endarterectomy is not available

13. A transient ischemic attack (TIA) patient with newly diagnosed patent foramen ovale (PFO) is being discharged on aspirin as secondary prevention. What condition would need to be present for this to be an appropriate plan of care?

   A. Urinary tract infection (UTI)
   B. Deep vein thrombosis (DVT)
   C. Diabetes mellitus (DM)
   D. Sequential compression device (SCD)

14. A stroke center serves a community that is predominantly Black (44%), with White (32%) and Hispanic (21%) populations coming in second and third. The hospital has limited personnel resources for community outreach. Which of the following would be the best use of a nurse's time/resources to ensure the highest rate of positive outcomes?

   A. Health fair at a local mall involving a dozen other community organizations
   B. Risk factor screening at the local African American community center
   C. Health talk at the local health club
   D. Distributing RAPIDO cards at a local elementary school

15. Identify the reason for older people to have increased risk of atrial fibrillation.

   A. Polypharmacy resulting in tachycardia/cardiac irritability
   B. Insulin resistance
   C. Myocardial hypertrophy
   D. Hypotension

16. Which of the following procedures carries greater risk of encephalitis?

   A. Carotid stenting
   B. Carotid endarterectomy
   C. Aneurysm clipping
   D. Aneurysm coiling

17. Before cardioversion of atrial fibrillation, what condition must be ruled out first?

   A. Deep vein thrombosis (DVT)
   B. Cardiac thrombus
   C. Tachycardia
   D. Pneumonia

(See answers next page.)

12. C) When the degree of stenosis is higher than 70% and there are anatomic or medical conditions present that increase risk of surgery

Patients with a high degree of stenosis but have either anatomical (history of neck trauma/scarring) or medical (severe lung disease, cardiac disease) conditions that make surgery risky, are recommended to be treated with stenting rather than endarterectomy. Patients older than 70 years are recommended to have endarterectomy. Neither endarterectomy nor stenting is recommended for stenosis less than 50%. Time frame and specific provider availability play no role in determining stent versus surgery.

13. B) Deep vein thrombosis (DVT)

While more studies are needed, the guidelines indicate that the research evidence supports an antithrombotic as treatment for PFO with DVT in patients who were not already on an anticoagulant for another reason. There is no correlation between UTI or DM and PFO as stroke risk. An SCD is a treatment modality, not a condition.

14. B) Risk factor screening at the local African American community center

With limited personnel and resources and the high percentage of Black people in the community, it is wise to focus outreach efforts on the highest risk population. Health fairs usually attract health-minded people and, while valuable, are not as valuable as focused screening at a community center. Health talks at local health clubs address those who are already health minded. Distribution of RAPIDO cards is also valuable, but not as much as focused screenings at an African American community center.

15. C) Myocardial hypertrophy

With age and chronic hypertension, stretching of the heart muscle is present, leading to atrial fibrillation. Polypharmacy, insulin resistance, and hypotension are not correlated with atrial fibrillation.

16. C) Aneurysm clipping

The invasive nature of aneurysm clipping creates the greatest risk of encephalitis. Carotid endarterectomy is an extracranial surgery, and so would not pose a risk of encephalitis. Stenting and coiling are done endovascularly, which would likely not lead to brain inflammation.

17. B) Cardiac thrombus

If cardiac thrombus is present, cardioversion to normal rhythm brings risk of embolism to the brain. DVT is not a risk for cardioversion. Tachycardia, as long as it is sinus tachycardia, does not pose a risk with cardioversion, nor does pneumonia.

18. Sleep apnea is considered a risk factor for stroke for what reason?

    A. Hypoxia
    B. Tachycardia
    C. Dysphagia
    D. Cardiomyopathy

19. Which is true of nonmodifiable risk factors for stroke?

    A. Men and women have similar incidence of stroke throughout their lifetime
    B. Black men under age 40 have less risk than Black women
    C. Half of all Hispanic men have risk factors for stroke
    D. Babies with birth weight under 6.5 lb. have three times the risk of stroke

20. Which type of prevention involves stopping the development of risk factors before they occur?

    A. Primordial prevention
    B. Tertiary prevention
    C. Primary prevention
    D. Secondary prevention

18. D) Cardiomyopathy

Cardiomyopathy is a result of stretching of the heart muscle with atrial fibrillation as a common result. Hypoxia and tachycardia from sleep apnea can strain the heart, but they are not the reason for stroke risk from sleep apnea. There is no correlation between sleep apnea and dysphagia.

19. C) Half of all Hispanic men have risk factors for stroke

Fifty percent of Hispanic men have heart disease, hypertension, and diabetes. The incidence of stroke between men and women varies across the lifetime. The risk of stroke in Black men is higher than Black women until age 70. A birth weight under 5.5 lb. carries twice the risk than above.

20. A) Primordial prevention

Primordial prevention, a key part of population health, involves preventing risk factor development in the first place. Primary prevention seeks to prevent the onset of specific diseases via risk reduction, that is, by altering behaviors that can lead to disease. Secondary prevention refers to measures taken to limit risk of another event, such as stroke or transient ischemic attack (TIA). Tertiary prevention refers to efforts to soften the impact of an ongoing illness or injury that has lasting effects by helping to manage long-term, complex health problems to improve as much as possible a person's ability to function, quality of life, and life expectancy.

REFERENCES

Adeoye, O., Nystrom, K. V., Yavagal, D. R., Luciano, J., Nogueira, R. G., Zorowitz, R. D., Khalessi, A. A., Bushnell, C., Barsan, W. G., Panagos, P., Alberts, M. J., Tiner, A. C., Schwamm, L. H., & Jauch, E. C. (2019). Recommendations for the establishment of stroke systems of care: A 2019 update. *Stroke, 50*(7), e187–e210. https://doi.org/10.1161/STR.0000000000000173

Ahmed, S. I., Javed, G., Bareeqa, S. B., Samar, S. S., Shah, A., Giani, A., Aziz, Z., Tasleem, A., & Humayun, S. H. (2019). Endovascular coiling versus neurosurgical clipping for aneurysmal subarachnoid hemorrhage: A systematic review and meta-analysis. *Cureus, 11*(3), e4320. https://doi.org/10.7759/cureus.4320

American Stroke Association & American Heart Association. (2020). *Stroke hero: What's your super power? Stroke hero toolkit.* Author. https://www.stroke.org/-/media/Stroke-Files/About-Stroke/Stroke-in-Children/Stroke-Heroes-Toolkit--FINAL--Digital.pdf

Arnett, D. K., Blumenthal, R. S., Albert, M. A., Buroker, A. B., Goldberger, Z. D., Hahn, E. J., Himmelfarb, C. D., Khera, A., Lloyd-Jones, D., McEvoy, J. W., Michos, E. D., Miedema, M. D., Muñoz, D., Smith, S. C., Virani, S. S., Williams, K. A., Yeboah, J., & Ziaeian, B. (2019). 2019 ACC/AHA guideline on the primary prevention of cardiovascular disease: A report of the American College of Cardiology/American Heart Association Task Force on Clinical Practice Guidelines. *Journal of the American College of Cardiology, 74*(10), e177–e232. https://doi.org/10.1016/j.jacc.2019.03.010

Béjot, Y., Delpont, B., & Giroud, M. (2016). Rising stroke incidence in young adults: More epidemiological evidence, more questions to be answered. *Journal of the American Heart Association, 5*(5), e003661. https://doi.org/10.1161/JAHA.116.003661

Benjamin, E. J., Virani, S. S., Callaway, C. W., Chamberlain, A. M., Chang, A. R., Cheng, S., Chiuve, S. E., Cushman, M., Delling, F. N., Deo, R., de Ferranti, S. D., Ferguson, J. F., Fornage, M., Gillespie, C., Isasi, C. R., Jiménez, M. C., Jordan, L. C., Judd, S. E., Lackland, D., ... Muntner, P. (2018). Heart disease and stroke statistics—2018 update: A report from the American Heart Association. *Circulation, 137*(12), e67–e492. https://doi.org/10.1161/CIR.0000000000000558

Gerber, Y. S., Rana, J. S., Jacobs Jr, D. R., Yano, Y., Levine, D. A., Nguyen-Huynh, M. N., Lima, J. A. C., Reis, J. P., Zhao, L., Liu, K., Lewis, C. E., & Sidney, S. (2021). Blood pressure levels in young adulthood and midlife stroke incidence in a diverse cohort. *Hypertension, 77*(5), 1683–1693. https://doi.org/10.1161/HYPERTENSIONAHA.120.16535

Goldstein, L. B., Bushnell, C. D., Adams, R. J., Appel, L. J., Braun, L. T., Chaturvedi, S., Creager, M. A., Culebras, A., Eckel, R. H., Hart, R. G., Hinchey, J. A., Howard, V. J., Jauch, E. C., Levine, S. R., Meschia, J. F., Moore, W. S., Nixon, J. V., & Pearson, T. A. (2011). Guidelines for the primary prevention of stroke: A guideline for healthcare professionals from the American Heart Association/American Stroke Association. *Stroke, 42*(2), 517–584. https://doi.org/10.1161/STR.0b013e3181fcb238

Howard, G., & Howard, V. J. (2020). Twenty years of progress toward understanding the Stroke Belt. *Stroke, 51*(3), 742–750. https://doi.org/10.1161/STROKEAHA.119.024155

Kernan, W. N., Viera, A. J., Billinger, S. A., Bravata, D. M., Stark, S. L., Kasner, S. E., Kuritzky, L., Towfighi, A., the American Heart Association Stroke Council, the Council on Arteriosclerosis, Thrombosis and Vascular Biology, the Council on Cardiovascular Radiology and Intervention, & the Council on Peripheral Vascular Disease. (2021). Primary care of adult patients after stroke: A scientific statement from the American Heart Assocation/American Stroke Association. *Stroke, 52*(9), e1–e14. https://doi.org/10.1161/STR.0000000000000382

Kleindorfer, D. O., Towfighi, A., Chaturvedi, S., Cockroft, K. M., Gutierrez, J., Lombardi-Hill, D., Kamel, H., Kernan, W. N., Kittner, S. J., Leira, E. C., Lennon, O., Meschia, J. F., Nguyen, T. N., Pollak, P. M., Santangeli, P., Sharrief, A. Z., Smith, S. C., Turan, T. N., & Williams, L. S. (2021). 2021 guideline for the prevention of stroke in patients with stroke and transient ischemic attack: A guideline from the American Heart Association/American Stroke Association. *Stroke, 52*(7), e364–e467. https://doi.org/10.1161/STR.0000000000000375

Kozak, R. (2021). RAPIDO—a new Spanish acronym to raise stroke awareness. *American Heart Association News.* https://www.heart.org/en/news/2021/03/12/rapido-a-new-spanish-acronym-to-raise-stroke-awareness

Meschia, J. F., Bushnell, C., Boden-Albala, B., Braun, L. T., Bravata, D. M., Chaturvedi, S., Creager, M. A., Eckel, R. H., Elkind, M. S. V., Fornage, M., Goldstein, L. B., Greenberg, S. M., Horvath, S. E., Iadecola, C., Jauch, E. C., Moore, W. S., & Wilson, J. A. (2014). Guidelines for the primary prevention of stroke: A statement for healthcare professionals from the American Heart Association/American Stroke Association. *Stroke, 45*(12), 3754–3832. https://doi.org/10.1161/STR.0000000000000046

Virani, S. S., Alonso, A., Aparicio, H. J., Benjamin, E. J., Bittencourt, M. S., Callaway, C. W., Carson, A. P., Chamberlain, A. M., Cheng, S., Delling, F. N., Elkind, M. S. V., Evenson, K. R., Ferguson, J. F., Gupta, D. K., Khan, S. S., Kissela, B. M., Knutson, K. L., Lee, C. D., Lewis, T. T., . . . Tsao, C. W. (2021). Heart disease and stroke statistics—2021 update: A report from the American Heart Association. *Circulation, 143*(8), e254–e743. https://doi.org/10.1161/CIR.0000000000000950

Case Studies

Cesar Velasco

CASE STUDY #1

Yulan Wu is a 74-year-old female who lost consciousness and collapsed in her home. Yulan's daughter, Samantha, did not witness her mother collapse but found her on the floor, appearing awake, confused, and slightly out of breath. Samantha initiated a call for emergency medical services (EMS) within 5 minutes of finding her mother on the floor, and the EMS team responded within 10 minutes. Upon arrival, an EMS paramedic acquired a finger-stick blood glucose measurement of 85 mg/dL and determined Yulan was having a stroke based on a positive Cincinnati Prehospital Stroke Scale, identifying facial droop and extremity weakness. At 14:00, Yulan is transported to the nearest comprehensive stroke center as an in-bound stroke alert with an estimated time of arrival (ETA) of 15 minutes. Her vital signs in route are blood pressure (BP) 170/95, heart rate (HR) 82 and irregular, respiratory rate (RR) 18, and blood oxygen saturation (SPO$_2$) 93% on room air (RA), and she is afebrile.

Upon presentation to the ED at 14:13, Yulan is greeted and triaged by the responding stroke team, consisting of an ED provider, a stroke neurologist, two ED nurses, and an ED pharmacist. Yulan is still apparently confused; therefore, Samantha is asked to provide information about her mother to the stroke team. She reports her mother telling Samantha that earlier in the week, Yulan experienced a brief 5-minute episode of right-sided numbness and tingling with slight confusion and slurred speech. When Samantha asked her mother if she had called her family physician about the episode, she shrugged it off saying, "It was nothing to worry about since the symptoms were gone." Samantha provides additional information that indicates Yulan has been treated for hypertension over the past 10 years but is noncompliant in taking her only prescribed medication, a diuretic. Additionally, she has no previous history of smoking, drinks socially, and is 10 lb. overweight for her stature. Yulan's National Institutes of Health Stroke Scale (NIHSS) score is a 10 for not being fully alert and mildly confused with a mild left facial droop and some effort against gravity in her upper and lower extremities. Computerized tomography/computerized tomographic angiogram (CT/CTA) is negative for a hemorrhage and indicates a thrombus in the M1 branch of the right middle cerebral artery. Current vital signs are BP 178/90, HR 84 and irregular, RR 20, and SPO$_2$ 94% on RA.

1. An acute emergency medical services (EMS) assessment and transport of a patient with suspected ischemic stroke should be similar to that of a level 1 trauma, utilizing limited time available for basic questioning and rapid physical assessment. What additional assessment, intervention, or question is important to help determine if Yulan will be eligible for acute treatment with intravenous (IV) thrombolysis and/or mechanical thrombectomy?
   A. Obtaining a 12-lead EKG to rule out atrial fibrillation
   B. Establishing a Glasgow Coma Scale (GCS) score
   C. Establishing a time when Yulan was last normal
   D. Insertion of bilateral 18-gauge peripheral IVs

1. C) Establishing a time when Yulan was last normal

Last known well (LKW) time is the date and time at which it was witnessed or reported that the patient was last known to be without symptoms of the current stroke or at her baseline state of health. The correct identification of a patient's LKW time is critical for determining a patient's eligibility for time-dependent acute ischemic stroke treatments with IV thrombolytic. An EKG is recommended if dysrhythmia is suspected but plays no role in treatment decision regarding thrombolysis or thrombectomy. A GCS score is not recommended for this stroke treatment decision. Bilateral 18-gauge peripheral IVs are valuable but are not part of this stroke treatment decision based on patient presentation.

2. Yulan has two significant risk factors for stroke. The first is a long history of hypertension. Which is the second?
   A. Underlying atrial fibrillation
   B. Prehospital finger-stick blood glucose of 85 mg/dL
   C. Weight of 10 lb. above normal
   D. Noncompliance in taking her diuretic

3. Yulan's previous episode of numbness, confusion, and slurred speech appears to be evidence of which other substantial risk factor for stroke?
   A. Hyperglycemia
   B. Atrial fibrillation (Afib)
   C. Transient ischemic attack (TIA)
   D. Excess alcohol use

4. It has been established that Yulan's last known well (LKW) time was 13:02, and she was found on the floor by her daughter at approximately 13:30. Based on her time of arrival to the ED, how many hours does the stroke team have to administer intravenous (IV) thrombolysis?
   A. 3 hours and 19 minutes
   B. 4 hours and 30 minutes
   C. 1 hour and 30 minutes
   D. 2 hours and 13 minutes

5. An order is placed for intravenous (IV) alteplase to be administered. Which of the following answers is correct?
   A. The nurse holds the drug and notifies the provider of this patient's hypertensive status requiring immediate treatment to reduce the risk of symptomatic intracerebral hemorrhage (ICH) post alteplase
   B. The nurse confidently administers IV alteplase as ordered
   C. The nurse waits for a point-of-care international normalized ratio (POC INR) result to determine the patient's clotting rate affected by her anticoagulant usage
   D. The nurse reviews the patient's medical record and notes an allergy to IV contrast and therefore requests an order for IV Benadryl before administering alteplase

6. After achieving a door-to-needle time of 45 minutes, the nurse's vascular stroke neurologist notifies the neurointervention team to inform them of Yulan's CT angiogram indicating a large-vessel occlusion (LVO) in the M1 right middle cerebral artery (MCA). Based on this discussion, this means:
   A. Yulan has up to 24 hours from last known well (LKW) time to receive a thrombectomy
   B. Yulan has up to 24 hours from IV alteplase infusion stop time to receive a thrombectomy
   C. Yulan is not eligible to receive a thrombectomy due to risk of hemorrhage after initiation of IV alteplase treatment
   D. A CT perfusion (CTP) study will be necessary to consider intervention on LVO patients within 6 hours from LKW time

(See answers next page.)

2. D) Noncompliance in taking her diuretic

Uncontrolled hypertension is the number one risk factor for stroke. The aim of prescribing a medication such as a diuretic is to assist in keeping an individual's blood pressure low and stable over many years. If patients like Yulan are noncompliant in taking their prescribed medication, their blood pressure will rise; therefore, so will their risk for stroke. There is no history of atrial fibrillation present. A blood sugar of 85 mg/dL is normal. Excess weight of 10 lb. is notable but doesn't represent as significant a risk factor as noncompliance with diuretics.

3. C) Transient ischemic attack (TIA)

A TIA is caused by a temporary blockage of blood flow to the brain, producing stroke-like symptoms, but no imageable damage. Patients like Yulan who have had one or more TIAs are almost 10 times more likely to have a stroke than someone of the same age and gender who has not. Hyperglycemia symptoms rarely include numbness or slurred speech. Symptoms of Afib are usually shortness of breath and palpitations. There is no history of excess alcohol use, and with her known risk factors, TIA is the most likely answer.

4. A) 3 hours and 19 minutes

A patient with acute ischemic stroke may receive treatment with IV thrombolytic therapy up to 4.5 hours from LKW time. Her LKW time was 13:02. 13:02 + 4:30 would put the end of her treatment window at 17:32. The question is asking how much time from arrival is left for treatment, and the answer is 17:32 to 14:13, or 3 hours and 19 minutes. The time of discovery by her daughter plays no role in the treatment decision.

5. B) The nurse confidently administers IV alteplase as ordered

Yulan's blood pressure is <185/110, and, therefore, it is safe to administer IV alteplase without risk of causing her to have symptomatic ICH post-therapy. Given her medication history, there would be no reason to wait for a POC INR result because Yulan is not reportedly on an anticoagulant. An allergy to IV contrast is not a contraindication to administer IV alteplase.

6. A) Yulan has up to 24 hours from last known well (LKW) time to receive a thrombectomy

The window of time for a neurointervention team to complete a mechanical thrombectomy on an acute ischemic stroke patient who meets criteria is up to 24 hours from LKW time. It is not based on the infusion time of thrombolytic. Recommendations for thrombectomy clearly indicate that thrombolysis is not a contraindication for thrombectomy and that for cases within 6 hours of LKW time, CTP is required.

Mr. Berg is a 65-year-old gentleman admitted for a left middle cerebral artery (MCA) stroke. His admitting National Institutes of Health Stroke Scale (NIHSS) score = 7, for a right sided facial droop, dysarthria, a mild expressive aphasia, and a mild right arm and right leg weakness. Mr. Berg's cognitive and communication skills are intact, and he expresses a desire to return home as soon as possible; however, Mr. Berg's wife and son express concern to the neurology provider regarding Mr. Berg's readiness for discharge. The neurologist provides a referral for stroke rehabilitation, and a multidisciplinary rehabilitation team is formed to assess Mr. Berg's rehabilitative needs, discuss the proper rehabilitation setting available, and develop a treatment strategy tailored to his specific medical needs.

The multidisciplinary rehab team informs Mr. Berg's family that early discharge to a community setting for ongoing rehabilitation may provide Mr. Berg with outcomes like those achieved in an inpatient rehabilitation facility. Based on 2016 American Heart Association/ American Stroke Association (AHA/ASA) guidelines for adult stroke rehabilitation and recovery, the early supported discharge (ESD) model of care links inpatient care with community services and allows certain patients to be discharged home sooner with support of the rehabilitation team. Eventually, this formalized plan is shared with Mr. Berg's spouse and son, and, together, it is decided to discharge him to an inpatient rehabilitation facility.

1. Evaluating a stroke patient's risk of complications is an important step in the overall recovery and discharge planning assessment. Among the most common complications are:
   A. Depressive disorder, cognitive delays, seizures, deep vein thromboses (DVTs), and frequent falls
   B. Cognitive delays, delirium, seizures, and agitation
   C. Falls, DVTs, pressure ulcers, swallowing dysfunction, bladder/bowel dysfunction, and depressive symptoms
   D. Dysphagia, urinary and bowel incontinence, DVTs, skin ulcerations, seizures, and agitation

2. Mr. Berg's stroke has left him with a residual neurological dysfunction that has affected his ability to swallow. Stroke is associated with several complications, among which feeding is a main issue. Dysphagia puts a stroke patient like Mr. Berg at risk of aspiration pneumonia, malnourishment, and other opportunistic infections, resulting in which of the following?
   A. Higher dose of acetaminophen and triple antibiotics
   B. Risk of cardiac failure and mechanical ventilation
   C. Extensive lab culture studies and use of broad-spectrum antibiotics
   D. Higher morbidity and mortality

3. While in the inpatient rehabilitation facility, Mr. Berg is frequently assessed for his swallowing ability. Before allowing Mr. Berg to eat, which of the following actions should the rehabilitative nurse take first?
   A. Check Mr. Berg's reflexes
   B. Request a soft diet with no liquids
   C. Place the patient in a high-Fowler's position
   D. Test the patient's ability to swallow with a small amount of coffee from his tray

1. C) Falls, DVTs, pressure ulcers, swallowing dysfunction, bladder/bowel dysfunction, and depressive symptoms

Not all stroke patients experience complications of cognitive delay. According to the National Heart, Lung, and Blood Institute's (NHLBI's) Family Health Study, data indicate that 6 months postischemic stroke, among survivors ≥65 years old, 50% had some hemiparesis, 30% were unable to walk without some assistance, 26% were dependent in daily activities, 19% had aphasia, 35% had symptoms of depression, and 26% were in a nursing home. Cognitive delays, delirium, seizures, and agitation are not considered common complications.

2. D) Higher morbidity and mortality

Dysphagia is one of the most common sequels of acute stroke, affecting as many as 70% of acute stroke survivors. The presence of dysphagia in stroke survivors has been associated with increased mortality and morbidities such as pulmonary complications, malnutrition, and dehydration. There is no guarantee of need for higher acetaminophen dose or triple antibiotics. There is no documented cardiac history, so cardiac failure resulting in mechanical ventilation is unlikely. Lab cultures would indicate specific antibiotics, with little need for broad-spectrum antibiotics.

3. C) Place the patient in a high-Fowler's position

Placing Mr. Berg in high-Fowler's position and having him tilt his head forward will help ease swallowing and further reduce his risk of aspiration. Checking reflexes has no impact on ensuring swallowing safety. A soft diet with no liquids may be safe, but stroke patients need hydration so this is not indicated. Using coffee for bedside swallowing evaluation is not recommended as it may be hot.

4. According to research, a majority of stroke recovery in patients like Mr. Berg may occur within the first 1 to 3 months and afterward may occur more slowly. Which factor has the greatest influence on the time course of recovery poststroke?
   A. Age—in most cases, younger patients demonstrate faster recovery
   B. Stroke severity—milder strokes reach maximal recovery sooner, while more severe strokes take longer to reach maximal recovery
   C. Location of stroke—left hemisphere strokes reach maximal recovery sooner than strokes that occur in the right hemisphere of the brain
   D. Inpatient rehabilitation—short bursts of early rehabilitation within a formalized facility, offered twice a week, may increase rapid recovery

5. How does Mr. Berg's admission National Institutes of Health Stroke Scale (NIHSS) score of 7 relate to his eventual discharge to an inpatient rehabilitation facility?
   A. It doesn't correlate with the research evidence since scores of 6 to 13 indicate likely discharge to a skilled nursing facility (SNF)
   B. It correlates with the research evidence since admission scores of 6 to 13 indicate likely discharge to an inpatient rehabilitation facility
   C. It doesn't correlate with the research evidence as the NIHSS is only scored on admission and too many factors impact discharge disposition for accurate prediction
   D. It correlates with the research evidence since a score of 7 to 9 indicates guaranteed acceptance to an inpatient rehabilitation facility

6. Which of the following is true regarding Mr. Berg's discharge to an inpatient rehabilitation facility?
   A. He can expect to be discharged to a nursing home for care following his rehabilitation stay
   B. He can expect to be discharged to home after 3 days of inpatient rehabilitation, which is average for poststroke recovery
   C. He can expect to have a once-weekly visit with his family to limit distractions in his therapy
   D. He can expect to receive a minimum of 3 hours of therapy per day to facilitate progressive recovery

4. B) Stroke severity—milder strokes reach maximal recovery sooner, while more severe strokes take longer to reach maximal recovery

If a stroke is mild, the brain damage may be minimal, resulting in a faster recovery. However, when a stroke is considered more severe, as determined by a high score on the National Institutes of Health Stroke Scale (NIHSS), recovery may take longer and require more intensive rehabilitative work. Age plays a minor role in stroke recovery, as young people with severe stroke would have longer stroke recovery despite their age. Location of stroke has been found to have minimal impact on recovery time. Short bursts twice a week of inpatient rehabilitation have not been shown to facilitate rapid recovery.

5. B) It correlates with the research evidence since admission scores of 6 to 13 indicate likely discharge to an inpatient rehabilitation facility

Patients with NIHSS scores of 6 to 13 are likely to be discharged to an inpatient rehab facility for mild to severe stroke symptom recovery. A score of 6 to 13 does not indicate discharge to an SNF. NIHSS is scored throughout the hospital stay and on discharge as well. The research evidence proved a wider range of 6 to 13 for inpatient rehabilitation, not only 7 to 9.

6. D) He can expect to receive a minimum of 3 hours of therapy per day to facilitate progressive recovery

It is a requirement of acute inpatient rehabilitation that patients receive a minimum of 3 hours of therapy per day. The duration of a patient's stroke rehabilitation depends on the severity of their stroke and related complications. The average rehab length of stay after stroke for Mr. Berg with a National Institutes of Health Stroke Scale (NIHSS) score of 7 is 13.9 days, so he will need more than 3 days of intensive therapy. There is no guarantee that he'll need skilled nursing after his rehab stay. A 3-day length of stay is not the average poststroke rehab stay. Other than COVID-19 or pandemic restrictions, inpatient rehabilitation encourages family involvement to facilitate transition to home.

Barry is a 52-year-old stroke survivor who attends monthly support group meetings at the outpatient rehab center. Upon meeting him, the nurse notes his right-sided facial droop and the limited use of his right arm, suggesting Barry had a stroke on the left hemisphere of his brain. The nurse begins a conversation with Barry and refers to the stormy and dreary weather at present time by saying, "It appears to be raining cats and dogs outside." Barry suddenly looks at the nurse with horror and remains speechless. Immediately, he turns around and anxiously makes his way toward a window.

1. Based on his response, the nurse suspects Barry has a condition suggesting he couldn't process the nurse's comment normally. What is the name of this condition?
   A. Dysarthria
   B. Expressive aphasia
   C. Apraxia of speech
   D. Receptive aphasia

2. Based on Barry's response to the nurse's statement of "it appears to be raining cats and dogs," the nurse suspects which lobe of his brain to be impacted by a stroke?
   A. Frontal
   B. Parietal
   C. Temporal
   D. Occipital

3. Within the human brain, which area is involved in speech production and which is involved in speech perception?
   A. Wernicke's area and Broca's area, respectively
   B. The cortex and the cerebellum, respectively
   C. The cerebellum and the cortex, respectively
   D. Broca's area and Wernicke's area, respectively

4. Many stroke survivors are left with problems with one of their arms. Barry exhibits a hemiplegia to his right upper extremity after his stroke and reports frequent spasticity, suggesting periods of tightness versus weakness in his right arm. Knowledge of his condition leads the nurse to assume Barry's arm may also have what condition?
   A. Numbness or limited feeling
   B. Xerosis cutis
   C. Burst blood vessels or bruising
   D. Hyperpigmentation

5. According to research conducted by the National Institute of Neurological Disorders and Stroke in 2020, a reported 15% to 30% of stroke survivors will have permanent disability. Barry and his partner were referred to the stroke support group by his rehabilitative clinician based on an American Heart Association/American Stroke Association (AHA/ASA) systematic review and meta-analysis that suggests which of the following can be improved or, at a minimum, maintained in stroke survivors when community interventions are available?
   A. Physical activity alone
   B. Depressive mood disorders alone
   C. Motor, cognitive, and psychosocial function
   D. Medication intake and follow-up clinic appointment compliance

(See answers next page.)

1. D) Receptive aphasia
Barry has difficulty understanding the meaning of words, in this case the expression "it appears to be raining cats and dogs," suggesting that Barry has a receptive aphasia. Dysarthria is a weakness in the muscles used for speech, which often causes slowed or slurred speech. Individuals with expressive aphasia have trouble speaking fluently, but their comprehension can be relatively preserved. Apraxia of speech is a problem with the motor coordination and initiation of speech.

2. C) Temporal
The temporal lobe, where Wernicke's area is located, is commonly associated with understanding language, memory retrieval, face recognition, perception, and processing of auditory information. The frontal lobe is where Broca's area, the motor speech area, is located. The parietal and occipital lobes do not contain speech/language areas.

3. D) Broca's area and Wernicke's area, respectively
The Broca's area is involved in speech production, whereas the Wernicke's area is involved in speech perception. The cortex is responsible for many higher-order brain functions that include sensation, voluntary motor function, perception, memory, association, and thought. The cerebellum is mainly responsible for balance and coordination of our body.

4. A) Numbness or limited feeling
Neurological patients with profound motor function loss can experience numbness on the affected side. Following stroke, motor recovery can be dictated by the degree of sensory disruption. Hyperpigmentation, bruising or bursting of blood vessels, and/or a development of dry skin (xerosis cutis) are not as common in most recovering stroke patients.

5. C) Motor, cognitive, and psychosocial function
Motor, cognitive, and psychosocial function can be improved or maintained, at a minimum, in stroke survivors when community interventions such as a support groups are made available. Support groups have been shown to be significant resources in teaching self-management skills to stroke survivors and caregivers who must often undertake the new challenge of one or more chronic conditions. These skills include having the confidence to deal with medical management, role management, and emotional management of their condition. Physical activity alone or depressive mood disorders alone do not cover all the benefits shown from support groups. Medication intake and appointment compliance were not seen as functions to impact, but rather the outcome of improved motor, cognitive, and psychosocial function.

6. Following stroke with hemiparesis, patients can develop contracture on the affected side. The nurse notes Barry has a right wrist contracture, which his partner reports as a barrier to his ability to independently complete activities of daily living such as dressing himself or combing his hair. All the following would be included in regular assessments of recovering stroke patients, except:
   A. Pain
   B. Motor function
   C. Psychological status
   D. Insurance referral

6. D) Insurance referral

An insurance referral is not part of a recovering stroke patient's regular assessments, but pain, motor function, and psychological status are.

● CASE STUDY #4

Mrs. Abdi is a 62-year-old who presented to the ED 2 months prior for a sudden onset of a severe headache. At the time, her husband reported she had a brief loss of consciousness and some confusion. In the ED, it was determined that the cause of her symptoms was linked to a small subarachnoid hemorrhage (SAH) seen on the CT scan. Subsequently, Mrs. Abdi required surgical intervention.

1. Based on the nurse's knowledge of her diagnosis, a subarachnoid hemorrhage (SAH) is most commonly caused by:
   A. Amyloid angiopathy
   B. Aneurysmal rupture
   C. Arteriovenous vascular malformation (AVM) rupture
   D. Arteriosclerotic vascular disease

2. 80% of hemorrhagic strokes, such as Mrs. Abdi's, are primarily caused by:
   A. An embolus
   B. A brain tumor
   C. A cerebral thrombus
   D. Uncontrolled hypertension

3. The nurse anticipates the following medical management orders except one. Which order is NOT anticipated?
   A. Limit stimulation and keep lights low and door shut
   B. Administration of fresh frozen plasma and vitamin K
   C. Administration of analgesic agent
   D. Application of sequential compression devices

4. Mrs. Abdi returned from the operating room with an external ventricular drain (EVD) in place to monitor for:
   A. Salt wasting syndrome
   B. Vasospasm
   C. Intracerebral pressure (ICP)
   D. Cerebral perfusion

5. Mrs. Abdi's plan of care will include which bed position?
   A. High-Fowler's
   B. Prone
   C. Supine
   D. Semi-Fowler's (head of bed at 15–30 degrees)

6. Given what the nurse knows of the cause for her subarachnoid hemorrhage (SAH), which of the following complications may occur?
   A. Cerebral hypoxia
   B. Vasospasm
   C. Increased intracerebral pressure (ICP)
   D. All of the above

1. B) Aneurysmal rupture

An SAH is most often caused by a ruptured aneurysm. Amyloid angiopathy would result in subdural hemorrhage. AVM rupture would result in intracerebral hemorrhage. Arteriosclerotic vascular disease would not necessarily result in any specific hemorrhage.

2. D) Uncontrolled hypertension

The most common cause of hemorrhagic stroke is uncontrolled hypertension. An embolus and thrombus would result in ischemic stroke. A brain tumor might have intracerebral hemorrhage as a complication but does not account for 80% of hemorrhagic strokes.

3. B) Administration of fresh frozen plasma and vitamin K

Administration of fresh frozen plasma and vitamin K is a measure taken to stop the progression of intracranial hemorrhage. There is no diagnostic evidence to suggest this patient is actively bleeding, and she was not on any anticoagulants that would have necessitated reversal of international normalized ratio (INR).

4. C) Intracerebral pressure (ICP)

The purpose of an EVD is to remove fluid from the ventricles of the brain, which can cause brain edema and hydrocephalus resulting in increased ICP. A basic metabolic panel (BMP) is used to monitor cerebral salt wasting, not an EVD. A transcranial Doppler ultrasound is used to determine cerebral blood flow and is used frequently in the evaluation of cerebrovascular vasospasm. Cerebral perfusion pressure is the net pressure gradient that drives oxygen delivery to brain tissue. This can be determined by calculating the difference between the mean arterial pressure (MAP) and the ICP in millimeters of mercury and does not require use of an EVD.

5. D) Semi-Fowler's (head of bed at 15–30 degrees)

Research suggests there may not be any benefit in sitting up or lying patients flat. However, a standard head of bed at 15 to 30 degrees (semi-Fowler's) appears to provide a safe positioning of the head for adequate perfusion or blood flow to the brain without causing harm. High-Fowler's represents too high a position for adequate perfusion. The prone position is not recommended in any poststroke recovery. Supine position would be used for patients with concerns for low intracerebral pressure (ICP).

6. D) All of the above

Common complications of SAH include the following: brain edema and increased ICP, rebleeding, and cerebral hypoxia from vasospasm and seizures.

George is a 63-year-old male who sustained a right-sided cerebellar hemisphere stroke 3 months ago. He is right hand dominant with a diagnosed history of uncontrolled hypertension and admits to being a smoker for 40+ years. George was trying to lose weight prior to having his stroke, but remains 30 lb. overweight from his recommended goal set by his primary care provider (PCP). He can no longer walk without using his cane and taking frequent breaks. A retired foreman for a construction company, George lives at home with his wife and their two dogs. George was referred to outpatient physiotherapy from a local rehab hospital following discharge to help improve his independence, mobility, and performance of activities of daily living.

During the medical history intake at the outpatient physiotherapy office, George speaks openly about his difficulty keeping his balance for long periods of time and notes that simple movements he would normally perform, such as feeding or walking his dogs, have felt more difficult to accomplish since he finds himself leaning toward the side. His wife expresses concern that George has been more isolated and depressed since returning home and thinks it is related to not being able to do the same independent tasks around the house that he could do prior to his stroke. "I can't even reach for things from the top shelf or help unload the dishwasher," he states with frustration. Presently, George uses a cane but is eager to get rid of it, although it has been helpful in preventing him from falling. His goals include regaining stability in his walking without an assistive device and being able to do simple tasks, such as emptying the dishwasher and being able to store dishes onto the top shelf of the kitchen cupboard.

1. During an objective physical and neurological assessment, George's gait is observed with use of his cane. Based on the nurse's knowledge of his right-sided cerebellar hemisphere stroke, which current state is expected?
   A. George will exhibit discoordination of his left leg and deviation to his left side as he walks forward
   B. George will exhibit discoordination of his right leg and deviation to his right as he walks forward
   C. George will exhibit a normal cadence and movement of his trunk as he walks forward using his cane for support
   D. George will exhibit a swaying motion with his hips bilaterally as he walks forward

2. Cerebellar strokes account for just 2.3% of overall cerebrovascular events. Clinically, patients will present with nonspecific symptoms such as:
   A. Slurred speech, facial droop, and upper and lower extremity weakness on one side of the body
   B. Headache, dizziness, facial droop, and numbness to one side of the body
   C. Dizziness, nausea, vomiting, unsteady gait, and headache
   D. Nystagmus, stiff neck, isolated facial numbness, and contralateral lower extremity weakness

3. When George was first seen in the ED for his cerebellar stroke, he was offered alteplase because he was within how many hours from his last known well (LKW) time?
   A. 3.5 hours
   B. 4 hours
   C. 4.5 hours
   D. 6 hours

(See answers next page.)   **227**

1. B) George will exhibit discoordination of his right leg and deviation to his right as he walks forward

Right-sided cerebellar strokes present with right-sided discoordination that may include difficulty walking or controlling motor movements on that same side. A discoordination of his left leg indicates left-sided cerebellar stroke, and his stroke was in the right cerebellum. George has described instability in walking, so he would not show a normal cadence yet. A bilateral swaying motion is very unlikely in unilateral discoordination.

2. C) Dizziness, nausea, vomiting, unsteady gait, and headache

Slurred speech, facial droop, and upper and lower extremity weakness on one side of the body is usually associated with a middle cerebral artery stroke, which accounts for approximately 80% of all ischemic strokes. Facial droop, numbness to one side of the body, nystagmus, stiff neck, isolated facial numbness, and contralateral lower extremity weakness are not considered common symptoms associated with a cerebellar stroke.

3. C) 4.5 hours

According to the 2019 American Heart Association/American Stroke Association (AHA/ASA) Guidelines for the Early Management of Patients with Acute Ischemic Stroke, patients with stroke symptom recognition within 4.5 hours of LKW time can benefit from intravenous (IV) thrombolytic administration.

4. The consulting neurologist informed George that the success rate of alteplase alone 90 days after receiving acute ischemic stroke treatment is around what percentage?
   A. 15%
   B. 21%
   C. 30%
   D. 42%

5. George's wife acknowledges his recovery has gradually improved, but she worries about his risk of having a secondary stroke. Given his medical history, what factor places George in the highest risk of having another stroke?
   A. Inadequate physical activity
   B. A history of smoking 40+ years
   C. Uncontrolled hypertension
   D. Obesity

6. To aid in preventing a second stroke, the nurse provides George with dietary education and references which of the following diets to assist him in achieving his weight loss goal and managing his elevated blood pressure?
   A. Lyon
   B. Mediterranean
   C. Keto
   D. Paleo

(See answers next page.)

4. C) 30%

According to the National Institutes for Neurological Diseases and Stroke (NINDS) and Stroke Tissue Plasminogen Activator (tPA) Stroke Study Group, as compared to patients who were given placebo, patients treated with intravenous (IV) alteplase were at least 30% more likely to have minimal or no disability at 3 months.

5. C) Uncontrolled hypertension

Inadequate physical activity, a history of smoking, uncontrolled hypertension, and obesity are all risk factors toward a secondary stroke; however, uncontrolled hypertension puts George at the biggest risk to experience another event.

6. B) Mediterranean

Numerous studies have confirmed the Mediterranean diet helps prevent heart disease and stroke. There is no Lyon diet, and while the keto and Paleo diets have been recognized as effective weight loss tools, it is the Mediterranean diet that is recommended consistently in stroke literature.

CASE STUDY #6

Mr. Lee is 72 years old and has been in inpatient rehabilitation for 2 weeks after his ischemic stroke. He is anticipated for discharge home soon. He was independent with activities of daily living prior to his stroke and has been widowed for 5 years. It has been suggested that he will need outpatient physical therapy to continue with his recovery as well as someone with him round-the-clock at least for the first few weeks due to cognitive gaps. His son lives in a neighboring state and is concerned about the need for round-the-clock care because he cannot fulfill that need.

1. What information can be shared with the concerned son regarding the plan for discharge to home?
   A. A family meeting with social services and care coordination has been scheduled to review options
   B. Round-the-clock care is not a requirement and only a suggestion if the son desires to return to his home state
   C. Examples of families who have moved to care for their loved ones
   D. Suggest a skilled nursing facility (SNF) as the better discharge disposition

2. Medical insurance copays for outpatient therapy appointments can be expensive and a barrier for many patients and family caregivers to comply with ongoing treatment throughout the rehabilitative phase. The nurse overhears Mr. Lee on the phone telling his son that he does not plan to keep his scheduled therapy appointments because he cannot afford the high copay. What is the best nursing action to take?
   A. Update the care team about the patient's decision and document noncompliance to ongoing therapy in the plan of care
   B. Inform the patient that the case manager will enroll him in a charitable treatment program
   C. Ask the primary therapist to speak with the patient and his family caregiver about the recommended number of therapy sessions necessary and offer the option of teaching him similar exercise activities to do at home on his own
   D. Tell the patient the structured therapy that has been ordered is not necessary since he is showing some improvement already

3. During a routine assessment, the nurse determines Mr. Lee is feeling down and is more reserved than in prior interactions. He seems indifferent to questions about his day and less interested in working with the physical and occupational therapy team members by asking to remain in bed. The nurse reports this change to the primary care team during morning rounds. What action can the nurse expect?
   A. An immediate psychiatric consult
   B. A discussion with the patient about current home medications and use of antidepressant
   C. Activation of nursing protocol, adding sertraline daily
   D. Steps toward suicide precautions

1. A) A family meeting with social services and care coordination has been scheduled to review options

A meeting with both members of the transitional care team will help Mr. Lee's son decide what steps he may want to take next. Social workers assist family in the process of adjusting to their family member's newly diagnosed stroke and disability for the purpose of facilitating the patient's return to the community, while the goal of care coordination is to assist in arranging appropriate and efficient delivery of health services available within or across a system. It is not a nursing function to determine if round-the-clock care is needed or to suggest a nursing home. The son may not have the ability to give up his job and move in with his father, and it is inappropriate to suggest this.

2. C) Ask the primary therapist to speak with the patient and his family caregiver about the recommended number of therapy sessions necessary and offer the option of teaching him similar exercise activities to do at home on his own

Securing the patient and the family caregivers' active involvement early in the rehabilitation process optimizes the patient's chances for recovery and community reintegration. Nursing can help present the primary therapists' recommendations through open conversation and providing both interactive and written materials of activities that can be done successfully at home. Updating the care team and documenting noncompliance can be taken; however, it does not address the patient or the family's concerns directly. Few communities have charitable treatment programs available, so it may not be a realistic remediation plan. It is not a nurse's role to determine if therapy is needed.

3. B) A discussion with the patient about current home medications and use of antidepressant

Individual patients will vary in how well they respond to challenging and demanding therapeutic approaches. A discussion with the patient about current home medications and use of antidepressants may be necessary. Only after a patient's unique needs and circumstances are determined can relevant specialists be incorporated for adjunct psychosocial therapy. There are no recommendations for nursing protocols to treat with an antidepressant. This patient hasn't exhibited risk for self-harm, so it is unadvised to take steps toward suicide precautions.

4. Mr. Lee's upper extremity and gait training needs have been met daily during his 14-day inpatient rehabilitation stay. With anticipation of Mr. Lee's discharge home, his son asks if his father's unaffected arm will still need to be in a sling for several hours a day. Which is the best response by his nurse?
   A. Application of the sling reduces the event of Mr. Lee from pulling out his naso-gastric (NG) tube
   B. The applied sling to the unaffected arm is to stimulate Mr. Lee's desire to be independent
   C. Constraint-induced movement therapy (CIMT) is an evidence-based therapy technique used to limit the use of the unaffected arm for designated periods of time throughout the day to increase the incentive to use the affected arm and has been effective in his father's case
   D. This technique forces the affected side to get stronger because the restraint reduces the muscle strength of the unaffected side

5. Additionally, Mr. Lee's son asks, "Why does my father complain of shoulder pain?" Which of the following answers will best answer his question?
   A. Stroke patients may commonly report pain depending on the area of the brain affected
   B. Mr. Lee may have fallen and injured his should as a result of the stroke, but it was not witnessed and therefore not reported
   C. A stroke patient with upper extremity paresis may experience shoulder pain due to the weight of the limb and reduced muscle, ligament, and tendon function around the affected shoulder
   D. A stroke patient with upper extremity paresis may experience shoulder pain dur-ing resting periods of constraint-induced movement therapy (CIMT) as a result of not maintaining the affected arm in a sling

6. Mr. Lee's son asks if any measures can be implemented to reduce his father's shoulder pain. Which is the best response?
   A. Administration of pain medication
   B. Implementation of proper alignment and positioning support of the affected arm when Mr. Lee is sitting, lying in bed, or ambulating
   C. When assisting him out of bed, it's suggested to avoid pulling on Mr. Lee's affected arm
   D. All of the above

4. C) Constraint-induced movement therapy (CIMT) is an evidence-based therapy technique used to limit the use of the unaffected arm for designated periods of time throughout the day to increase the incentive to use the affected arm and has been effective in his father's case

CIMT is specialized in practicing to use the affected limb and aims at decreasing the nonuse of the affected limb that can occur after a stroke. The purpose of immobilizing the unaffected limb is not to prevent tube displacement or to stimulate independence. Restraining the unaffected limb is not to the point of reducing the muscle strength of that limb.

5. C) A stroke patient with upper extremity paresis may experience shoulder pain due to the weight of the limb and reduced muscle, ligament, and tendon function around the affected shoulder

According to the American Heart Association/American Stroke Association (AHA/ASA), about 84% of stroke survivors with arm weakness develop shoulder pain associated with shoulder subluxation and motor weakness of the affected limb. This pain is usually a result of a weak rotator cuff muscle, which connects the upper arm bone to the shoulder blade. Because of the upper extremity paresis, Mr. Lee's muscles are not maintaining shoulder joint alignment during arm movement, which causes him discomfort. Poststroke arm/shoulder pain is not a result of specific areas of the brain affected. While it's possible that Mr. Lee might have fallen, it is far less likely than subluxation as the cause of the pain. There is no evidence of shoulder pain in the affected limb with CIMT.

6. D) All of the above

Pain medication, proper alignment, positioning support of the affected arm, and avoiding pulling on the affected arm will all serve as measures to help reduce pain and further limit damage to his muscle and joints.

According to The Joint Commission, substandard hand-off reporting can cause serious or fatal consequences including, but not limited to, delay in treatment, inappropriate treatment, care omission, increased length of stay, readmissions, increased costs, inefficient care from initial workup, and minor and/or major patient harm. Nurse hand-off reporting during change of shift is an equally critical process, crucial in protecting a stroke patient's safety. Throughout the nursing hand-off report, it's important to deliver precise, up-to-date, and pertinent information to the receiving nurse.

During hand-off report at 19:00, a nurse is told that their 54-year-old female stroke patient failed the ED bedside nursing swallow screen after her initial evaluation at approximately 11:00 this morning. As a result, the patient's ordered dose of 81 mg of aspirin by mouth was held. She arrives to the acute care unit in stable condition with mild right-sided facial palsy and slurred speech, which she had for 2 days prior to arrival. Her CT scan indicates a small hypodense area of the left middle cerebral artery (MCA) territory, indicating an ischemic stroke. She is presently alert and oriented x3 and in stable condition with no focal upper or lower weakness on bedside neurological examination. Her previous medical history includes hypertension, type 2 diabetes, and high cholesterol, for which she is taking nicardipine, metformin, and simvastatin. Plan of care includes MRI and cardiac workup. Current vitals are heart rate (HR) 116 irregular, blood pressure (BP) 155/85, respiratory rate (RR) 18, and blood oxygen saturation (SPO$_2$) 98%.

1. On admission the patient is designated as NPO, or nothing by mouth, because she is exhibiting swallowing difficulties. What is this condition called?
   A. Dysarthria
   B. Dysphagia
   C. Dysphasia
   D. Dystaxia

2. Speech pathology will not be available to see this newly admitted patient until 07:00 the next morning. The resident physician has asked if the patient has received her antithrombotic medication as ordered. The nurse recalls from evening shift hand-off report that this medication was held owing to the patient failing the bedside nursing swallow screen. What is their best response?
   A. Antithrombotics are to be given by end of hospital day 2, so the nurse has time to administer this ordered medication after the patient is cleared by speech pathology
   B. Antithrombotics need to be given early for best patient outcomes; therefore, the nurse requests for the resident physician to change the order for suppository
   C. Antithrombotics are only necessary for small vessel stroke diagnosis
   D. Antithrombotics need to be given early for best patient outcomes, so the nurse will crush the tablet into apple sauce and feed it to the patient

3. Within the first 24 hours, this patient exhibits a new onset of atrial fibrillation on the cardiac monitor. She is started on a beta-blocker medication to help slow her heart rate at rest and during activity. Given her previous medical history, the newly ordered beta blocker may cause what side effect?
   A. Hypoglycemia
   B. Hypotension
   C. Hypothermia
   D. Hypotonia

1. B) Dysphagia

Dysphagia is a medical term for difficulty in swallowing foods or liquids, putting patients at greater risk of aspirating. Dysarthria is slowed or slurred speech caused by a weakness in the muscles used for speech. Dysphasia is a language disorder affecting a person's ability to comprehend and generate speech. Dystaxia is an impairment of balance or coordination, linked to damage of the brain, nerves, or muscles.

2. B) Antithrombotics need to be given early for best patient outcomes; therefore, the nurse requests for the resident physician to change the order for suppository

According to American Heart Association/American Stroke Association (AHA/ASA) guidelines, early antithrombotic treatment is linked to better patient outcomes and a reduction of recurrent stroke and other cardiovascular events. However, dysphagia patients with swallowing difficulty who are ordered PO (by mouth) antithrombotics should have modified medication orders for a different route, such as suppository or via nasogastric (NG) tube. With fluctuation of stroke patient status, putting off an evidence-based treatment is unwise and not best practice. Antithrombotics are not only needed for small vessel disease—they are recommended on admission for all ischemic stroke patients. With a failed bedside swallow screen, nothing should be given orally until cleared by the speech and language pathologist; therefore, the best course of action is to change the order to a suppository.

3. B) Hypotension

Beta-blocker medication may have the side effect of lowering blood pressure. Beta blockers have no impact on blood sugar, body temperature, or muscle tone.

4. At 19:00 shift change, a nurse and the departing day-shift nurse completed a joint neurological exam, the purpose of the exam is so that each provider can establish an agreed-upon status for that patient. At the time, the patient was deemed alert and oriented x3, with mild right-sided facial palsy with slurred speech and a normal motor and sensory examination of all four extremities. At 23:00, the nurse enters the patient's room to return her to bed after spending several hours in her chair watching television. A neurological examination indicates the patient is alert and oriented x3, however she exhibits a complete paralysis of her right face, garbled speech, and flaccid right upper extremity. Presently, the cardiac monitor indicates heart rate (HR) 65, blood pressure (BP) 90/75, respiratory rate (RR) 14, and blood oxygen saturation (SPO_2) 92% on room air. Which would be the best action to take next?
   A. Return the patient to bed, notify the provider, check a finger stick blood glucose (FSBG), and prepare the patient for a stat MRI of the head and a fluid bolus
   B. Safely return the patient back into bed and check a FSBG and record it
   C. Place the patient back into bed in a semi-Fowler's position, place her on 2 L of nasal cannula oxygen, and recheck her blood pressure
   D. Return the patient to bed, ensure the head of the bed is flat, check a FSBG and BP, and notify the provider

5. A nursing colleague assisting in this intervention suspects the patient's worsening of neurological symptoms are a result of:
   A. Being overly tired from the exertion of getting out of bed after a long physical therapy session
   B. Hypoxia, due to the demand of oxygen with exertion
   C. The patient experiencing postural hypotension while sitting in her chair for a lengthy period and causing an exacerbation of her baseline stroke symptoms
   D. The patient is showing signs of depression and cognitive decline associated with subacute stroke

6. Which of the following is correct regarding the importance of getting this patient back to bed quickly?
   A. The oxygen tubing does not reach from the wall source to the bedside chair
   B. Patients who become acutely depressed after a stroke are less likely to cooperate with a neurological exam
   C. Patients who have experienced a stroke require more rest in the first 72 hours than the average patient
   D. Cerebral autoregulation can be impaired in patients who have had a stroke, making them more likely to decline neurologically with extreme low and high blood pressure (BP) readings

4. D) Return the patient to bed, ensure the head of the bed is flat, check a FSBG and BP, and notify the provider

The best action to take is to safely return this patient to bed, ensuring the head of bed is flat to counter her low BP (90/75), which may produce stroke-like symptoms as a result of poor perfusion to the brain. In addition, the FSBG is acquired to rule out hypoglycemia, which is another common stroke-mimic. Stat MRI is not the imaging modality used in emergent situations. Simply recording the fingerstick glucose result is not adequate in an emergent situation. Semi-Fowler's position does not facilitate cerebral perfusion and should be avoided.

5. C) The patient experiencing postural hypotension while sitting in her chair for a lengthy period and causing an exacerbation of her baseline stroke symptoms

An extended period of postural hypotension in stroke patients can further impair cerebral blood flow, increase stroke size, or hinder recovery. Fatigue does not explain the new deficits noted, and the patient hasn't been exerting herself recently to result in hypoxia. The new deficits noted are not signs of depression or cognitive decline.

6. D) Cerebral autoregulation can be impaired in patients who have had a stroke, making them more likely to decline neurologically with extreme low and high blood pressure (BP) readings

Autoregulation impairment in the presence of moderate to severe ischemic stroke may render penumbral brain tissue particularly vulnerable to alterations in systemic BP and overall perfusion to the brain. The patient needs to be supine, regardless of oxygen supply. The new deficits are unrelated to depression. The rationale for getting a symptomatic patient back to bed immediately is unrelated to a patient needing more rest.

Malcom, a 43-year-old African American male, was found on the bathroom floor in an altered mental state by his wife. She called 911 immediately. Initial emergency medical services (EMS) examination determined Malcom was lethargic and nonsensical in his speech. His initial vital signs included heart rate (HR) 88, blood pressure (BP) 210/105, respiratory rate (RR) 18, and blood oxygen saturation (SPO_2) of 93% on room air. Malcom's previous history includes hypertension, diabetes, and deep vein thrombosis (DVT) for which he was on warfarin. Emergent CT scan of his brain revealed a 2 mm x 2.5 mm hemorrhage in the left posterior parietal lobe. He was admitted to the ICU for acute management and monitoring by neurosurgical services. Subsequent MRI indicated no surgical intervention at this time and would require follow-up in the outpatient setting.

1. Prior to his hemorrhagic stroke, Malcom was placed on warfarin to manage his deep vein thrombosis (DVT) diagnosis. DVT can cause a stroke only if there is a presence of:
   A. Atrial fibrillation
   B. Patent foramen ovale (PFO)
   C. Mitral valve regurgitation
   D. Endocarditis

2. During his hospital stay, Malcom's wife was confused about his clinical diagnosis, given that intraparenchymal hemorrhage (IPH) is synonymous with which of the following terms?
   A. Intraventricular hemorrhage (IVH)
   B. Subarachnoid hemorrhage (SAH)
   C. Intracerebral hemorrhage (ICH)
   D. Intradural hemorrhage

3. The most common cause of intraparenchymal hemorrhage (IPH) is:
   A. Extreme hyperglycemia linked to Malcom's diabetes, causing damage to the blood–brain barrier
   B. Extreme hyperthermia, causing capillary leakage in his newly discovered arterio-venous malformation (AVM)
   C. Aneurysmal rupture, causing high intracerebral pressure (ICP)
   D. Hypertension, causing arterial wall stiffness and rupture

4. Arteriovenous malformations (AVMs) can result in an intraparenchymal hemorrhage (IPH) likely related to which of the following reasons?
   A. Arteries and veins connecting directly rather than the usual route of arteries to arterioles, to capillaries, to venules, to veins
   B. Connection of underdeveloped veins to arteries
   C. Vascular anomalies located in the circle of Willis
   D. Chronic hypertension fusing together arteries with veins

(See answers next page.)   **239**

1. B) Patient foramen ovale (PFO)

According to a 2018 article in *Stroke*, because venous thrombosis is more common among adults and venous thrombi generate numerous migrating emboli, right-to-left shunting due to a PFO can expose patients to substantial acute ischemic stroke risk. Atrial fibrillation, mitral valve regurgitation and endocarditis have no correlation with DVT and increased risk of stroke.

2. C) Intracerebral hemorrhage (ICH)

IPH or ICH refers to nontraumatic bleeding into the brain parenchyma, i.e., tissue. IVH is bleeding into the fluid-filled areas, or ventricles, surrounded by the brain. SAH refers to bleeding into the space between the pia and the arachnoid membranes. An intradural hemorrhage is generally synonymous with subdural hemorrhage, in which blood collects between the dura mater and the arachnoid mater.

3. D) Hypertension, causing arterial wall stiffness and rupture

A nontraumatic IPH is commonly a result of hypertensive damage to the brain's blood vessel walls. Extreme hyperglycemia will eventually cause vascular damage but not as commonly as hypertension. Hyperthermia is not a related cause for this condition. Aneurysmal rupture would result in subarachnoid hemorrhage (SAH), rarely intracerebral hemorrhage (ICH).

4. A) Arteries and veins connecting directly rather than the usual route of arteries to arterioles, to capillaries, to venules, to veins

An AVM can put extreme pressure on the walls of the affected veins, which results in making these vessels more thin or weak. Eventually, this may cause the AVM to rupture and bleed into the brain tissue. Even well-developed veins that connect directly to arteries are at risk of rupture due to lack of muscular walls. Vascular anomalies located in the circle of Willis are likely to be aneurysms. Chronic hypertension does not fuse arteries with veins; rather, it places vessels such as these at risk for rupture.

5. What are the American Heart Association/American Stroke Association recommendations for safe restart of anticoagulation therapy in Malcom's case?
   A. After 1 month, it should be safe for any patient to resume oral anticoagulation
   B. Resumption of Malcom's anticoagulation therapy should be held for at least 1 week
   C. Low-dose intravenous (IV) anticoagulation should be started within 48 hours
   D. If after 24 hours an inpatient MRI confirms he is stable, he may resume oral anticoagulation

6. At the time of discharge from the rehabilitation hospital, Malcom and his wife are reviewing instructions of what to do if he develops stroke symptoms after he returns home. The nurse determines Malcom and his wife understand his instructions based on the following answer.
   A. "I should drive to the ED immediately"
   B. "I should take my blood pressure and report high findings to my family doctor"
   C. "I should call 911 right away"
   D. "I should make sure I bring my medications with me to the ED"

(See answers next page.)

5. B) Resumption of Malcom's anticoagulation therapy should be held for at least 1 week

Optimal timing to resume anticoagulation therapy after an intraparenchymal hemorrhage (IPH) is still unknown; however, earlier than 1 week is not recommended, regardless of MRI results. Both early (<2 weeks) and late (>4 weeks) restart of therapy should be determined after extensive evaluation of risks for IPH recurrence and thromboembolism.

6. C) "I should call 911 right away"

Given Malcom's diagnosis and risk for a subsequent stroke, it is important for him and his wife to call 911 immediately if new symptoms are noted. A recurrent stroke is a time-sensitive medical emergency, and prehospital paramedics are highly trained clinicians in the acute management of stroke. Driving to the ED should not be considered because Malcom should utilize prehospital services by calling 911. Taking blood pressure after developing stroke symptoms does not address emergent nature of the indication. By responding that they will bring medications to the ED, they have not fully addressed the core of the issue—to respond quickly to the emergent indication.

A team of stroke-certified nurses have volunteered to educate the public on how to reduce the risk of stroke by participating in a local community health fair. During the event, the volunteer nursing staff engage with folks as they walk by the hospital's health fair booth, quizzing participants to identify warning signs associated with stroke. One woman from the community stops by the booth and states she has had a transient ischemic attack (TIA) in the past year, "but they didn't find a cause of my symptoms."

1. Which of the following statements by this community member would be most concerning to the volunteer nurse?
   A. "I occasionally drink 2 beers a day, especially on weekends, and have been a 1 pack per day smoker for 10 years"
   B. "My boyfriend asks if it is ok to still smoke marijuana around me"
   C. "I smoke 1 pack per day and take an oral contraceptive"
   D. "I'm not going to continue taking that daily aspirin, it'll make me feel like an old lady"

2. When asked if she is following up with her primary care provider (PCP), she says yes, noting as well that she is confused because her provider told her that she couldn't have had a transient ischemic attack (TIA) because nothing was seen on her imaging. What is the best nursing response?
   A. There can be confusion regarding TIA, but the hallmark of TIA is that the symptoms are transient and nothing is seen on imaging, so you are correct when you say you had a TIA
   B. You may need to find another PCP because they are wrong about it not being a TIA
   C. You need to be followed by a neurologist because PCPs aren't expert enough to understand the difference between TIA and stroke
   D. There can be confusion regarding TIA, but the hallmark of TIA is that there are tiny infarcts seen on MRI, so your PCP is correct

3. Upon listening to the nurse, the young woman considers her current risk but states she's been healthy all her life except for her recent transient ischemic attack (TIA). "Anyway, I thought people in their 60s and men and women as old as my 85-year-old grandmother have strokes." Based on this statement, the volunteer nurse informs the young woman that there has been a 44% increase of stroke incidence among which age group?
   A. Ages 12 to 18 years
   B. Ages 25 to 44 years
   C. Ages 50 to 64 years
   D. Ages 85 to 98 years

4. All the following are this woman's nonmodifiable risk factors for stroke EXCEPT which one?
   A. Age
   B. Gender
   C. Atrial fibrillation
   D. Race/ethnicity

1. C) "I smoke 1 pack per day and take an oral contraceptive"

The volunteer nurse should be concerned with the community member's statement of smoking 1 pack per day in addition to using oral contraceptives. Smoking while using oral contraceptives can lead to a greater risk of stroke and heart attacks. The extreme risk of the combination of smoking and oral contraceptives makes it a more worrisome statement than comments about secondhand marijuana use, alcohol and cigarette consumption, and unwillingness to take daily aspirin.

2. A) There can be confusion regarding TIA, but the hallmark of TIA is that the symptoms are transient and nothing is seen on imaging, so you are correct when you say you had a TIA

During community outreach education, it is not unusual to have community members report questionable advice from their PCPs, and care must be taken in giving a response. By the information provided, this person did have a TIA since there were no changes on her MRI, and it seems that her PCP is incorrect. It is not appropriate to tell her that she needs to find another provider or to tell her that PCPs cannot understand TIA and stroke.

3. B) Ages 25 to 44 years

There has been a rise in stoke incidence in people aged 25 to 44 years. Multiple suspected causes for this increase include the prevalence of type 2 diabetes, high cholesterol, and obesity in high-income countries like the United States. Additionally, the use of cigarettes and the abuse of alcohol and recreational drugs are frequent among young people and have tended to increase over time.

4. C) Atrial fibrillation

Risk factors are conditions that increase our risk of developing a disease like stroke. Stroke risk factors are either modifiable, meaning measures can be taken to change them, or nonmodifiable, meaning they cannot be changed. Atrial fibrillation is the only risk factor listed that can be reduced or stopped by taking prescribed medications, receiving electrical shock (cardioversion), or having minimally invasive surgery (ablation).

5. The community health fair this year was being held at the urban recreation center near the state capital. Based on the demographic picture of community members in attendance, the group of volunteer nurses make it a goal to inform which racial group about their high incidence of, and mortality from, stroke due to the higher prevalence of hypertension, obesity, and diabetes?
   A. Hispanic/Latino Americans
   B. African Americans
   C. Whites
   D. Asian/Pacific Islanders

6. When asked by participating community members about how much physical activity is necessary to reduce their risk factor for stroke, the nursing volunteers reference the American Heart Association (AHA) guidelines of:
   A. A minimum of 40 minutes/day of moderate to vigorous aerobic activity daily
   B. A minimum of 60 minutes/day of moderate aerobic activity twice a week
   C. A minimum of 40 minutes/day of moderate to vigorous aerobic activity three to four times a week
   D. 20 minutes of vigorous aerobic activity twice a day, three times a week

5. B) African Americans
According to the Centers for Disease Control and Prevention (CDC), African Americans have nearly double the risk of a stroke over Whites/Caucasians, Pacific Islanders, and Hispanics. Although Hispanics have seen a rise in death rates since 2013, their rates are still lower than those of African Americans.

6. C) A minimum of 40 minutes/day of moderate to vigorous aerobic activity three to four times a week
The AHA guidelines of at least 40 minutes/day of moderate to vigorous aerobic activity three to four times a week are recommended for primary stroke prevention. When making this recommendation, it should be stressed as part of an overall strategy in preventing stroke, but even more so in persons with other risk factors.

Josefina is a 33-year-old female who presented to the ED via emergency medical services (EMS) transport. She was running outside with her roommate when she reported a sudden onset of a "thunderclap" headache. Her roommate called EMS immediately when Josefina abruptly stopped running and lowered herself to the ground and verbalized sudden severe headache and extreme photophobia. EMS arrived to find Josefina with her head in her hands and responding slowly to initial examination questions. During transport, she became more lethargic, and upon presentation to the ED she exhibits agitation and writhing in pain with her eyes closed. Josefina is oriented to self and place and capable of verbalizing that her head hurts but will not open her eyes or answer questions about events leading to her arrival to the ED. She is able to follow only simple commands and will move all extremities to pain. Her vitals include a temperature of 37 °C (98.6 °F); she is tachycardic and hypertensive with heart rate (HR) 110 and blood pressure (BP) 150/100. Her lungs are clear with respiratory rate (RR) 20 and blood oxygen saturation (SPO$_2$) at 98% on room air (RA). Head CT revealed a large subarachnoid hemorrhage.

1. A patient with any type of intracranial hemorrhage may present with coma, rapidly declining level of consciousness (LOC), or seizure. Therefore, in cases such as this, the priority is:
   A. Assessing a baseline Glasgow Coma Scale (GCS) to determine the next step in care
   B. Checking a finger stick blood glucose (FSGB) to rule out a stroke mimic
   C. Addressing her ABCDs: airway, breathing, circulation, and disability
   D. Acquiring a stat CT scan of the head

2. In patients with significant intracranial hemorrhage, it's important to be able to recognize Cushing's triad, as this is a sign of impending brain herniation. Cushing's triad describes the physiologic response to rapidly increasing intracerebral pressure (ICP) and imminent brain herniation. Its features include:
   A. Bradycardia
   B. Hypertension
   C. Abnormal respiratory patterns
   D. All of the above

3. Which neurological assessment by the nurse is most important in this situation?
   A. Glasgow Coma Scale (GCS)
   B. National Institutes of Health Stroke Scale (NIHSS)
   C. Modified Rankin Scale (mRS)
   D. Cranial nerves

4. During rounds, the critical care team reviews Josefina's history closely with her, explaining that recent exertion, history of hypertension, excess alcohol intake, and cigarette smoking are risk factors for subarachnoid hemorrhage (SAH). But they point out that the strongest predictor of SAH is:
   A. Family history
   B. Gender
   C. Age
   D. Glasgow Coma Scale (GCS)

1. C) Addressing her ABCDs: airway, breathing, circulation, and disability

Priority should be airway management in a patient presenting with coma, rapidly declining level of consciousness, or seizure. In these scenarios, a patient may not be able to maintain their airway, breathe on their own, or both. Baseline GCS is not required for determining the next step in care, and these symptoms do not represent hypoglycemia/hyperglycemia as stroke mimics. A CT scan of the head is important but is pointless without stabilization first.

2. D) All of the above

Bradycardia, hypertension, and abnormal respiratory patterns are the three symptoms that make up Cushing's triad.

3. B) National Institutes of Health Stroke Scale (NIHSS)

In the setting of acute stroke, the NIHSS is essential and is required for all certified stroke centers. The GCS has limited value in stroke and is not recommended or required. The mRS score is valuable but not as critical as the NIHSS and is not required on admission. Cranial nerve assessment is not appropriate in an emergency stroke setting.

4. A) Family history

A family history of SAH is strongly associated with a risk of SAH. To prevent the onset of SAH at a younger age, more attention should be given to individuals with any family member (first-degree relatives) suffering SAH episodes, and education should be given regarding modifiable risk factor control. Gender and age play a lesser role in risk of SAH. GCS plays no role.

5. A classic presenting symptom of a subarachnoid hemorrhage (SAH) is an acute onset of "thunderclap" headache that may be accompanied by a loss of consciousness, vomiting, neck stiffness, or seizure activity. Most SAH are due to:
   A. Ruptured artery in the middle cerebral artery (MCA) hemisphere
   B. Rupture of a saccular aneurysm
   C. Shearing of bridging veins between the dura and arachnoid mater
   D. Hypertensive vasculopathy

6. Josefina's level of consciousness (LOC) deteriorates, and she is intubated for airway protection. She is taken to CT, where her noncontrast head CT reveals a subarachnoid hemorrhage (SAH). Her blood pressure (BP) is 217/108. Neurosurgery is consulted with anticipation of an intraventricular device placement to monitor her intracerebral pressure (ICP). Which acute interventions would occur next?
   A. Start of a nicardipine infusion to manage her BP and hypertonic saline to lower her ICP
   B. Laying her head flat and preparing the patient for a stat lumbar puncture (LP)
   C. Allow permissive hypertension to ensure cerebral perfusion
   D. Initiation of therapeutic hypothermia

(See answers next page.)

5. B) Rupture of a saccular aneurysm

SAH is commonly caused by a brain aneurysm. A ruptured artery in the hemisphere would result in intracerebral hemorrhage (ICH). Shearing of bridging veins would result in a subdural hemorrhage. Hypertensive vasculopathy most commonly results in ICH.

6. A) Start of a nicardipine infusion to manage her BP and hypertonic saline to lower her ICP

Intravenous (IV) nicardipine is commonly used to reduce elevated BP in acute hemorrhagic stroke care management. Laying a patient flat would unnecessarily increase her BP and potentially worsen her neurological condition. Permissive hypertension and the initiation of therapeutic hypothermia are not part of the clinical guidelines for managing SAH.

BIBLIOGRAPHY

Arnold, M., Liesirova, K., Broeg-Morvay, A., Meisterernst, J., Schlager, M., Mono, M.-L., El-Koussy, M., Kägi, G., Jung, S., & Sarikaya, H. (2016). Dysphagia in acute stroke: Incidence, burden and impact on clinical outcome. *PLoS One*, *11*(2), e0148424. https://doi.org/10.1371/journal.pone.0148424

Béjot, Y., Delpont, B., & Giroud, M. (2016). Rising stroke incidence in young adults: More epidemiological evidence, more questions to be answered. *Journal of the American Heart Association*, *5*(5), e003661. https://doi.org/10.1161/JAHA.116.003661

Camicia, M., Wang, H., DiVita, M., Mix, J., & Niewczyk, P. (2016, March). Length of stay at inpatient rehabilitation facility and stroke patient outcomes. *Rehabilitation Nursing*, *41*(2), 78–90. https://doi.org/10.1002/rnj.218

Caplan, L. R. (2005). Cerebellar infarcts: Key features. *Revue Neurologique Disorders*, *2*(2), 51–60. PMID: 19813298. https://pubmed.ncbi.nlm.nih.gov/19813298/

Howard, V. J., & McDonnel, M. N. (2015). Physical activity in primary stroke prevention: Just do it! *Stroke*, *46*(6), 1735–1739. https://doi.org/10.1161/STROKEAHA.115.006317

Li, Y.-G., & Lip, G. Y. H. (2018). Anticoagulation resumption after intracerebral hemorrhage. *Current Atherosclerosis Reports*, *20*(7), Article 32. https://doi.org/10.1007/s11883-018-0733-y

Okamoto, K., Horisawa, R., Kawamura, T., Asai, A., Ogino, M., Takagi, T., & Ohno, Y. (2003). Family history and risk of subarachnoid hemorrhage: A case-control study in Nagoya, Japan. *Stroke*, *34*(2), 422–426. https://doi.org/10.1161/01.str.0000053851.17964.c6

Saver, J. L., Mattle, H. P., & Thaler, D. (2018). Patent foramen ovale closure versus medical therapy for cryptogenic ischemic stroke: A topical review. *Stroke*, *49*(6), 1541–1548. https://doi.org/10.1161/STROKEAHA.117.018153

Smithard, D. G., Smeeton, N. C., & Wolfe, C. D. A. (2007). Long-term outcome after stroke: Does dysphagia matter? *Age and Ageing*, *36*(1), 90–94. https://doi.org/10.1093/ageing/afl149

Practice Exam

1. In which situation is it appropriate to administer intravenous (IV) thrombolysis to an intracerebral hemorrhage (ICH) stroke patient in the ED?
   A. If symptom onset was greater than 24 hours ago
   B. If the CT angio indicates that the blood collection is less than 20 mL
   C. It is not appropriate to administer IV thrombolysis to an ICH patient in the ED
   D. After the provider has provided informed consent from the patient/family

2. Identify the FALSE statement regarding acute stroke–ready hospital (ASRH) certification requirements.
   A. They must have 24/7 imaging capability with images read within 24 hours
   B. They must have 24/7 laboratory capability
   C. They must have 24/7 intravenous (IV) thrombolytic capability
   D. They must have 24/7 provider availability, including neurological consultation

3. The definition of transient ischemic attack (TIA) has changed from time-based to tissue-based for what reason?
   A. Inconsistencies in obtaining accurate time of onset/resolution
   B. Increased number of slices seen on CT and MRI
   C. To avoid confusion with use of ministroke to describe TIA
   D. To avoid confusion with angina pectoris

4. Which population has been found to be less likely to call 911 with acute stroke symptoms?
   A. Pacific Islander
   B. Caucasian
   C. Black
   D. Hispanic

5. The upper limit of 160 mmHg is applicable to which of these stroke patients?
   A. 34-year-old subarachnoid hemorrhage (SAH) patient with no history of hypertension
   B. 60-year-old ischemic stroke patient with history of intracerebral hemorrhage (ICH)
   C. 75-year-old ICH patient with history of hypertension
   D. 86-year-old ischemic stroke patient with no history of hypertension

6. Frequent nursing rounds are recommended to prevent which of the following events?
   A. Patients falling from beds or chairs
   B. Patients falling asleep too often during the day and then not sleeping at night
   C. Patients eating too slowly, allowing food to get cold
   D. Patients drinking a lot and needing to go to the toilet more often

7. According to the National Institute of Neurological Disorders and Stroke (NINDS) ED-based stroke care time recommendations, what is the time frame for patients to be seen by an ED provider?
   A. Door-to-physician <2 minutes
   B. Door-to-physician <6 minutes
   C. Door-to-physician <10 minutes
   D. Door-to-physician <20 minutes

8. An ED patient weighing 250 lbs has been ordered to receive intravenous (IV) alteplase. The ED nurse will calculate and administer which dose?
   A. 102.4 mg
   B. 90 mg
   C. 113.6 mg
   D. 100 mg

9. Which of the following represents the vessels of the circle of Willis?
   A. Middle cerebral arteries, anterior cerebral arteries, posterior cerebral arteries, and posterior communicating arteries
   B. Internal carotid arteries, anterior cerebral arteries, anterior communicating artery, posterior cerebral arteries, and posterior communicating arteries
   C. Middle cerebral arteries, posterior cerebral arteries, posterior communicating arteries, and vertebral arteries
   D. Middle cerebral arteries, internal carotid arteries, anterior communicating arteries, posterior cerebral arteries, and vertebral arteries

10. Identify the reason for frequent groin checks and peripheral pulse checks on a postop coiling patient.
    A. Early identification of arterial dissection with retroperitoneal hemorrhage
    B. Early detection of arterial thrombosis with restricted perfusion pattern
    C. Early detection of failure/migration of closure device
    D. All of the above

11. Treatment of hyponatremia in a subarachnoid hemorrhage (SAH) patient would involve fluid restriction only in which situation?
    A. Cerebral salt wasting
    B. Hemoconstriction
    C. Syndrome of inappropriate antidiuretic hormone secretion (ADH)
    D. Hypertonicity

12. Socioeconomic factors associated with increased risk of stroke include which of the following?
    A. Lack of transportation, poverty, and low educational achievement
    B. Food insecurity and urban setting
    C. Poverty, food security, and rural setting
    D. Unreliable transportation, poverty, and high educational achievement

13. Transcranial and deep brain stimulation represent which of the following key purposes of poststroke therapy?
    A. Inhibition of task initiation
    B. Compensatory training
    C. Inhibition of neurospasticity
    D. Facilitation of neuroplasticity

14. Which group of risk factors has been attributed to 90% of strokes?
    A. Obesity, smoking, poor diet, physical inactivity, hypertension
    B. Obesity, diabetes, poor diet, hypertension, physical inactivity
    C. Hypertension, atrial fibrillation (Afib), diabetes, physical inactivity, poor diet
    D. Afib, carotid stenosis, hypertension, diabetes, physical inactivity

15. A patient with a ruptured cerebral aneurysm most likely had which type of stroke?
    A. Intraventricular hemorrhage
    B. Subarachnoid hemorrhage
    C. Intracerebral hemorrhage
    D. Intracranial hemorrhage

16. Compensatory strategies for patients with extinction do NOT include which of the following?
    A. Visual scanning
    B. Body rotation
    C. Immobilization
    D. Colored armband on affected limb

17. Indicate which cranial nerve(s) (CNs) innervate the eyes.
    A. CN III
    B. CN VI
    C. Both CN III and VI
    D. Neither of them

18. Which of the following would be considered a penetrating artery?
    A. Proximal middle cerebral artery (MCA)
    B. Proximal posterior cerebral artery (PCA)
    C. Proximal vertebral artery
    D. None of the above

19. Which of the following is NOT a certified stroke center designation?
    A. Thrombectomy-capable stroke center
    B. Comprehensive stroke center
    C. Thrombolytic-ready stroke center
    D. Primary stroke center

20. Which of the following is responsible for the first recommendations for primary stroke centers (PSCs)?
    A. Det Norske Veritas (DNV)
    B. Healthcare Facilities Accreditation Program (HFAP)
    C. The Joint Commission (TJC)
    D. Brain Attack Coalition (BAC)

21. Which of the following describes a speech difficulty that would be seen in a cerebellar stroke patient?
    A. Dystonia
    B. Aphasia
    C. Dysgraphia
    D. Dysarthria

22. Which of the following is true regarding stroke readmissions tracked by the Centers for Medicare & Medicaid Services (CMS)?
    A. Scheduled readmissions for carotid endarterectomy (CEA) or carotid stent (CAS) are not included since they are planned
    B. There is a penalty for organizations with all-cause readmissions above the national average
    C. Hospitals are extending lengths of stay to avoid readmission penalties
    D. All of the above

23. Which of the following poststroke patients would be most at risk of harm if they lived alone?
    A. Left-handed patient with discharge National Institutes of Health Stroke Scale (NIHSS) of 3 for facial droop (1) and right arm weakness (2)
    B. Right-handed patient with discharge NIHSS of 1 for upper limb ataxia
    C. Left-handed patient with discharge NIHSS of 5 for gaze palsy (1), facial droop (1), sensory loss (1), right arm weakness (1), and right leg weakness (1)
    D. Right-handed patient with discharge NIHSS of 2 for level of consciousness (LOC) question (1) and LOC command (1)

24. An acute stroke patient in the ED has a blood pressure (BP) of 240/102 and a history of chronic, uncontrolled hypertension. The stroke nurse suspects which of the following diagnoses?
    A. Ischemic stroke
    B. Intracerebral hemorrhage
    C. Subarachnoid hemorrhage
    D. Any of the above

25. When is it appropriate to hold the chest x-ray (CXR) until patient is out of the ED?
    A. When the ED is overflowing
    B. It is part of stroke care guidelines to wait until day 2
    C. If the patient is stable and without pulmonary symptoms
    D. It is never appropriate to delay the CXR

26. Treatment of hemorrhagic stroke patients with which of the following medication types is no longer a level A recommendation by the American Heart Association/American Stroke Association (AHA/ASA)?
    A. Antiseizure medications for seizure prevention
    B. Antibiotics for urinary tract infection (UTI)
    C. Antiemetics for vomiting
    D. Antipyretics for hyperthermia

27. In addition to sterile technique during suctioning, what nursing function has been shown to reduce the incidence of ventilator-associated pneumonia?
    A. Placing the ventilated patient in a negative air flow room
    B. Prompt administration of prophylactic antibiotics
    C. Ensuring the suction catheter reaches deep into each bronchus
    D. Diligent, regular oral care

28. Which is true of primary and secondary risk factor management?
    A. Secondary prevention blood pressure (BP) management has a systolic BP (SBP) goal that is 10 mmHg lower than primary prevention
    B. Low-density lipoprotein (LDL) goals are the same for primary and secondary prevention
    C. International normalized ratio (INR) goals are the same for primary and secondary prevention in patients with nonvalvular atrial fibrillation (Afib)
    D. Body mass index (BMI) goal is 25 kg/m^2 as primary prevention and 23 kg/m^2 as secondary prevention

29. Which of the following is true regarding anterior and posterior circulation?
    A. Anterior circulation originates from the basilar arteries
    B. Posterior circulation originates from the vertebral arteries
    C. The right anterior and posterior circulation originate from the brachiocephalic artery
    D. The posterior cerebral artery is part of the anterior circulation

30. A stroke survivor who does not recognize the left side of their body had damage to which part of their brain?
    A. Right frontal lobe
    B. Right parietal lobe
    C. Right cerebellar lobe
    D. Right temporal lobe

31. The stroke nurse would suspect retroperitoneal hemorrhage in which of these patients?
    A. Post–carotid endarterectomy patient with nausea and hypotension
    B. Postthrombectomy patient with diaphoresis and lower abdominal and back pain
    C. Post–aneurysm coiling patient with shortness of breath and hypoxia
    D. Post–carotid stenting patient with new-onset hemiparesis and aphasia

32. How can the stroke nurse know that dissection of the left carotid caused their patient's stroke rather than a cardiac source simply by looking at the plain head CT?
    A. Scattered pattern of strokes in bilateral hemispheres
    B. Pattern of multiple strokes in one side of the cerebellum
    C. Pattern of multiple strokes in the same hemisphere
    D. Scattered pattern of strokes throughout the cerebrum and cerebellum

33. What is the rationale for the Centers for Medicare & Medicaid Services (CMS) and the American Heart Association/American Stroke Association (AHA/ASA) recommendations that systems of care be accountable for poststroke outcomes?
    A. Systems of care can address the continuum of care with greater efficiency
    B. Continue the success shown by stroke center quality standards compliance
    C. Primary care provider (PCP) professional organizations have been unwilling to cooperate with quality measures
    D. Both A and B

34. Which of the following represents a significant risk for stroke among young adults?
    A. Dual utilization of vaping and marijuana
    B. Combination of oral tobacco with alcohol
    C. Mixing oral contraceptives and smoking
    D. Alcohol abuse while pregnant

35. Primordial prevention is represented by which of the following scenarios?
    A. Providing stroke education to high school students with type 2 diabetes
    B. Providing stroke education to college students who play football
    C. Providing stroke education to adults in the stroke recovery group
    D. Providing stroke education to seniors on warfarin for atrial fibrillation (Afib)

36. Horner's syndrome is characterized by which of the following?
    A. Headache, nuchal rigidity, and nausea
    B. Ptosis, anhidrosis, and meiosis
    C. Nystagmus, vertigo, and vomiting
    D. Photophobia, ptosis, and vertigo

37. Which antithrombotic will NOT be prescribed for an ischemic stroke patient who reports frequent headaches as a baseline?
    A. Rivaroxaban (Xarelto)
    B. Dipyridamole/aspirin (Aggrenox)
    C. Clopidogrel (Plavix)
    D. Dabigatran (Pradaxa)

38. A stroke alert patient arrives within 2 hours of symptom onset. Past medical history includes peripheral vascular disease for which he takes aspirin and clopidogrel, a concussion 10 years ago, and minor surgery on his right foot 14 days ago. Blood pressure (BP), labs, and head CT are normal. National Institutes of Health Stroke Scale (NIHSS) score is 3—aphasia (1), hemiparesis (2). Identify the contraindication for receiving intravenous (IV) thrombolytic.
    A. Current use of aspirin and clopidogrel
    B. Arrival within 2 hours
    C. Recent minor surgery
    D. None of the above

39. Which nursing action would be appropriate when caring for a patient with extinction?
    A. Approach them from the right side
    B. Place call bell on the patient's left side
    C. Speak loudly and slowly into their left ear
    D. Have patient sit on right side of bed for all meals

40. Which of the statements below is true regarding dysphagia screening of stroke patients?
    A. It continues to be one of the STK (stroke) measures
    B. It should be done on admission and whenever there has been a change in level of consciousness (LOC)
    C. It is not needed if the provider says it's not necessary
    D. It need only be done by nursing on admission to the hospital, after that by speech therapists

41. Which of the following is NOT an on-scene function by emergency medical services (EMS) according to the Mission: Lifeline® Stroke Severity-Based Stroke Triage Algorithm for EMS?
    A. Obtain Chem 7 lab panel
    B. Perform stroke screen
    C. Stabilize ABCs
    D. Interview witnesses

42. Which of the following tools used on admission has proven valid as a discharge disposition predictor?
    A. Barthel Index (BI)
    B. Glasgow Coma Scale (GCS)
    C. ABCD2
    D. National Institutes of Health Stroke Scale (NIHSS)

43. Which of the following is true regarding blood pressure (BP) management of an acute ischemic stroke patient?
    A. There is no guideline for lower limit of systolic BP (SBP) because hypotension is not a concern
    B. The guidelines recommend SBP no lower than 140 mmHg
    C. The guidelines recommend SBP no lower than 160 mmHg
    D. There is no guideline for lower limit of SBP, but patients with history of hypertension may not tolerate lower BP

44. At 10:16 a.m., emergency medical services (EMS) delivered a suspected acute stroke patient to the ED. In prenotification, they had reported left facial droop, along with left arm weakness, and last known well (LKW) time of 6:10 a.m. Admission National Institutes of Health Stroke Scale (NIHSS) score was 2, and then 0 at 15 minutes after arrival. Medical history includes hypertension treated with lisinopril. CT was negative, and blood sugar was 107. At the 30-minute check, the patient is noted to have a facial droop and left arm weakness with NIHSS of 5. Which of the following is the correct action?
    A. Continue to monitor the patient, as it might be a transient ischemic attack (TIA) and will likely return to 0
    B. Continue to monitor the patient, since it is too late for thrombolysis
    C. Administer intravenous (IV) thrombolytic as ordered according to their weight
    D. Call in the endovascular team in anticipation of mechanical thrombectomy

45. ED nurses assigned to work on improving door in, door out (DIDO) times for their hospital would be working at which level of stroke center?
    A. Primary stroke center (PSC)
    B. Acute stroke–ready hospital (ASRH)
    C. Both A and B
    D. Neither A nor B

46. Which of the following is NOT a cardioembolic source for stroke?
    A. Large patent foramen ovale (PFO)
    B. Endocarditis
    C. Atrial fibrillation (Afib)
    D. Sinus tachycardia

47. Describe the distinction between primary and primordial prevention.
    A. Primary prevention is a subtype of primordial prevention, just specific to stroke
    B. Primordial prevention cannot be measured, but primary prevention can
    C. Primordial prevention = prevention of conditions before they start; primary prevention = prevention of stroke in the setting of risk factors like diabetes or hypertension
    D. Primary prevention = prevention of conditions after they start; primordial prevention = successful reversal of the condition

48. Stroke nurses working on process improvement for safely mobilizing stroke patients might utilize any of the following EXCEPT which one?
    A. Six Sigma
    B. Plan, Do, Study, Act (PDSA)
    C. Root cause analysis
    D. Define, Measure, Analyze, Improve, Control (DMAIC)

49. Which group has similar stroke incidence to Caucasians, but whose rising risk factors are anticipated to increase the stroke incidence considerably?
    A. Hispanic women
    B. Hispanic men
    C. Black men
    D. Both A and B

50. A patient with a hemorrhagic stroke as the result of a ruptured aneurysm would most likely have which type of aneurysm?
    A. Mycotic
    B. Fusiform
    C. Saccular
    D. None of the above

51. At the 30-day stroke clinic visit, the provider notes their stroke patient's improving functional recovery, with the patient's National Institutes of Health Stroke Scale (NIHSS) score rising from 8 to 3—the remaining deficits being left arm weakness (2) and sensory loss (1). The provider informs the patient that they are clearing them for return to work. The patient responds that their job was as a court stenographer and they were let go already because they cannot type fast enough with their left hand, and, frankly, they don't believe they'll ever be able to. What is the appropriate response by the provider?
    A. Recommend the patient see an attorney
    B. Consult vocational rehabilitation services
    C. Consult psychiatric services
    D. Remind that patient that if they really want to regain their job, they have to work harder in therapy

52. During their 1-week primary care provider (PCP) visit, a stroke patient reports that they've started to take their partner's gemfibrozil in addition to their atorvastatin because they want to make sure their cholesterol really is controlled. Which is the best response by the provider?
    A. Let's get you your own prescription as you should never take another person's prescription
    B. Evidence does not support fibrates for cholesterol control, so please stop the gemfibrozil and give the atorvastatin a chance to work
    C. While evidence does support fibrates for cholesterol control, the combination with statins increases your risk of liver toxicity six-fold, so please call us with any muscle aches/cramps
    D. As long as you feel OK, that's a practical approach and saves you some money; let's check your liver profile to be sure you're OK

53. Which of the following is true of the circle of Willis?
    A. A complete circle of Willis serves as protection against stroke
    B. An incomplete circle of Willis is a rare phenomenon
    C. An incomplete circle of Willis is a common phenomenon
    D. The circle of Willis is not complete until age 5

54. Which of these patients will the stroke nurse anticipate having an adjustment in their warfarin dose?
    A. 80-year-old lacunar stroke patient with admission international normalized ratio (INR) 1.2
    B. 60-year-old embolic stroke patient with INR 1.8
    C. 70-year-old hemorrhagic stroke patient with INR 1.6
    D. 50-year-old atrial fibrillation (Afib) stroke patient with INR 2.8

55. A stroke patient who only eats the food on the right side of their plate and only recognizes things on their right side is showing signs of which of the following?
    A. Extinction
    B. Hemianopia
    C. Apraxia
    D. Cortical blindness

56. Which of the following conditions presents a risk of both stroke and Alzheimer's disease?
    A. Cavernous angioma
    B. Vasculitis
    C. Moyamoya
    D. Amyloid angiopathy

57. What is the mechanism that makes subarachnoid hemorrhage (SAH) patients more susceptible to cardiac arrhythmias?
    A. The proximity of the SAH to the medulla
    B. The release of catecholamines
    C. The extent of cerebral salt wasting
    D. The extent of cerebral edema

58. In a community presentation on stroke prevention, a young woman says that her mother and grandmother had strokes due to aneurysm rupture. What is the stroke nurse's best response to her?
    A. If you haven't had any headaches you're OK, but please call your primary care provider (PCP) if you ever have a bad headache
    B. If your mother and grandmother use hormone replacement, you should avoid that
    C. If you haven't had imaging done, please talk to your PCP about that and blood pressure (BP) control
    D. If you don't get your aneurysm fixed now, it may be too late as you are at increased risk

59. An ischemic stroke patient's imaging on day 2 reveals hemorrhagic transformation. Which of the following would indicate that the nurse should expect to see symptoms of increasing intracerebral pressure (ICP)?
    A. Postdural hemorrhage
    B. Parenchymal hemorrhage
    C. Petechial hemorrhage
    D. Precentriole hemorrhage

60. A stroke patient who had been discharged home to live with their son after a 14-day inpatient rehabilitation stay has been admitted to a nursing home after just 3 weeks at home. Which of the following could be the reason?
    A. The son had a car accident and broke his hip
    B. The son realized that he doesn't want to be a long-term caregiver
    C. The patient doesn't like that their son is rarely home, thus not providing their meals and meds consistently
    D. All of the above

61. For which of these patients would abdominal wound care be included in their daily plan of care?
    A. Intraparenchymal hemorrhage (IPH) patient with an external ventricular drain (EVD)
    B. Ischemic stroke patient with a hemicraniectomy
    C. Subarachnoid hemorrhage (SAH) patient with endovascular coiling
    D. Transient ischemic attack (TIA) patient with carotid endarterectomy

62. Which of these subarachnoid hemorrhage (SAH) scores is based on symptoms present rather than amount of blood on imaging?
    A. World Federation of Neurosurgical Societies (WFNS) score
    B. Hunt and Hess score
    C. Fisher scale
    D. None of the above

63. Damage to the precentral gyrus would produce which symptoms?
    A. Limb weakness
    B. Limb numbness
    C. Dysarthria
    D. Extinction

64. Which of these phrases would be used regarding a procedure that received class IIA recommendation?
    A. It is reasonable
    B. It is recommended
    C. It is not recommended
    D. It is potentially harmful

65. Although not approved by the U.S. Food and Drug Administration (FDA) for use in acute ischemic stroke, which thrombolytic is being used around the United States and is administered as an intravenous (IV) bolus over 5 seconds?
    A. Tenecteplase
    B. Abciximab
    C. Aripiprazole
    D. Alteplase

66. Significant reduction in door-to-needle time for thrombolytic has been the result of which of the following?
    A. Use of CT angiogram (CTA)
    B. Reduced cost of thrombolytic agents
    C. Use of telemedicine
    D. Education of emergency medical services (EMS)

67. Which of the following is true regarding stroke units in certified stroke centers?
    A. They must be distinct areas of the hospital where all stroke patients are cared for
    B. They have been shown to reduce in-hospital mortality
    C. They must be overseen by a certified vascular neurologist
    D. They have been shown to reduce discharges to home

68. Vascular dissection would be best described by which of the following?
    A. Fusion of two cerebral vessels as a result of chronic vasculitis through which blood passes back and forth between them
    B. A weakened area in the wall of the vessel resulting in a ballooning out
    C. A tear in the inner lining of the vessel allowing blood to collect between the layers and blood clots to form along the edges of the tear
    D. A buildup of plaque causing occlusion of the vessel

69. What is the rationale for emergency medical service (EMS) providers to receive education about transient ischemic attack (TIA)?
    A. The symptoms may be attributed to another less significant cause and might not be transported with as much urgency
    B. Patients may refuse to be transported to a hospital if symptoms abate, so EMS need to educate the patient about the importance of a workup with TIA
    C. Although the symptoms disappear in a short period of time, they represent a risk for subsequent stroke
    D. All of the above

70. A febrile ischemic stroke patient on oral anticoagulation should be given which these antipyretic treatments?
    A. Acetaminophen
    B. Aspirin
    C. Ibuprofen
    D. Ice bath

71. Studies have shown that even just a 1% increase in the number of health professionals in this role can reduce inpatient rehab length of stay (LOS) by 6%. Which role is it?
    A. Physiatrists
    B. Nurses
    C. Therapists
    D. Social workers

72. What is the reason for providers in the ED to ask patients if they could live with their deficit?
    A. To determine if hospice consult is warranted in patients with severe deficits
    B. To determine their baseline risk for depression in patients with mild/improving symptoms
    C. To determine if admission is warranted in patients with mild/improving symptoms
    D. To determine if thrombolytic treatment is warranted in patients with mild/improving symptoms

73. A middle cerebral artery (MCA) patient with a "poor bony window" may have trouble getting reliable results from which of these diagnostic tests?
    A. Transthoracic echocardiogram (TTE)
    B. Transesophageal echocardiogram (TEE)
    C. Electrocardiogram (ECG)
    D. Transcranial Doppler (TCD)

74. A patient who presents with symptoms of nausea, vomiting, vertigo, nystagmus, tachycardia, dysarthria, dysphagia, imbalance, and crossed signs would be displaying which of the following?
    A. Horner's syndrome
    B. Cryptogenic syndrome
    C. Wallenberg's syndrome
    D. Gyral syndrome

75. Identify the mechanism for atrial fibrillation (Afib) to cause a stroke.
    A. Clots form in the atria as a result of blood stagnating
    B. Rapid, irregular rate results in muscle fatigue
    C. Clots form in the ventricles and are pumped out to the brain
    D. Rapid rate results in valve insufficiency and endocarditis

76. In calculating a transient ischemic attack (TIA) patient's short-term risk of stroke, which tool would be used?
    A. ABCD2 score
    B. Modified Rankin Scale (mRS) score
    C. CHA_2DS_2-VASc score
    D. Barthel Index (BI) score

77. Pneumonia secondary to aspiration is a complication of stroke that can be prevented if what is done by emergency medical services (EMS)/ED staff?
    A. Hypoxia screen followed by supplementary oxygen
    B. Comprehensive assessment of lung sounds prior to oral intake
    C. Deep breathing and coughing every hour
    D. Nil per os (NPO) until dysphagia screen

78. The provider orders a transesophageal echocardiogram (TEE) instead of a transtho-
    racic echocardiogram (TTE) on a stroke patient with a new heart murmur. Which of
    the following statements is appropriate to tell the patient?
    A. TTE involves swallowing a big tube, which isn't necessary for you
    B. TEE provides better visualization of the heart structures than TTE
    C. TEE is simpler and takes less time than a TTE
    D. While TTE provides better visualization of the heart structure, the provider must
       not be too concerned about that murmur

79. Which of the following conditions is being extensively studied to determine its cause-
    and-effect relationship with stroke?
    A. Menopause
    B. Sleep apnea
    C. Hypothyroidism
    D. Heat exhaustion

80. Contracture of the arm is a long-term functional limitation and is often painful. During
    the acute and early postdischarge period, what condition do therapists and patients
    work hard to overcome to reduce the incidence of contracture?
    A. Spasticity
    B. Muscle atrophy
    C. Hypoflexion
    D. Ataxia

81. When describing the results of a thrombectomy procedure that was documented as
    Thrombolysis In Cerebral Infarction (TICI) 3, which term is accurate?
    A. Reocclusion of the vessel
    B. Restoration of the thrombus
    C. Recanalization of the vessel
    D. Removal of the bifurcation

82. Which of the following is a benefit of emergency medical services (EMS) bypassing a
    primary stroke center (PSC) with a suspected stroke patient?
    A. Less time to thrombectomy treatment
    B. Greater demand for EMS services
    C. Faster dispatch time
    D. None of the above

83. Stroke incidence has increased among people aged 25 to 44 years and decreased
    among people over age 55. Which of the following accounts for this shift?
    A. Increase in risk factors in childhood/Increased control of blood pressure (BP) and
       cholesterol in older adults
    B. Decrease in physical activity in childhood/Decrease in alcohol abuse in older
       adults
    C. Increase in vaping in childhood/Increase in physical activity in older adults
    D. Decrease in smoking in childhood/Increase in smoking in older adults

84. Which of the following are the optimal time and tool for stroke depression screening?
    A. During the acute hospital stay, using the Patient Health Questionnaire-9 (PHQ-9)
    B. Within first 7 days postdischarge, using any of the tools
    C. There has been no established optimal time/tool for stroke depression screening
    D. During the 30-day follow-up visit, using the combine results of Centers for Epidemiologic Studies-Depression (CES-D) and Hamilton Rating Scale for Depression (HDRS)

85. Knowing the cause of stroke is essential for the stroke team in developing the most appropriate secondary prevention strategy. What other term might the stroke nurse encounter when referring to the cause of stroke?
    A. Stroke sequelae
    B. Stroke etiology
    C. Stroke activator
    D. Stroke instigator

86. Which of the following patients would NOT be considered for endovascular clot removal?
    A. Large-vessel occlusion (LVO) patient arriving within 3 hours who received intravenous (IV) alteplase
    B. LVO patient arriving within 24 hours with penumbra evident on imaging
    C. LVO patient arriving within 12 hours with no penumbra evident on imaging
    D. LVO patient arriving within 6 hours who is taking Eliquis

87. How many of the original 10 stroke performance measures are now STK (stroke) measures?
    A. 10
    B. 9
    C. 8
    D. None of them

88. Identify one of the critical actions by emergency medical services (EMS) in acute stroke care.
    A. Establishing last known well (LKW) time
    B. Establishing last meal content
    C. Establishing time of last primary care provider (PCP) visit
    D. Establishing minimum of three phone numbers for contact

89. Which of the following would the stroke nurse expect to see in the physical therapist's notes on safety education regarding falls for a stroke patient with hemiparesis who is going home?
    A. Patient was instructed to group all physical activities into the morning and then remain sitting through the afternoon
    B. Patient was instructed to plan the living space to keep furniture close together so they have something to hold onto
    C. Patient was instructed in techniques for getting up after falling
    D. Patient was instructed to be careful not to fall

90. What is the main reason that most subarachnoid hemorrhage (SAH) patients have length of stay (LOS) of 10 to 14 days?
    A. Vasospasm occurs between 4 and 10 days
    B. Patients aren't conscious enough for therapy until about day 10
    C. Ventilator support is required for 8 to 10 days
    D. Hydrocephalus occurs between day 8 and day 10

91. During the 30-day telemedicine visit via two-way audio-video connection, a stroke patient's 80-year-old partner expresses concern over the patient's 10-lb weight loss since discharge. The partner states that they cook all the patient's favorite things, but they barely take a bite and fall asleep in their chair. The partner notes they have trouble getting the patient safely to bed. What is the appropriate response by the provider?
    A. Order Ensure supplement and a consult for a percutaneous endoscopic gastrostomy (PEG) tube
    B. Validate the partner's frustration and reassure them that they are doing everything they can
    C. Offer to call 911 for transport to a nearby hospital for evaluation
    D. Offer to make recommendations for area nursing homes to give the partner respite from the caregiver burden

92. An ED thrombolytic patient received intravenous (IV) labetalol 10 mg for blood pressure (BP) of 190/84 at 2:30 p.m. At the next check, the patient is drowsy and slow to respond with BP 135/76. What is the best action?
    A. Do a neurological assessment and document that along with the BP
    B. Document the new BP, noting that the labetalol was effective
    C. Do a neurological assessment and notify provider of suspected hypoperfusion
    D. Ask them if they are feeling okay and offer a cool compress to help them wake up

93. A 70-year-old acute stroke–ready hospital (ASRH) ED ischemic stroke patient's temperature is recorded as 39 °C (102.2 °F). What is the next step for the ED nurse?
    A. Record the temperature and administer pro re nata (PRN) acetaminophen as ordered
    B. Record the temperature and prepare to induce therapeutic hypothermia
    C. Record the temperature and ask the patient if they've had any recent cold/flu symptoms
    D. Record the temperature and prepare for transfer to a thrombectomy-capable stroke center (TSC)

94. What would be the most likely discharge destination for a patient with a Hunt and Hess score of 5?
    A. Acute inpatient rehabilitation
    B. Day rehabilitation program
    C. Home with outpatient therapy
    D. Hospice

95. Identify the role of gamma knife in primary and secondary stroke prevention.
    A. It is used in primary prevention to obliterate intracranial carotid stenosis
    B. It is helpful in potentiating the effect of intravenous (IV) thrombolytic in clot dissolution
    C. It is only used in secondary prevention due to the increased risk
    D. It is used in arteriovenous malformation (AVM) patients who are not candidates for surgery or endovascular therapy

96. Why does the stroke nurse have a patient close their eyes during parts of the National Institutes of Health Stroke Scale (NIHSS) assessment?
    A. Closing the eyes facilitates neurological rest
    B. Closing the eyes eliminates visual cues
    C. Closing the eyes reduces anxiety of being tested
    D. The NIHSS assessment is done with patients eyes open at all times

97. What is the most appropriate schedule of neuro assessment and vital sign monitoring on day 3 after intravenous (IV) thrombolytic and thrombectomy?
    A. Every 8 hours while awake because they are stable
    B. Every 4 hours because stroke patients' symptoms may fluctuate during the first few days
    C. Every 1 hour because they received IV thrombolytic in the ED
    D. Every 2 hours because their hemoglobin A1C was 7

98. The Cincinnati Prehospital Stroke Scale includes all but which of the following?
    A. Arm drift
    B. Facial symmetry
    C. Speech ability
    D. Swallow ability

99. At the 30-day follow-up appointment, a subarachnoid hemorrhage (SAH) patient reports that they have stopped therapy because the therapist wanted them to use utensils with built-up handles and they didn't like the feel of it. Now the patient is ready to try it again. What type of therapy would the provider consult?
    A. Adapted living therapy
    B. Physical therapy
    C. Cognitive therapy
    D. Occupational therapy

100. A patient who awakens from knee surgery with numbness and weakness of their left arm and an imaged ischemic stroke has most likely experienced which of the following?
    A. Cryptogenic stroke
    B. Silent stroke
    C. Watershed stroke
    D. Transient ischemic attack (TIA)

101. It may surprise some stroke nurses that which type of therapy has been widely, and successfully, used in poststroke rehabilitation?
    A. Wii-habilitation therapy
    B. Deep immersion therapy
    C. Pac-habilitation therapy
    D. Aversion therapy

102. Which of the 10 original performance measures are NOT part of the current STK (stroke) measures?
    A. Dysphagia screening, antithrombotic by day 2
    B. Smoking cessation, rehab assessment
    C. Smoking cessation, dysphagia screening
    D. Dysphagia screening, stroke education

103. Why do some providers refer to lacunar strokes as *pure motor* or *pure sensory* strokes?
   A. With the territory of infarct being so large, it only impacts either motor or sensory fibers
   B. With the territory of infarct being scattered, it rarely impacts more than one type of fiber
   C. With the territory of infarct being so small, it is possible to only impact motor or sensory fibers
   D. None of the above; lacunar strokes are synonymous with transient ischemic attack (TIA)

104. The care team is developing the discharge plan with a patient. How does their preadmission modified Rankin Scale (mRS) of 3 impact the plan?
   A. It does not impact the discharge plan; it only impacted the inpatient plan of care
   B. It indicates that the discharge plan should be for a skilled nursing facility (SNF) if younger than 65, inpatient rehabilitation facility (IRF) if over 65
   C. It indicates that the patient had a prior hospitalization for stroke
   D. It indicates that goals for functional recovery will likely not be for full independence

105. Successful endovascular intervention is represented by which of the following Thrombolysis In Cerebral Infarction (TICI) scores?
   A. 3, 2b
   B. 0, 1
   C. 2a, 2b
   D. 1, 2a

106. Which of the following would be considered infratentorial as opposed to supratentorial?
   A. Anterior lobe cerebellum
   B. Posterior Broca's area
   C. Internal basal ganglia
   D. Anterior hypothalamus

107. The stroke nurse is preparing his patient for an upcoming CT angiogram (CTA). Which of the following statements is correctly included in his patient education?
   A. This test will involve a strong magnet, so as long as you don't have a pacemaker, you're OK
   B. This test is the same as an MRI, it's just easier to schedule
   C. This test is being done to get a look at your blood vessels
   D. This test will help us to determine if you need intravenous (IV) thrombolytic

108. When a stroke patient is said to have *extended* their stroke, what has occurred?
   A. Their length of stay (LOS) has exceeded 5 days
   B. Part/all of their penumbra has infarcted
   C. Their deficits have not resolved within 7 days
   D. Part/all of their tentorium has infarcted

109. A patient with which of the following would NOT be told they had interruption of cerebral blood flow?
A. Cerebral embolus
B. Cerebral thrombosis
C. Cerebral vasospasm
D. Cerebral vasodilation

110. What makes bedridden stroke patients especially susceptible to skin breakdown?
A. Cerebral perfusion deficits result in peripheral perfusion deficits
B. Motor and sensory deficits inhibit their ability to adjust their position or feel the pain of pressure points
C. Bedrest and motor deficits inhibit their ability to cough and deep breathe
D. Multiple intravenous (IV) sites and dysarthria inhibit their ability to move around and alter their position

111. The difference between the Cincinnati Prehospital Stroke Scale and the Cincinnati Prehospital Stroke Severity Scale is which of the following?
A. The Cincinnati Prehospital Stroke Scale establishes the probability of stroke, and the Cincinnati Prehospital Stroke Severity Scale confirms that is stroke
B. The Cincinnati Prehospital Stroke Scale is performed in the eastern United States, while the Cincinnati Prehospital Stroke Severity Scale is performed across the western United States
C. The Cincinnati Prehospital Stroke Scale establishes the probability of stroke, and the Cincinnati Prehospital Stroke Severity Scale establishes the probability of large-vessel occlusion (LVO)
D. None of the above; they are the same scale

112. The stroke nurse notices that their ischemic stroke patient is harder to arouse today (day 2), and now, in addition to the facial droop and left arm weakness the patient was admitted with yesterday, their left leg is weak. What is the most likely explanation?
A. Their penumbra has enlarged to include the leg area of the motor strip
B. Their blood pressure (BP) was allowed to fluctuate during the previous shift
C. Their blood sugar is over 200
D. They have been wakened often during the night and are sleep deprived

113. Which is true regarding the use of supplemental oxygen for ED stroke patients?
A. Provide to intracerebral hemorrhage (ICH) patients with O_2 saturation less than 95% in the presence of high intracerebral pressure (ICP)
B. Only administer to ischemic stroke patients in the presence of shortness of breath
C. Limit use to hemorrhagic stroke patients with O_2 saturation less than 88%
D. Provide to all stroke patients with O_2 saturation less than 92%

114. Endovascular flow diversion would be best described to a subarachnoid hemorrhage (SAH) patient by which of the following?
A. It is a cylindrical, flexible, and self-expanding object that is positioned across the aneurysm neck to keep blood from going in and out of the aneurysm
B. It is the same as the stents used in cardiac patients and helps to keep the vessel open, so it is left in place
C. It is a flexible plug, similar to putty at body temperature, that is positioned in the neck of the aneurysm to prevent blood from going in and out of the aneurysm
D. It is a technique in which the operator uses a suction catheter to pull in the bulging aneurysmal sac in order to obliterate it and remove it endovascularly

115. Which of the following stroke patients would be treated with anticoagulant for secondary prevention?
  A. 66-year-old female with CHA_2DS_2-VASc score of 2 and modified Rankin Scale (mRS) score of 4
  B. 80-year-old male with ABCD2 score of 5 and CHA_2DS_2-VASc score of 0
  C. 56-year-old female with Hunt and Hess score of 2 and mRS score of 3
  D. 48-year-old male with National Institutes of Health Stroke Scale (NIHSS) score of 7 and ABCD2 score of 3

116. Which of the following patients would the stroke nurse be able to reassure that the treatment they received has been shown to improve functional outcomes by 30%?
  A. Ischemic stroke patient with mechanical clot removal
  B. Hemorrhagic stroke patient with minimally invasive intracerebral hemorrhage (ICH) removal
  C. Ischemic stroke patient with intravenous (IV) thrombolysis
  D. Hemorrhagic stroke patient with aneurysm coiling as opposed to clipping

117. What is the relationship between a patent foramen ovale (PFO) and deep vein thrombosis (DVT) as a mechanism for embolic stroke?
  A. DVT becomes lodged in the PFO and sends clots to the brain
  B. DVT passes through the PFO and flows out to the brain
  C. Multiple DVT are required to pass through the PFO and flow out to the brain
  D. There is no relationship, they separately represent risk of embolic stroke

118. Which of the following represents a distinction between primary stroke center (PSC) and thrombectomy-capable stroke center (TSC) hospital capabilities?
  A. 24/7 capability for emergent evaluation and administration of intravenous (IV) thrombolytic
  B. Compliance with all STK (stroke) measures
  C. 24/7 capability to admit most stroke patients
  D. 24/7 capability to perform mechanical clot retrieval

119. Wernicke's aphasia would be diagnosed by which of the following presentations?
  A. Inability to understand instructions or questions
  B. Inability to sing a song or write a note
  C. Inability to say the words they want to say
  D. Inability to say anything

120. Which is true of primary prevention strategies?
  A. Opportunities are limited to the community and primary care settings
  B. It is impossible to measure the effectiveness
  C. They are not covered by most insurance
  D. The ED is an excellent opportunity for primary prevention

121. Why does the stroke nurse have orders to treat a temperature above normal?
  A. Hyperthermia is associated with uncontrolled hypertension and worse outcomes
  B. Hyperthermia decreases metabolic demand and makes the brain sluggish
  C. Hyperthermia suppresses mitochondrial activity and reduces platelet formation
  D. Hyperthermia is associated with increased metabolic needs and worse outcomes

122. Which of the following is a stroke mimic?
   A. Seizure
   B. Bell's palsy
   C. Complex migraine
   D. All of the above

123. Which of the following is true of middle cerebral artery (MCA) syndrome?
   A. Motor and sensory loss of the face and arm
   B. Motor and sensory loss of the leg
   C. Sensory loss of the legs along with imbalance
   D. Motor loss of speech along with imbalance

124. In hand-off report, the stroke nurse learns that their hemorrhagic stroke patient received thrombolytic earlier that day, which was not questioned. Should the nurse have questioned it?
   A. No, because they knew that small, ruptured aneurysms were treated with thrombolytic
   B. Yes, because hemorrhagic stroke patients should never receive thrombolytic
   C. Yes, because the reporting nurse may have made a dangerous medication error
   D. No, because they knew that this patient had developed intraventricular hemorrhage

125. Faster mobilization of ED resources is facilitated by what emergency medical services (EMS) action?
   A. Quicker ambulance dispatch
   B. Obtaining blood glucose enroute
   C. Enroute prenotification
   D. Obtaining EKG on scene

126. Which of the following represents telemedicine services in the postacute stroke realm?
   A. On-site clinic visit with vascular neurologist
   B. Telephone follow-up by clinical pharmacist
   C. Home visit by home health aide
   D. None of the above

127. What is the rationale for maintaining the neck in midline position for acute stroke patients?
   A. It facilitates improved swallowing function to prevent dysphagia
   B. It facilitates venous drainage and reduces intracerebral pressure (ICP)
   C. It supports proper alignment and prevents stress headaches
   D. It encourages proper posture for more rapid progress after discharge

128. A cerebellar stroke patient has begun to vomit and is unable to hold themselves upright in bed. Indicate the best action for the nurse to take next.
   A. Help them into the left lateral recumbent position
   B. Prepare for stat chest x-ray (CXR)
   C. Insert an oral airway and lower their head
   D. Insert nasogastric (NG) tube and call a ventilator

129. Indicate the value of obtaining a preadmission modified Rankin Scale (mRS) score on a stroke patient.
    A. It provides a baseline functional score and helps to establish goals for recovery
    B. There is no value in a preadmission functional score; it is only the discharge score that matters
    C. Along with the ABCD2 score, it helps to determine who will qualify for inpatient rehab
    D. Patients with mRS of ≥3 indicates discharge will be to a skilled nursing facility (SNF)

130. An ED ischemic stroke patient's blood sugar is recorded as 198. What is the ED nurse's next step?
    A. Recheck it in an hour and record, and if still over 160, administer insulin 12 units
    B. Recheck it and record it, and, if still over 180, notify provider
    C. Recheck it and if still over 140, initiate an insulin drip per protocol
    D. Recheck it and record it, and if still under 200, no need to act

131. Which is NOT true of last known well (LKW) time and time of discovery with acute stroke patients?
    A. The LKW time indicates the last time they were known to be normal
    B. The LKW time is always the time of discovery
    C. The time of discovery is the same as LKW time with a witnessed onset
    D. The time of discovery indicates the time someone found them with symptoms

132. What is the rationale for sequential compression devices (SCDs) rather than thrombo-embolic deterrent (TED) stockings to be used on acute stroke patients?
    A. SCDs are easier to apply and easier to ambulate with
    B. TED stockings cost more and need to be washed daily
    C. TED stockings are associated with more harm than good in stroke patients
    D. SCDs are easier to store and deliver to nursing units

133. What ataxia score would a stroke patient receive on the National Institutes of Health Stroke Scale (NIHSS) with the following presentation: their right leg drifted slightly but did not touch the bed, and they were unable to perform the heel/shin maneuver? The patient was able to do it successfully on the unaffected side.
    A. 2—Present in both upper and lower limbs
    B. 0—Absent
    C. 1—Present in upper or lower limb
    D. They would only be tested for ataxia on the left side due to weakness in their limbs

134. Which of the following patients would a nurse answering a call bell know had a decompressive hemicraniectomy?
    A. 40-year-old with limited visitors and a helmet on
    B. 66-year-old with shades drawn and lights low
    C. 50-year-old with a nicardipine drip and external ventricular drain (EVD)
    D. 80-year-old with ventilator and ventriculoperitoneal (VP) shunt

135. What role does the Glasgow Coma Scale (GCS) play in assessment of a stroke patient?
    A. It is the most reliable assessment tool for stroke patients
    B. If the GCS is abnormal, the National Institutes of Health Stroke Scale (NIHSS) is performed
    C. It is commonly used, but not recommended
    D. It is interchangeable with the NIHSS

136. To which patient would the stroke nurse be more likely to provide education to and prepare for insertion of a left atrial appendage occlusive device?
    A. 45-year-old intracerebral hemorrhage (ICH) patient with arteriovenous malformation (AVM)
    B. 70-year-old ICH patient with atrial fibrillation (Afib)
    C. 68-year-old ischemic stroke patient with Afib
    D. 51-year-old subarachnoid hemorrhage (SAH) patient with aneurysm

137. The stroke nurse notes that today's transcranial Doppler (TCD) reading of cerebral blood flow dropped below normal range. What is normal range?
    A. 10 to 30 mL/100 g/min
    B. 30 to 40 mL/100 g/min
    C. 45 to 60 mL/100 g/min
    D. 65 to 75 mL/100 g/min

138. Describe the relationship between migraine with aura and ischemic stroke.
    A. Migraine is both a stroke risk and result of stroke
    B. Migraine is both a stroke mimic and a stroke risk
    C. Migraine is a stroke mimic only
    D. Migraine is a result of stroke

139. Which one of these stroke patients requires oral anticoagulation according to the American Heart Association/American Stroke Association's (AHA/ASA's) secondary prevention guidelines?
    A. Patient with a small patent foramen ovale (PFO)
    B. Patient with a small subarachnoid hemorrhage (SAH)
    C. Patient with no known cause
    D. Patient with atrial fibrillation (Afib)

140. A patient with a proximal middle cerebral artery (MCA) occlusion can be expected to have which of the following procedures?
    A. Decompressive craniectomy
    B. Endovascular embolization
    C. Hematoma evacuation
    D. Ventriculoperitoneal shunt

141. Indicate which is true of the relationship between cancer and stroke.
    A. Stroke survivors have a 10-year increased risk of brain tumors at the infarct site
    B. Cancer and some chemotherapeutic agents are prothrombotic
    C. Cancer is responsible for 30% of strokes
    D. Stroke survivors are recommended to have annual head CTs to screen for brain tumors

142. Which part of shift handoff is most essential to ensure consistency?
    A. A review of the medical record
    B. A joint neurological assessment
    C. A detailed documentation of the previous neurological condition
    D. A detailed report of the day's events

143. Which member of the healthcare team would be more likely to document a Barthel Index (BI) score on a stroke patient?
    A. Social worker
    B. Med review pharmacist
    C. Patient advocate
    D. Physical therapist

144. Effective strategies for communication with a patient with receptive aphasia would NOT include which of the following?
    A. Raising your voice until they indicate understanding
    B. Pausing between sentences to allow time to process
    C. Supplementing speech with gestures
    D. Use of simple drawings

145. In the intervention suite, a potential large-vessel occlusion (LVO) patient has become restless, with oxygen level dropping from 94% to 84% and blood pressure (BP) rising to 180/90. Which is more likely to be happening?
    A. Patient is frightened and needs to be reassured that they will be OK
    B. Patient has chronic obstructive pulmonary disease (COPD) and this is normal, but they may need to be restrained
    C. Patient is decompensating and needs to be intubated and sedated
    D. Pulse ox equipment needs to be replaced

146. Which patient would be scheduled for a lower extremity ultrasound for development of a definitive primary prevention treatment plan?
    A. 50-year-old medical assistant with patent foramen ovale (PFO)
    B. 60-year-old paramedic with 77% carotid stenosis
    C. 62-year-old nurse with bilateral posterior cerebral artery (PCA) aneurysms
    D. 56-year-old provider with uncontrolled atrial fibrillation (Afib)

147. The majority of intraparenchymal hemorrhages occur in which area of the brain?
    A. Basal ganglia
    B. Frontal lobe
    C. Brain stem
    D. Occipital lobe

148. The midbrain, pons, and medulla are collectively known as which of the following?
    A. Homunculus
    B. Brainstem
    C. Basal ganglia
    D. Foramen magnum

149. Which thrombectomy device has the highest recommendation from the American Heart Association/American Stroke Association (AHA/ASA)?
  A. Penumbra clot disrupters
  B. Stent recoilers
  C. Endovascular thrombolyis
  D. Stent retrievers

150. Studies have shown that the higher death rate from stroke in the Stroke Belt is attributable to which of the following?
  A. Heredity and lifestyle
  B. Limited access to care
  C. Alcoholism and sleep apnea
  D. Both A and B

151. What is the primary advantage of an organization adding a mobile stroke unit to their fleet?
  A. A mobile stroke unit is cheaper than a fully equipped ambulance
  B. A mobile stroke unit eliminates demand for a stop in the ED
  C. A mobile stroke unit enables faster door-to-needle and door-to-puncture times
  D. A mobile stroke unit eliminates need for pharmacy support in the ED

152. What makes posterior stroke more challenging to diagnose by symptoms than middle cerebral artery (MCA) territory stroke?
  A. Symptoms are identical whether cerebellar or occipital
  B. Posterior strokes impact short-term memory and patients cannot report symptoms consistently
  C. Posterior strokes produce the inability for patients to recognize symptoms
  D. Symptoms are not classic hemispheric symptoms, and sometimes there can be crossed signs

153. During discharge education for an ischemic stroke patient, the patient's partner comments that they just read that the risk of recurrent stroke is only 8% the first year, then drops to 2% after that, so the stroke nurse need not go into detail. What is the stroke nurse's best response?
  A. While that rate doesn't seem to be high, being one of the 8% could be devastating to your partner
  B. Many of these secondary prevention measures carry benefit beyond just stroke prevention, such as preservation of cognition and prevention of vascular disease in the heart
  C. The patient's best chance of preventing recurrence is in understanding the plan of care, so let's just take a few minutes to prepare as best we can
  D. All of the above

154. In triaging, which ED ischemic stroke patient with a blood sugar recorded as 210 mg/dL would be most critical to treat to bring it under control?
  A. Diabetic patient with recent hemoglobin (Hgb) A1C of 7%
  B. Nondiabetic patient who received intravenous (IV) thrombolytic
  C. Nondiabetic patient with blood pressure (BP) 180/86
  D. Diabetic patient with slurred speech

155. Who has the most responsibility for poststroke care and quality improvement efforts to resolve gaps in care?
   A. The discharging hospital stroke team
   B. The primary care provider (PCP)
   C. The patient and caregiver
   D. All of the above

156. Which of the following is described as having slow blood flow?
   A. Clipped aneurysm
   B. Thrombolysis In Cerebral Infarction (TICI) 3 middle cerebral artery (MCA)
   C. Cavernous angioma
   D. None of the above

157. Which of the following therapies provides the advantages of allowing patients to experience situations without the limits of their disabilities as well as immediate feedback?
   A. Transcranial magnetic stimulation (TMS)
   B. Virtual reality (VR) therapy
   C. Constraint-induced movement therapy (CIMT)
   D. Robotic therapy

158. Nursing care consistent with which of the following has been shown to reduce 90-day death and dependency by 16%?
   A. FeSS
   B. ASCVD
   C. PDSA
   D. PTSD

159. What is the main reason nurses get a patient back to bed from the chair quickly when their stroke symptoms worsen?
   A. To prevent them from falling out of the chair and getting injured
   B. To facilitate rapid administration of intravenous (IV) thrombolytic
   C. To facilitate quicker transfer to litter for stat head CT
   D. To get them into a supine position to facilitate cerebral perfusion

160. On day 10 of acute inpatient rehabilitation, a right hemisphere ischemic stroke patient has been making good progress, and discharge home is planned for the within the next few days. They just showed up for their morning therapy session with blood dripping from their left hand. When asked, they have no idea what happened and report no pain. Another patient overhears and says they saw the patient bump hard into a doorway but didn't seem fazed by it. Describe the next steps for the care team.
   A. Assess and bandage the wound, then remind the patient to be more careful
   B. Assess and bandage the wound, then alter plan of care to emphasize strategies for addressing extinction
   C. Assess and bandage the wound, then send the patient back to their room as they are unsafe for therapy
   D. Assess and bandage the wound, then page the provider to cancel discharge plans

161. The quality director for the ED has set a goal for how long stroke patients should remain in the ED before admission to the hospital. What is it?
    A. Less than 3 hours
    B. Between 6 and 12 hours
    C. Less than 5 hours
    D. Between 12 and 18 hours

162. What impact can a stroke nurse anticipate from a minimally invasive device used to evacuate their patient's intracerebral hemorrhage (ICH)?
    A. Use of a helmet for 6 weeks to protect their brain
    B. Complete bedrest with head of bed flat for 24 hours
    C. Increased headache compared to patients without evacuation of ICH
    D. Shorter length of stay (LOS) compared to patients without evacuation of ICH

163. What is the rationale for proceeding with endovascular intervention if there is no one available to provide informed consent?
    A. The patient will die without it, so proceed in order to preserve life
    B. It is standard of care for large-vessel occlusion (LVO), so it can be done under the premise of emergency consent
    C. It is not permitted to proceed without informed consent
    D. If three providers agree/document that it is essential, it is permitted

164. What is the rationale for doing a lumbar puncture (LP) on a subarachnoid hemorrhage (SAH) patient?
    A. When SAH is present, but not evident on imaging, LP will show presence of blood
    B. When intraventricular hemorrhage is suspected as well, LP will show cerebrospinal fluid (CSF)
    C. When there is concern for vasospasm, LP will show fluctuating pressure
    D. LP is only indicated in intracerebral hemorrhage (ICH) patients

165. Evidence-based practice is best defined by which of the following?
    A. Practice developed from evidence of what is preferred by the medical director
    B. Practice developed as a result of the citations from the latest stroke certification visit summary
    C. Practice developed from results of research
    D. Practice developed from latest editorials in *The New England Journal of Medicine*

166. Which preventable poststroke complication is a common reason for readmission and eventual institutionalization in a nursing home?
    A. Urinary tract infection (UTI)
    B. Depression
    C. Subluxation
    D. Osteoporosis

167. Which poststroke complication would the stroke clinic nurse be addressing when they encouraged ambulation and adequate hydration?
    A. Pneumonia
    B. Constipation
    C. Spasticity
    D. Osteoporosis

168. Hyperextensions of the neck and chiropractic manipulation have been associated with the risk of which of the following?
   A. Vessel dissection
   B. Third nerve palsy
   C. Vessel spasm
   D. Sudden sinus headache

169. An acute stroke–ready hospital (ASRH) ED patient's CT scan reveals a large subarachnoid hemorrhage (SAH). What is the ED nurse's best next action?
   A. Monitor level of consciousness (LOC) and prepare for intubation
   B. Prepare them for admission to the neuro ICU
   C. Monitor blood pressure (BP) and administer pro re nata (PRN) labetolol if >200
   D. Monitor LOC and notify provider if pulse ox <100%

170. According to the Mission: Lifeline® Stroke Severity-Based Stroke Triage Algorithm for EMS, what is to be done with a large-vessel occlusion (LVO)–suspected patient if the nearest comprehensive stroke center (CSC) or thrombectomy-capable stroke center (TSC) is 45 minutes away?
   A. Prenotify that CSC/TSC and transport
   B. Prenotify the nearest certified stroke center and transport
   C. Ask the patient if they want to go to a certified stroke center
   D. Prenotify the nearest urgent care center and transport

Practice Exam: Answers

1. **C) It is not appropriate to administer IV thrombolysis to an ICH patient in the ED**

   The only time thrombolysis is given to an ICH patient is if there is blood in the ventricle, and it would be given via external ventricular drain (EVD), not IV. There are no time- or volume-based recommendations, as IV thrombolysis is contraindicated for ICH patients anywhere. Informed consent is not appropriate for a contraindicated treatment.

2. **A) They must have 24/7 imaging capability with images read within 24 hours**

   ASRHs must have emergent images for evaluation of treatment of acute stroke and must be read within 30 to 45 minutes, not within 24 hours. They are required to have 24/7 laboratory and thrombolytic capability and around-the-clock provider availability.

3. **B) Increased number of slices seen on CT and MRI**

   By increasing the number of slices, and thinning the slices, even tiny lacunar infarcts are now visible. In the previous time-based definition, small lacunar infarct symptoms might only last a few hours and then resolve, leading to an inaccurate TIA diagnosis. The change of definition is not due to inconsistencies in obtaining accurate time of onset and resolution, not to avoid confusion with the use of ministroke to describe TIA, nor to avoid confusion with angina pectoris, the pain associated with myocardial infarction.

4. **C) Black**

   Black populations activate 911 significantly less often than other racial groups.

5. **A) 34-year-old subarachnoid hemorrhage (SAH) patient with no history of hypertension**

   The upper limit of 160 mmHg is for all SAH patients. The upper limit for the ischemic stroke patient with a history of ICH would be determined by the provider. The upper limit for ICH patients is 140 mmHg. The upper limit for an ischemic patient with no history of hypertension is 220 mmHg, or 185 mmHg if thrombolytic is considered.

6. **A) Patients falling from beds or chairs**

   Frequent nursing rounds are essential to prevent patient falls. They may be helpful in keeping patients more awake, but that is not why they are recommended. Frequent rounds are not recommended to make patients eat more quickly or to keep them from drinking and needing to go to the toilet. They are, however, beneficial in ensuring that patients can get to the toilet safely more often if needed.

7. **C) Door-to-physician <10 minutes**

   The NINDS recommendations indicate that the patient should be seen by a physician in less than 10 minutes and seen by a stroke team member in less than 15 minutes.

8. **B) 90 mg**

   This patient weighs 113.6 kg and 0.9 mg/kg = 102.4 mg; however, 90 mg is the max dose to be given to anyone, regardless of weight.

9. **B) Internal carotid arteries, anterior cerebral arteries, anterior communicating artery, posterior cerebral arteries, and posterior communicating arteries**

   The middle cerebral artery is connected to the circle of Willis but is not part of it. The circle of Willis is made up of the internal carotid arteries, anterior cerebral arteries, anterior communicating artery, posterior cerebral arteries, and posterior communicating arteries.

10. **D) All of the above**

    Postop coiling patients need frequent groin checks and peripheral pulse checks because they had large artery access and are at risk of artery dissection with retroperitoneal hemorrhage, arterial thrombosis with restricted perfusion pattern, and failure/migration of closure device.

11. **C) Syndrome of inappropriate antidiuretic hormone secretion (ADH)**

    Syndrome of inappropriate ADH involves euvolemia or hypervolemia, and the treatment is fluid restriction. Cerebral salt wasting involves hypovolemia and would require fluid therapy. Hemoconstriction indicates increased specific gravity and would require fluid therapy. Hypertonicity indicates excessive muscle tone and would not require fluid restriction or therapy.

12. **A) Lack of transportation, poverty, and low educational achievement**

    Lack of transportation, poverty, and low educational achievement are all socioeconomic factors that are associated with increased risk of stroke. Urban setting is not associated with increased risk of stroke, a rural setting is. Food security is not associated with increased risk of stroke, food insecurity is. High educational achievement is not associated with increased risk of stroke.

13. **D) Facilitation of neuroplasticity**

    Repetitive stimulation over the area of infarction facilitates the brain's ability to rewire itself, thus supporting and improving neuroplasticity. Inhibition of task initiation would not be a purpose of this therapy. Compensatory training refers to therapies to encourage work-arounds to increase independence. There is no evidence that brain stimulation impacts neurospasticity.

14. **A) Obesity, smoking, poor diet, physical inactivity, hypertension**

    While diabetes and Afib are also significant risk factors, studies have shown that they are not among the five that account for 90% of strokes: obesity, smoking, poor diet, physical inactivity, and hypertension.

15. **B) Subarachnoid hemorrhage**

    The majority of ruptured aneurysms are within the subarachnoid space, causing a subarachnoid hemorrhage. Intraventricular hemorrhage is generally an extension of a subarachnoid hemorrhage or intracerebral hemorrhage. Intracerebral hemorrhage is the result of a ruptured blood vessel, not an aneurysm. Intracranial hemorrhage refers to any intracranial bleeding, including subdural hemorrhage.

16. **C) Immobilization**

    Immobilization is not a compensatory strategy for patients with extinction. Visual scanning, body rotation, and placing a brightly colored armband on the affected limb are all examples of compensatory strategies for patients with extinction.

17. **C) Both CN III and VI**

    CN III (oculomotor) controls the pupil, upper eyelid, and eye muscles that allow for visual tracking and gaze fixation. CN VI (abducens) controls lateral movement of the eyes. Both the CN III and CN VI innervate the eyes.

18. **D) None of the above**

    Penetrating arteries are smaller distal branches of the large cerebral arteries that penetrate the pia mater and the brain tissue. The proximal MCA, proximal PCA, and proximal vertebral artery are not considered penetrating arteries as they do not follow this definition.

19. **C) Thrombolytic-ready stroke center**

    There is no thrombolytic-ready stroke center, as all levels of stroke centers must be thrombolytic capable. Thrombectomy-capable stroke centers (TSCs), comprehensive stroke centers (CSCs), and primary stroke centers (PSCs) are all certified stroke center designations.

20. **D) Brain Attack Coalition (BAC)**

    The BAC wrote *Recommendations for Primary Stroke Centers* in 2000, which outlines the first recommendations for PSCs. The certifying bodies such as DNV, HFAP, and TJC developed certification standards for certified centers based on those recommendations.

21. **D) Dysarthria**

    Dysarthria is slurred speech that is a sign of cerebellar dysfunction that would be seen in a cerebellar stroke patient. Dystonia is involuntary muscle contractions, aphasia is the inability to say/write the correct word, and dysgraphia is difficulty with writing. None of these would be seen in a cerebellar stroke patient.

22. **B) There is a penalty for organizations with all-cause readmissions above the national average**

    The CMS tracks all-cause readmissions, including scheduled readmissions, and penalizes organizations who exceed the national average. All-cause readmissions include even planned readmissions. There is no published evidence that hospitals are extending lengths of stays to avoid readmission penalties.

23. **D) Right-handed patient with discharge NIHSS of 2 for level of consciousness (LOC) question (1) and LOC command (1)**

    Cognitive deficits represent safety risks for living alone due to inability to reliably use the telephone if help is needed, to take medications safely, and to manage appliances such as the stove safely. A patient with an NIHSS of 2 for LOC question (1) and LOC command (1) will have cognitive issues that will put them at risk for harm if they live alone. Patients with mild physical limitations are at a lower risk as long as their cognition is intact.

24. **D) Any of the above**

    Hypertension is the most common cause of all strokes. Hypertension can cause ischemic strokes as a result of vascular stiffness and narrowing and can also cause hemorrhagic strokes as a result of vascular stiffening and brittleness.

25. **C) If the patient is stable and without pulmonary symptoms**

    CXRs can be useful if emergent pulmonary or cardiac concerns are evident but should not delay stroke intervention regardless of how busy the ED is; it should be done if patient's condition warrants it. The guidelines do not dictate that the CXR be done on a specific day. It is appropriate and recommended that if the patient is stable, the CXR should be delayed until after the emergent stroke work is completed.

26. **A) Antiseizure medications for seizure prevention**

    Antiseizure medications are associated with side effects that often outweigh the benefit and are no longer recommended by the AHA/ASA. Antibiotics for UTI, antiemetics for vomiting, and antipyretics for hyperthermia are still recommended for these patients.

27. **D) Diligent, regular oral care**

    Diligent and regular oral care has been shown to reduce ventilator-associated pneumonia. Suction should be done at the level of the epiglottis, not bronchus. Prophylactic antibiotics and negative air flow rooms are not associated with decreased incidence of ventilator-associated pneumonia.

28. **C) International normalized ratio (INR) goals are the same for primary and secondary prevention in patients with nonvalvular atrial fibrillation (Afib)**

    With regard to primary and secondary risk factor prevention, INR goals are the same in nonvalvular Afib, but differ for valvular Afib. SBP and BMI goals are the same whether primary or secondary prevention. Low density lipoprotein (LDL) goals differ significantly between primary and secondary prevention.

29. **C) The right anterior and posterior circulation originate from the brachiocephalic artery**

    The right-side cerebral circulation originates from the brachiocephalic artery, also known as the innominate artery, which is connected to the aorta. The anterior circulation originates from the common carotid on the left, and the brachiocephalic on the right. The posterior circulation originates from the subclavian on the left, and the brachiocephalic on the right. The posterior cerebral artery is part of the posterior circulation.

30. **B) Right parietal lobe**

    Extinction is the result of right parietal lobe dysfunction, not frontal, cerebellar, or temporal lobe damage.

31. **B) Postthrombectomy patient with diaphoresis and lower abdominal and back pain**

    Retroperitoneal hemorrhage is a complication of endovascular procedures with groin access in which the catheter punctures the arterial wall; the symptoms are diaphoresis and lower abdominal and back pain from the pressure of the retroperitoneal blood. Carotid endarterectomy only involves the neck. Aneurysm coiling and stent patients could have retroperitoneal hemorrhage, but the symptoms provided do not indicate it.

32. C) Pattern of multiple strokes in the same hemisphere

In dissection, clots can form along the intimal tear, then break off and flow to the brain. Multiple strokes in one hemisphere provide a clue that the source was from the carotid since they each supply just one hemisphere. A pattern of strokes in both hemispheres would indicate that the source was cardiac, and as the clots left the heart, they could travel up either side to the brain. Multiple cerebellar strokes would indicate vertebral or basilar dissection. Scattered pattern of strokes throughout the cerebrum and cerebellum would be exceptionally rare and be indicative of an overwhelming vasculitis.

33. D) Both A and B

The CMS and AHA/ASA recommend that systems of care involve prehospital, acute care, postacute, and community collaboration, and are familiar with the value of compliance with quality standards for stroke patients. This is because both institutions dictate that systems of care can address the continuum of care with greater efficiency. There is no evidence that PCP professional organizations are not cooperative with quality measures.

34. C) Mixing oral contraceptives and smoking

Studies have shown that the combination of hormone therapy and smoking increases stroke risk at any age. There is no definitive evidence regarding increased stroke risk and the combination of vaping and marijuana, the combination of oral tobacco and alcohol, or alcohol abuse while pregnant.

35. B) Providing stroke education to college students who play football

Primordial prevention involves education to prevent the development of risk factors. Providing stroke education to students with type 2 diabetes or to seniors on warfarin for Afib are examples of primary prevention since risk factor is already present. Providing stroke education to adults in a stroke recovery group represents secondary prevention since the group has already had stroke.

36. B) Ptosis, anhidrosis, and meiosis

Ptosis (droopy eyelid), anhidrosis (absence of hemifacial sweating), and meiosis (pupil constriction) are the classic triad of Horner's syndrome and are seen with carotid artery dissection.

37. B) Dipyridamole/aspirin (Aggrenox)

With 40% of patients who take dipyridamole/aspirin combo (Aggrenox) complaining of headache, it would not be wise to prescribe it for someone with baseline frequent headaches. If a patient has frequent headaches, they can still take rivaroxaban (Xarelto), clopidogrel (Plavix), or dabigatran (Pradaxa).

38. D) None of the above

Minor foot surgery 14 days ago is not an exclusion for alteplase. The recommendations state that even major surgery in the last 14 days can be considered, but selection is patient specific. It is safe to give IV thrombolysis to patients on aspirin and clopidogrel; they are oral antithrombotics. Oral anticoagulants, not antithrombotics, are contraindicated. IV thrombolysis is safe up to 4.5 hours from symptom onset, and this patient arrived within 2, so it is within the window for IV thrombolysis.

39. **A) Approach them from the right side**

Extinction is a result of right parietal lobe dysfunction, so they are not aware of the left side. Approaching them and call bell placement should both occur on the right side. Speaking loudly and slowly is always a good approach with hospitalized patients, but not necessarily into a specific ear. Having the patient sit on a particular side of the bed for meals has no impact on the deficit of extinction.

40. **B) It should be done on admission and whenever there has been a change in level of consciousness (LOC)**

The dysphagia screening is a nursing function that should be done on admission and whenever there is reason to believe that the patient's ability to swallow may have changed. It is no longer one of the STK measures but is required to be done at certified stroke centers. It is required even if the provider says it's not necessary. Speech therapists perform much more detailed assessment of patients' swallow, not just a simple screening as done by nurses.

41. **A) Obtain Chem 7 lab panel**

The only blood test done by EMS is glucose, which can be done enroute, not on-scene. Stabilization of airway, breathing, circulation (ABC), performing a stroke screen, and briefly getting information from witnesses are all on-scene functions.

42. **D) National Institutes of Health Stroke Scale (NIHSS)**

Research has proven that NIHSS score on admission is valid in predicting discharge disposition. The BI is not done on admission; the GCS is used to indicate depth of coma and decreased level of consciousness, not discharge disposition; and the ABCD2 score is used in triaging transient ischemic attack (TIA) patients in the ED.

43. **D) There is no guideline for lower limit of SBP, but patients with history of hypertension may not tolerate lower BP**

There is no specific guideline for lower limits of SBP; however, care should be taken with treating hypertension that the BP is not made too low for the patient. Hypotension is a concern, so it is incorrect to say that it is not. The upper BP limit for intracerebral hemorrhage (ICH) is 140 mmHg and the same for subarachnoid hemorrhage (SAH) is 160 mmHg.

44. **C) Administer intravenous (IV) thrombolytic as ordered according to their weight**

If the patient's symptoms have resolved, the NIHSS would be 0 and they would be considered normal, or well. If symptoms return, that becomes the new LKW time and the clock starts again. When symptoms return, treatment should be initiated as evidence has shown that thrombolytic given in TIA or stroke mimic does not cause harm. There is no indication of large-vessel occlusion (LVO) and no need for endovascular team.

45. **C) Both A and B**

Since both PSC and ASRH EDs transfer some patients to higher levels of care, they are required to report their DIDO times.

46. **D) Sinus tachycardia**

    Sinus tachycardia is still sinus rhythm, so there is no quivering of the atria that allows clots to form. A large PFO allows blood to pass back and forth between atria and allows blood to pool. Endocarditis is often associated with clot formation on infected tissue. Afib involves ineffective atrial pumping, allowing blood to pool.

47. **C) Primordial prevention = prevention of conditions before they start; primary prevention = prevention of stroke in the setting of risk factors like diabetes or hypertension**

    Primordial prevention is the prevention of conditions before they start; primary prevention is the prevention of stroke in the setting of risk factors like diabetes, hypertension, and so on. Primary prevention is not a subtype of primordial prevention. Both primordial and primary prevention are difficult to measure. Primordial prevention does not refer to successful reversal of the condition.

48. **C) Root cause analysis**

    Root cause analysis is the process of taking an event, usually an adverse outcome, and analyzing every aspect that led up to it to find the cause. The purpose is to then make sure that it does not happen again. Six Sigma, PDSA, and DMAIC are methodologies for evaluating processes to eliminate defects.

49. **D) Both A and B**

    Hispanic men and women are expected to see a 29% rise due to increasing incidence of heart disease, hypertension, and diabetes. Black men have a higher incidence than Caucasian or Hispanic populations.

50. **C) Saccular**

    Saccular aneurysms comprise 80% to 90% of all cerebral aneurysms. Mycotic aneurysms are associated with an infectious source. Fusiform aneurysms are much less common, ~10% of cerebral aneurysms.

51. **B) Consult vocational rehabilitation services**

    Vocational rehabilitation services will provide therapy and support for possible change in job type. Recommending an attorney or psychiatric services or simply telling the patient to work harder are not appropriate in this situation.

52. **B) Evidence does not support fibrates for cholesterol control, so please stop the gemfibrozil and give the atorvastatin a chance to work**

    The PCP should tell the patient that fibrates' effect on cholesterol control are not supported and that atorvastatin should be given the chance to work. Fibrates are not recommended, and the combination does increase liver toxicity by six-fold. Therefore, offering the patient the gemfibrozil or letting them continue to take it is not indicated. Since it has only been a week since the patient has begun atorvastatin, it is too soon to measure impact on the liver.

53. **C) An incomplete circle of Willis is a common phenomenon**

    Up to 75% of the population has an incomplete circle of Willis, and no correlation with increased stroke risk has been found. The circle of Willis is developed in utero.

54. **B) 60-year-old embolic stroke patient with INR 1.8**

    Therapeutic INR range for most anticoagulated stroke patients is 2.0 to 3.0, and that patient hadn't reached therapeutic range yet. Lacunar stroke patients are not treated with anticoagulants. Hemorrhagic patients are rarely treated with anticoagulants. The 50-year-old patient has hit therapeutic range and doesn't need a dose adjustment.

55. **A) Extinction**

    Extinction is the result of right parietal lobe damage and is characterized by the inability to recognize or be aware of the left side of their body or things on their left side. Hemianopia is the loss of half of the visual field, it would not prohibit someone from recognizing things on their left side. Apraxia is the inability to initiate voluntary movement or speech. Cortical blindness is loss of vision due to brain abnormality.

56. **D) Amyloid angiopathy**

    Amyloid angiopathy involves deposits of protein in small arteries of the brain resulting in progressive narrowing and ischemia. Accumulation of these proteins can occlude vessels and is a precursor to Alzheimer's disease. Cavernous angioma, vasculitis, and moyamoya are not associated with Alzheimer's disease.

57. **B) The release of catecholamines**

    Catecholamine release can trigger arrhythmias, tachycardia, hypertension, and increased troponins, which are manageable and reversible. The reasons for the release of catecholamines are still unknown but common with SAH. The proximity of the medulla to the SAH is not the mechanism, nor is cerebral salt wasting or cerebral edema.

58. **C) If you haven't had imaging done, please talk to your PCP about that and blood pressure (BP) control**

    Family history of aneurysms increases risk of stroke. This young woman should be screened and have tight BP control. It is inappropriate and inadequate to simply state that headache is the only symptom of stroke due to aneurysm rupture or that hormone therapy is the cause. There is no proof that the woman has an aneurysm.

59. **B) Parenchymal hemorrhage**

    Parenchymal hemorrhage (PH) is characterized as either parenchymal hemorrhage 1 (PH1; <30% volume of space-occupying blood) or parenchymal hemorrhage 2 (PH2), which is defined as >30% volume of space-occupying blood and would result in increased ICP. Postdural and precentriole hemorrhage are not actual terms. Petechial hemorrhages are not space occupying and would have minimal effect on ICP.

60. **D) All of the above**

    Caregiver inability or unwillingness to be long-term caregivers is a leading cause of stroke patient institutionalization.

61. **B) Ischemic stroke patient with a hemicraniectomy**

    Hemicraniectomy patients' bone flaps can be stored in the freezer or in the subcutaneous tissue of the abdomen. EVD, endovascular coiling, and carotid endarterectomy do not involve the abdomen.

62. **B) Hunt and Hess score**

    The Hunt and Hess score is based on symptoms present. The Fisher scale is based on the amount of blood present. The WFNS score is based on the Glasgow Coma Scale (GCS) and motor deficit.

63. **A) Limb weakness**

    The precentral gyrus is the area of the frontal lobe where the motor strip is located. Damage would produce weakness. Numbness would result from damage to the postcentral gyrus where the sensory strip is located. It is right behind the precentral gyrus but located in the parietal lobe. Dysarthria would result from damage to the cerebellum. Extinction would result from damage to the parietal lobe, not the sensory strip portion.

64. **A) It is reasonable**

    Class IIA indicates that a procedure/treatment is reasonable and can be effective. Class I indicates that it is recommended. Class III indicates that it is not recommended and potentially harmful.

65. **A) Tenecteplase**

    Tenecteplase is being used around the country due to the evidence that it is effective/safe and very easy to administer compared to alteplase. Abciximab is a glycoprotein IIb/IIIa inhibitor used in interventional cardiology to inhibit platelet aggregation. Aripiprazole is an antipsychotic used in schizophrenia. Alteplase is a thrombolytic approved by the FDA and administered over 60 minutes.

66. **C) Use of telemedicine**

    The use of telemedicine brings expert consultants into the community ED and has resulted in faster evaluation and a significant reduction in door-to-needle time. Treatment with thrombolytic is not dependent on CTA. The cost of thrombolytics has no impact on the treatment times. Education of EMS may have helped to reduce treatment time by better prenotification, but not as significantly as the use of telemedicine.

67. **B) They have been shown to reduce in-hospital mortality**

    Stroke units have been shown to reduce in-hospital mortality, length of stay (LOS), and increase discharges to home. They are not required to be a distinct area of the hospital and are not required to be overseen by a certified vascular neurologist. They have, in fact, been shown to increase discharges to home, not reduce them.

68. **C) A tear in the inner lining of the vessel allowing blood to collect between the layers and blood clots to form along the edges of the tear**

    These small blood clots commonly break off and travel upstream, blocking smaller blood vessels, resulting in multiple small infarcts. A fusion of two cerebral vessels because of chronic vasculitis describes a vascular fistula. A weakened area in the wall of the vessel resulting in a ballooning out describes an aneurysm. A buildup of plaque causing vessel occlusion describes a thrombus.

69. **D) All of the above**

Educated EMS providers will be better able to recognize that TIA symptoms should not be ignored and can help to inform the patient about the importance of a workup. EMS education of TIA can help to correctly identify emergent situations, allow EMS to educate patients about the condition, and prevent a subsequent stroke from occurring.

70. **A) Acetaminophen**

Acetaminophen has a very weak antiplatelet effect and only at very high doses. A febrile ischemic stroke patient on oral anticoagulation can be given this medication. Ibuprofen and aspirin have a stronger antiplatelet effect and should not be given for antipyretic therapy to patients on oral anticoagulants since they could exacerbate the anticoagulant effect. An ice bath is not indicated.

71. **B) Nurses**

Evidence shows that certified rehabilitation nurses provide higher quality of care that results in better outcomes for the patients. There has been no reported evidence of such an impact with physiatrists, therapists, or social workers.

72. **D) To determine if thrombolytic treatment is warranted in patients with mild/improving symptoms**

Patients with symptoms that are mild or rapidly improving historically did not get thrombolytic, and studies showed their symptoms often worsened. Most providers now can justify ordering it for these patients if they answer that they cannot live with the deficit regardless of how mild. Hospice consult is not based on patient response to this question, nor is baseline depression status, nor admission status.

73. **D) Transcranial Doppler (TCD)**

TCD is done through the temporal bony window and is used to monitor the MCA and the anterior cerebral artery (ACA). TTE involves looking at the heart through the chest wall. TEE involves looking at the heart through the esophageal wall. ECG involves recording the electrical activity of the heart through leads on the chest.

74. **C) Wallenberg's syndrome**

Wallenberg's syndrome is indicative of posterior stroke from vertebrobasilar insufficiency. The crossed signs refer to the mix of left and right deficits possibly due to the motor fibers coming together at the brainstem to pass through the foramen magnum. Horner's syndrome involves ptosis, anhidrosis, and meiosis. Cryptogenic syndrome and gyral syndrome do not exist.

75. **A) Clots form in the atria as a result of blood stagnating**

Blood pools in the quivering atria, which allows clot formation. Blood does not pool in the ventricles. Muscle fatigue alone does not cause Afib. Endocarditis is inflammation of valves, not the result of rapid rate.

76. **A) ABCD2 score**

The ABCD2 score predicts short-term risk of stroke in patients with TIA. mRS is used for measuring functional ability. CHA_2DS_2-VASc score is used to calculate atrial fibrillation patients' stroke risk. BI score is another measure of functional ability.

77. **D) Nil per os (NPO) until dysphagia screen**

Screening for dysphagia prior to any oral intake has been shown to reduce aspiration pneumonia incidence. Hypoxia screening followed by supplementary oxygen, a comprehensive assessment of lung sounds, and deep breathing and coughing every hour will not help to prevent aspiration pneumonia.

78. **B) TEE provides better visualization of the heart structures than TTE**

For a closer look at heart structures, the TEE eliminates having to look through the ribs and chest muscles. TEE, not TTE, involves swallowing a tube. TEE is not simpler than TTE. TTE does not provide better visualization than TEE.

79. **B) Sleep apnea**

Sleep apnea has been shown to be common in stroke survivors, and there is suspicion that it may also increase risk of stroke. There is no evidence of a relationship between stroke and menopause, hypothyroidism, or heat exhaustion.

80. **A) Spasticity**

Unresolved spasticity limits joint movement and results in pain and contracture. Muscle atrophy is a result of disuse of the limb, not a cause of contracture. Hypoflexion refers to reduced flexion of a joint and would not result in contracture. Ataxia refers to abnormal, uncoordinated movements and would not result in contracture.

81. **C) Recanalization of the vessel**

Recanalization refers to occluded vessels that have been reopened, restoring circulation to the ischemic area. When a procedure is documented as TICI of 3, the result is recanalization. Reocclusion indicates a vessel that had been reopened and is now blocked again. Restoration of the thrombus refers to a thrombus redeveloping at an area that had been cleared of a thrombus previously. The removal of the bifurcation would indicate removal of an area where two vessels intersect.

82. **A) Less time to thrombectomy treatment**

Bypassing a PSC would reduce thrombectomy time if the patient has a large-vessel occlusion (LVO). Bypass also reduces demand for another ambulance to pick up the patient at a PSC to go to a higher level of care. Dispatch time is unaffected by bypassing a PSC.

83. **A) Increase in risk factors in childhood/Increased control of blood pressure (BP) and cholesterol in older adults**

Evidence suggests that the increase in stroke incidence in young adults is due to sedentary lifestyle, excessive portion size, and excessive fast food intake, resulting in an increase of type 2 diabetes in childhood. There is no evidence of reduction in alcohol abuse in older adults. There is no evidence of a link between vaping and stroke. Smoking is linked to increased stroke risk.

84. **C) There has been no established optimal time/tool for stroke depression screening**

Despite numerous studies, there has been no established optimal time/tool for stroke depression screening. The PHQ-9, CES-D, and HDRS are valid tools for depression screening in the general population, but not specific to stroke and not in the acute setting, although many organizations use the PHQ-9 tool in the acute setting.

85. **B) Stroke etiology**

Stroke etiology refers to the cause of stroke and is absolutely essential to development of effective secondary prevention. Stroke sequelae refer to the resulting deficits of the stroke. Stroke activator and stroke instigator are not medical terms.

86. **C) LVO patient arriving within 12 hours with no penumbra evident on imaging**

The lack of penumbra on imaging indicates that the stroke is completed, and there is no viable tissue to salvage by removing the clot. The acceptable time frame for intervention is 24 hours. IV alteplase and novel oral anticoagulants such as Eliquis are not barriers to endovascular intervention for LVO patients.

87. **C) 8**

Eight are stroke (STK) measures. Dysphagia screening and smoking cessation are no longer considered to be STK measures.

88. **A) Establishing last known well (LKW) time**

Establishing the LKW time is one of the critical actions by EMS and facilitates treatment decisions. The content of last meal and last PCP visit date are not essential in acute stroke care. Establishing a phone number for contact is essential, but there is no need for a minimum of three of them.

89. **C) Patient was instructed in techniques for getting up after falling**

Patients with hemiparesis are at increased risk of falling, and it would be helpful for them to be instructed on safe techniques for getting up again. Patients are instructed to intersperse activities with rest periods throughout the day, not to plan them all in the morning. It is incorrect to instruct the planned living space to feature furniture close together because this patient will need more than just holding onto furniture to get around; there will need to be room for that assistance. There is no value in simply telling a patient to be careful not to fall.

90. **A) Vasospasm occurs between 4 and 10 days**

Vasospasm, which can result in delayed ischemia, is commonly seen between 4 and 10 days and can occur up to 21 days after stroke. Many SAH patients begin therapy within the first few days of hospitalization. Ventilator support is not necessary for all SAH patients and only for as long as patient condition warrants. Hydrocephalus is not a risk unless blood has gotten into the ventricles.

91. **C) Offer to call 911 for transport to a nearby hospital for evaluation**

Malnutrition is a threat to recovery and needs to be addressed. The extreme case of somnolence may be an indication of a bigger problem and needs to be assessed. The patient's caregiver cannot provide the level of care and risks harm to both themself and the patient without intervention. Without a comprehensive evaluation of the patient, it is inappropriate to order nutritional support. Validation and reassurance are inadequate in this situation, as is recommending a respite stay in a nursing home.

92. **C) Do a neurological assessment and notify provider of suspected hypoperfusion**

    Patients with history of hypertension can have poor tolerance for "normal" BP. Further neurological assessment is warranted, along with notification of the provider. Given the presentation, proper recourse must include notification, so simply performing and documenting a neurological assessment or documenting the new BP is not advised. Asking the patient if they are okay and waking them up does nothing to address their state.

93. **A) Record the temperature and administer pro re nata (PRN) acetaminophen as ordered**

    A temperature greater than 38 °C (100.4 °F), regardless of cause, should be treated. Therapeutic hypothermia is not recommended in most acute stroke patients; normothermia is recommended. Recent cold/flu symptoms have no bearing on whether the high temperature should be treated. Transfer from an ASRH to a TSC is not warranted based on this information.

94. **D) Hospice**

    A Hunt and Hess score of 5 indicates coma, making hospice the most likely discharge destination. A patient in a coma would likely not be placed in an acute inpatient rehabilitation or day rehab program, nor will they be discharged home with outpatient therapy.

95. **D) It is used in arteriovenous malformation (AVM) patients who are not candidates for surgery or endovascular therapy**

    Gamma knife's focused radiation is used for AVM patients who cannot tolerate surgery or endovascular therapy, as well as following surgery or endovascular therapy to eliminate any remaining lesion. It is not used in carotid stenosis treatment or as adjunct to IV thrombolytic. If it is done prior to AVM bleeding, it is the primary prevention of stroke, and if done after bleeding, it is secondary prevention.

96. **B) Closing the eyes eliminates visual cues**

    Closing the eyes during the extinction exam eliminates the patient being able to see when/where they are being touched. Neurological rest is not necessary during the brief NIHSS assessment. Closing the eyes does not impact anxiety about the test. The NIHSS is not done entirely with eyes open.

97. **B) Every 4 hours because stroke patients' symptoms may fluctuate during the first few days**

    Patients with acute stroke are at risk of neurological fluctuation or deterioration during their acute stay and should be monitored frequently. Therefore, a correct schedule is every 4 hours. Every 8 hours is not recommended because it is too infrequent for stroke patients. Every hour schedule for post-IV thrombolytic is only required up to 24-hours postadministration. Hemoglobin A1C does not impact the monitoring schedule.

98. **D) Swallow ability**

    Arm drift, facial symmetry, and speech ability are the components of the Cincinnati Prehospital Stroke Scale.

99. **D) Occupational therapy**

Occupational therapists provide support for improving the ability to do day-to-day functions, also called activities of daily living (ADLs), such as feeding, dressing, or bathing oneself. Adapted living therapy is a term used mainly in psychotherapy. Physical therapy focuses on mobilization and strength. Cognitive therapy focuses on attention and calculation, recall, and language skills.

100. **C) Watershed stroke**

Watershed strokes occur when distal arterial beds are not perfused adequately. During surgery with anesthesia, blood pressure can fluctuate below what the patient can tolerate, raising the risk for inadequate perfusion. Cryptogenic strokes refer to strokes for which no cause is found, which would be rare postop. Silent strokes refer to strokes found on imaging for which there was no symptomatology. TIA refers to symptoms of stroke without any imaged stroke.

101. **A) Wii-habilitation therapy**

Wii-hab or Wii-habilitation therapy has been widely used as it provides variety and immediate feedback. Immersion therapy is used in resolution of phobias. Pac-habilitation does not exist. Aversion therapy is designed to pair unwanted behavior with an unpleasant experience such as pain and is not used in stroke rehabilitation.

102. **C) Smoking cessation, dysphagia screening**

Smoking cessation and dysphagia screening were not endorsed by the National Quality Forum in 2008. Dysphagia screening was not endorsed due to the lack of a valid, reliable, standardized screening tool or process supported by research, although it is recognized as an important aspect of prevention of aspiration pneumonia. Smoking cessation was not endorsed as it was deemed to have already been met by organizational initiatives and through documentation of teaching or counseling provided.

103. **C) With the territory of infarct being so small, it is possible to only impact motor or sensory fibers**

Lacunar strokes impact a very small territory that may only affect one type of fiber. A large infarct would impact more than just motor or sensory fibers. Lacunar strokes are not synonymous with scattered strokes, nor are they synonymous with TIA.

104. **D) It indicates that goals for functional recovery will likely not be for full independence**

Preadmission mRS is an indication of function prior to this hospitalization and may be a result of injury or other debilitating conditions; it should guide expectations and therapy goals for the care team. It is incorrect to say that an mRS of 3 does not affect the care plan. There is no evidence that the preadmission mRS or age dictate the level of postdischarge destination. Prior stroke is just one of the possibilities for a preadmission mRS of >0, not a necessary reason.

105. **A) 3, 2b**

Only 2b (full, but slow perfusion) and 3 (complete perfusion) are considered successful reperfusion. 2a indicates less than 2/3 perfusion, 1 indicates penetration with minimal perfusion, and 0 indicates no perfusion.

106. **A) Anterior lobe cerebellum**

    The cerebellum is located below the tentorial fold of the dura mater and would be considered infratentorial. The other structures are located above the tentorial fold of the dura mater and are considered supratentorial.

107. **C) This test is being done to get a look at your blood vessels**

    The "A" in CTA, or magnetic resonance angiography (MRA), stands for *angio* and refers to blood vessels. CTA does not involve a strong magnet, like MRI. An MRI looks at the brain tissue, not vessels. Decisions regarding thrombolytic therapy are based on plain CT, not CTA.

108. **B) Part/all of their penumbra has infarcted**

    If all or part of the penumbra is not preserved in the first hours, it will also infarct, making the core larger, referred to as extension of a stroke. It does not refer to LOS, deficit resolution, or tentorium infarction.

109. **D) Cerebral vasodilation**

    Cerebral vasodilation is the expansion of the lumen of the vessels, so it would not interrupt cerebral blood flow. A thrombus or embolus would be capable of interruption of flow, and vasospasm can narrow the vessel to the point of interruption of blood flow.

110. **B) Motor and sensory deficits inhibit their ability to adjust their position or feel the pain of pressure points**

    Motor and sensory deficits make them much more vulnerable to skin breakdown, as they cannot adjust their position and do not feel pain where breakdown may be occurring. Cerebral perfusion deficits do not result in peripheral perfusion deficits. Coughing and deep breathing do not impact skin integrity. Dysarthria does not impact ability to move and alter position.

111. **C) The Cincinnati Prehospital Stroke Scale establishes the probability of stroke, and the Cincinnati Prehospital Stroke Severity Scale establishes the probability of large-vessel occlusion (LVO)**

    The emergency medical services (EMS) perform Cincinnati Prehospital Stroke Scale on anyone with stroke symptoms, and then the Cincinnati Prehospital Stroke Severity Scale is performed on those patients to determine if there is suspected LVO and to guide which stroke center to transport them to. Although both have been referred to with the acronym CPSS, they are two different scales. The Cincinnati Prehospital Stroke Severity Scale does not confirm a stroke. Geography does not play a factor in the use of these scales.

112. **A) Their penumbra has enlarged to include the leg area of the motor strip**

    Once swelling develops around the core of the stroke, there can be drowsiness and additional deficits noted. With proper medical support, the swelling will dissipate, and the additional deficits will resolve. BP fluctuation, unless it was extremely high or low, would not result in new deficits. A blood sugar over 200 or sleep deprivation of one night would not likely result in these new deficits.

113. **D) Provide to all stroke patients with O$_2$ saturation less than 92%**

Evidence-based guidelines indicate that for best oxygenation of the brain, an O$_2$ saturation of less than 92% should be supplemented with oxygen, regardless of type of stroke.

114. **A) It is a cylindrical, flexible, and self-expanding object that is positioned across the aneurysm neck to keep blood from going in and out of the aneurysm**

Endovascular flow diversion is a "flow diverter" in that it is impervious and blocks the flow of blood from entering or leaving the aneurysmal sac. It is not same as cardiac stents, it is not a flexible plug, nor is it an aneurysm removal device.

115. **A) 66 year-old female with CHA$_2$DS$_2$-VASc score of 2 and modified Rankin Scale (mRS) score of 4**

A CHA$_2$DS$_2$-VASc score of >1 for men and >2 for women indicates risk in patients with atrial fibrillation (Afib) so anticoagulation is recommended. A CHA$_2$DS$_2$-VASc score of 0 does not indicate anticoagulation. The Hunt and Hess score is a hemorrhagic determiner, not a guide for anticoagulation. The ABCD2 score is a transient ischemic attack (TIA) scoring tool that will not give any indication about anticoagulation treatments.

116. **C) Ischemic stroke patient with intravenous (IV) thrombolysis**

Evidence has shown that ischemic stroke patients who receive IV alteplase have 30% better functional outcome than those who do not received it. There is no evidence that mechanical clot removal, minimally invasive ICH removal, or aneurysm coiling show such an improved functional outcome on their respective populations.

117. **B) DVT passes through the PFO and flows out to the brain**

Even a single DVT, when mobile, can pass through the PFO and flow out to the brain causing an embolic stroke. It would be rare for DVT to become lodged in a PFO, and it would not send clots to the brain. Without a PFO, a DVT could not present a risk of embolic stroke.

118. **D) 24/7 capability to perform mechanical clot retrieval**

TSCs are PSCs with the additional capability of performing mechanical clot retrieval. 24/7 capability for emergent evaluation and treatment are required for all levels of stroke centers. Compliance with all stroke measures and 24/7 capability to admit most stroke patients are required for PSCs, TSCs, and comprehensive stroke centers (CSCs).

119. **A) Inability to understand instructions or questions**

Understanding instructions or questions is part of receptive speech, the function of Wernicke's area. Singing and speaking are examples of motor speech, the function of Broca's area.

120. **D) The ED is an excellent opportunity for primary prevention**

Primary prevention opportunities exist in the community, primary care, and ED settings. It is difficult, but not impossible, to measure effectiveness of prevention strategies. Diabetes management, blood pressure (BP) meds, anticoagulants, and so on are covered by insurance.

121. **D) Hyperthermia is associated with increased metabolic needs and worse outcomes**

    Under conditions of hyperthermia, metabolic needs increase as individual cells attempt to maintain ionic balance. Hyperthermia is not associated with uncontrolled hypertension, and it does not suppress mitochondrial activity or platelet function.

122. **D) All of the above**

    Seizure, Bell's palsy, and complex migraine are mimics of stroke.

123. **A) Motor and sensory loss of the face and arm**

    The MCA supplies blood to the middle portion of the motor and sensory strips, which controls the face and arm. The anterior cerebral artery (ACA) supplies the top of the motor and sensory strip, which controls the leg. Imbalance is a result of cerebellar dysfunction, and it is supplied by the basilar artery, not the MCA.

124. **D) No, because they knew that this patient had developed intraventricular hemorrhage**

    When blood gets into the ventricles, it can coagulate on the arachnoid villi, clogging the flow of cerebrospinal fluid, resulting in hydrocephalus. Administration of thrombolytic via a ventriculostomy catheter has been effective in dissolving the clots and preventing hydrocephalus. Ruptured aneurysms are not treated with thrombolytic. Hemorrhagic stroke patients do not receive thrombolytic systemically, but it is indicated via ventriculostomy when blood has gotten into the ventricles.

125. **C) Enroute prenotification**

    Enroute prenotification of the arrival of a suspected stroke is important for the EMS so that the CT scanner can be cleared and the stroke team can be ready to assess on arrival. Quicker ambulance dispatch and blood glucose enroute are important but don't impact mobilization of ED resources. An EKG should not be done on-scene in suspected stroke.

126. **B) Telephone follow-up by clinical pharmacist**

    Telemedicine services include both telephone and two-way audio-video communication, not in-person visits or in-home visits.

127. **B) It facilitates venous drainage and reduces intracerebral pressure (ICP)**

    Midline positioning facilitates venous drainage, which will help to reduce ICP. Positioning to improve swallow safety involves head tuck to slow liquid passage, or chin extension to promote food passage. Maintaining the midline position may help to prevent stress headaches; however, there is no evidence to support that in the stroke population. Midline positioning has not been shown to impact progress after discharge.

128. **A) Help them into the left lateral recumbent position**

    Placing the patient in the left lateral recumbent position is the most appropriate action to take right away to protect against aspiration. A stat CXR may be beneficial eventually if the patient becomes symptomatic, but it is not an immediate intervention. As long as the patient is conscious, an oral airway would not be appropriate. The patient may eventually need to be intubated, but there are not enough indicators for that yet.

129. **A) It provides a baseline functional score and helps to establish goals for recovery**

Knowledge of prestroke functional independence facilitates realistic discharge goals, providing a baseline functional score and establishing goals for recovery. If they were functionally dependent before, they may not be appropriate for inpatient rehab. The age, blood pressure (BP), clinical features, duration of symptoms, diabetes (ABCD2) score only is used for triaging transient ischemic attack (TIA) patients. A patient with a preadmission mRS of 3 could have their home equipped for their needs and enough support to care for them already, so it does not necessarily indicate discharge to an SNF.

130. **B) Recheck it and record it, and, if still over 180, notify provider**

The recommended range for blood sugar in ischemic stroke patients is 150 to 180. Waiting an hour to recheck is not recommended, and the upper limit is not 200, 160, or 140. The first step after rechecking would be to notify the provider.

131. **B) The LKW time is always the time of discovery**

The time of discovery involves someone finding them with symptoms, and the LKW time is the last time the patient was known to be normal. The only time that is the same as LKW time is with a witnessed onset.

132. **C) TED stockings are associated with more harm than good in stroke patients**

Most stroke patients cannot apply TED stockings themselves and may have sensory or communication deficits putting them at risk of not being aware/not being able to tell someone that they aren't fitting right. This puts the patient at risk of injury, which outweighs any possible benefit. SCDs are easier to apply, but not easier to ambulate with. The cost of the TED stockings would not prohibit their use if it were appropriate. SCDs are not easier to store.

133. **C) 1—Present in upper or lower limb**

The rules for scoring ataxia in the NIHSS state that you should only score an inability as ataxia if the inability to perform the task is out of proportion to the patient's weakness. This patient would have scored a 1 in motor for lower extremity drift, which is not enough weakness to defer testing for ataxia in that limb. Their inability to do the heel/shin maneuver should be scored as a 1, and they would be tested on both sides as usual.

134. **A) 40-year-old with limited visitors and a helmet on**

Patients with decompressive hemicraniectomies often wear helmets to protect the area where the bone flap is missing. Shades drawn and lights low could indicate several types of patients with increased intracerebral pressure (ICP). Nicardipine drip and EVD are used on several types of patients with increased ICP. Ventilator support and VP shunt also are not specific to hemicraniectomy.

135. **C) It is commonly used, but not recommended**

The GCS was developed in 1974 to evaluate the depth of decreased consciousness and coma in the head injury population. The motor component only tests for best effort, so a stroke patient with hemiparesis could still get a normal motor score owing to being able to demonstrate motor strength with the unaffected limb. Therefore, it does not have high reliability with the stroke population. It is not used as a precursor to the NIHSS, and it is not used interchangeably with the NIHSS. The NIHSS is the recommended assessment tool in stroke.

136. **B) 70-year-old ICH patient with atrial fibrillation (Afib)**

     Afib patients who are at risk for anticoagulants are candidates for the atrial append-age occlusive device to prevent blood pooling. The ICH patient with an AVM and the SAH patient with an aneurysm would not benefit from atrial appendage closure. The ischemic stroke patient would be treated with anticoagulant and only consider the atrial appendage closure if there is intolerance/failure of anticoagulation.

137. **C) 45 to 60 mL/100 g/min**

     Normal TCD reading of cerebral blood flow is 45 to 60 mL/100 g/min. Irreversible damage occurs when it drops below 10 mL/100 g/min.

138. **B) Migraine is both a stroke mimic and a stroke risk**

     Complex migraines represent a stroke mimic, whereas migraine with aura represents a stroke risk. There is no evidence of migraine being the result of stroke.

139. **D) Patient with atrial fibrillation (Afib)**

     Patients with Afib should receive oral anticoagulation to prevent further clot forma-tion. Research has shown that patients with small PFO only require aspirin therapy. Oral anticoagulation is not indicated for SAH patients. For strokes without a known cause, anticoagulation is not indicated.

140. **A) Decompressive craniectomy**

     Proximal occlusion of a vessel deprives all distal areas of circulation, resulting in large territory ischemic stroke, which carries high risk of cerebral edema. Endovascular embolization, hematoma evacuation, and ventriculoperitoneal (VP) shunt are proce-dures done on hemorrhagic stroke patients.

141. **B) Cancer and some chemotherapeutic agents are prothrombotic**

     Cancer and some chemotherapeutic agents are prothrombotic, meaning they increase the likelihood of forming clots. There is no increased risk of brain tumors after stroke. Cancer is not responsible for 30% of strokes. There is no recommendation for stroke survivors to have any screenings for brain tumors.

142. **B) A joint neurological assessment**

     Joint neurological assessment between the off-going and on-coming nurse is essential to ensure consistency. Medical record review, detailed documentation of neurological condition, and detailed report of day's events are valuable, but not as important as a joint neurological assessment.

143. **D) Physical therapist**

     The BI is a measurement of physical functional ability and is not scored by the pro-vider or nurse. Rather, it would be scored by the physical therapist. It would not be scored by the social worker, pharmacist, or patient advocate.

144. **A) Raising your voice until they indicate understanding**

     Receptive aphasia is the difficulty with understanding speech or reading, not the inability to hear. Pausing between sentences to allow time to process, supplementing speech with gestures, and using simple drawings can all be effective strategies to com-municate with a receptive aphasia patient.

145. **C) Patient is decompensating and needs to be intubated and sedated**

For endovascular intervention, patients need to be able to lie still. In this situation, the patient will need to be intubated and sedated, so preparation for that is correct. Frightened patients will rarely show a 10 point drop in O_2 saturation. The described behavior is not normal for COPD patients. The patient is symptomatic, so there is no reason to distrust the pulse oximetry reading.

146. **A) 50-year-old medical assistant with patent foramen ovale (PFO)**

The recommendation for management of PFO is antithrombotics; however, it is raised to anticoagulants if deep vein thrombosis (DVT) is present with the PFO. Lower extremity ultrasound is not indicated in treatment planning in carotid stenosis, cerebral aneurysms, or Afib.

147. **A) Basal ganglia**

Fifty percent of intraparenchymal hemorrhages occur in the basal ganglia, whereas 33% occur in the cerebral hemispheres. Few occur in the occipital lobe or the brainstem.

148. **B) Brainstem**

The midbrain, pons, and medulla make up the brainstem, which connects to the spinal cord at the foramen magnum. The homunculus is the diagram that depicts which parts of the body are controlled by the motor and sensory strips. The basal ganglia serve as a connector between the cortex and the brainstem.

149. **D) Stent retrievers**

Penumbra clot disrupters and endovascular thrombolysis alone do not have the same success rate as stent retrievers. Stent retrievers have the highest recommendation from the AHA/ASA. There is no such thing as a stent recoiler.

150. **D) Both A and B**

Heredity (race), lifestyle factors (smoking), and limited access to care have been found to account for the higher mortality rate in the Stroke Belt. Alcoholism and sleep apnea are thought to be related to stroke incidence, but a link to increased mortality has not been found.

151. **C) A mobile stroke unit enables faster door-to-needle and door-to-puncture times**

Mobile stroke units facilitate faster processes prearrival, which reduces ED workload and likely improves patient outcomes. Mobile stroke units are more expensive than ambulances, largely due to the onboard CT scanner. Patients transported/treated on a mobile stroke unit still require evaluation in the ED for possible large-vessel occlusion (LVO) as well as pharmacy support for other emergent treatment such as antihypertensives.

152. **D) Symptoms are not classic hemispheric symptoms, and sometimes there can be crossed signs**

Posterior circulation strokes do not produce such classic symptoms as hemispheric strokes and are often misdiagnosed, particularly in younger people who are not expected to have strokes. Cerebellar and occipital symptoms are not identical. Short-term memory and patients' ability recognize stroke symptoms are not impacted by posterior strokes.

153. **D) All of the above**

At every opportunity, it is important to share information about stroke prevention. It should be noted that 8% does not mean that risk for stroke will not occur. It should also be noted that secondary prevention of stroke can promote a general healthy lifestyle, and the best way to prevent a stroke recurrence is to understand and follow the plan of care.

154. **B) Nondiabetic patient who received intravenous (IV) thrombolytic**

Blood sugar control is particularly important in the setting of thrombolytic therapy as high sugars have been associated with poor outcomes in those patients. All ischemic stroke patients, regardless of diabetic status, are recommended to have blood sugars maintained between 150 and 180, but those who received thrombolytic need it even more.

155. **D) All of the above**

The most successful models for poststroke recovery involve collaboration between the discharging hospital stroke team, the PCP, and the patient and caregiver.

156. **C) Cavernous angioma**

Cavernous angioma is composed of large, adjacent capillaries with slow flow. Clipped aneurysms have no flow. TICI 3 cerebral arteries have full flow.

157. **B) Virtual reality (VR) therapy**

VR therapy provides a variety of experiences like sports and immediate feedback that makes the session more enjoyable resulting in patients willing to participate in longer sessions. TMS, CIMT, and robotic therapy do not minimize the impact of disability during treatment.

158. **A) FeSS**

FeSS stands for fever, sugar, swallow. When these nursing-controlled aspects of care have been compliant with guideline recommendations, patient outcomes are improved. ASCVD stands for arteriosclerotic cardiovascular disease, which is not a protocol for care of stroke patients. PDSA stands for Plan, Do, Study, Act, a process improvement method utilized in many quality improvement programs, and is not a protocol for care of stroke patients. PTSD stands for posttraumatic stress disorder, not a protocol for care of stroke patients.

159. **D) To get them into a supine position to facilitate cerebral perfusion**

Stroke patients who sit out in a chair for extended periods of time during first week or so may be at risk of decreased cerebral perfusion, which would manifest in worsening stroke symptoms. Getting them back to bed would prevent falling out of the chair, but this action does not need to be done "quickly" when returning a patient to bed for safety. IV thrombolytic would only be done after CT, so they would have already been in bed for that treatment; it would facilitate quicker transfer to a litter, but the best answer is to facilitate cerebral perfusion.

160. **B) Assess and bandage the wound, then alter plan of care to emphasize strategies for addressing extinction**

The patient is displaying signs of extinction with being unaware of their left side. The patient and caregiver need to be taught strategies to keep them safe and to increase awareness of their left side. Reminding the patient to be more careful, sending the patient back to their room, or paging the provider to cancel discharge plans are inadequate for keeping this patient safe as they don't directly address the underlying problem.

161. **A) Less than 3 hours**

The American Heart Association/American Stroke Association (AHA/ASA) guidelines include recommendation for the ED length of stay (LOS) benchmark to be 3 hours or less. The intent is for the patient to be quickly admitted to a stroke unit where staff is specifically educated and trained to meet the needs of the stroke patient.

162. **D) Shorter length of stay (LOS) compared to patients without evacuation of ICH**

The benefits of evacuation of ICH with minimally invasive devices is that there is maximum clot removal, which reduces cerebral edema, which would shorten LOS. Helmets and keeping the head of the bed flat are not indicated. There is no evidence of increased headache.

163. **B) It is standard of care for large-vessel occlusion (LVO), so it can be done under the premise of emergency consent**

It became a standard of care for LVO because evidence has proven that while there is risk, it is a better option than allowing the large vessel territory to infarct, so it can be done under the premise of emergency consent. Although death is possible in this procedure, it is not certain. It is possible to proceed with endovascular intervention without informed consent regardless of how many providers agree.

164. **A) When SAH is present, but not evident on imaging, LP will show presence of blood**

LPs are only used in SAH if imaging doesn't support but suspicion is high. LPs are useful in intraventricular hemorrhage diagnosis, are not used in vasospasm detection, and are not indicated for ICH detection.

165. **C) Practice developed from results of research**

Evidence-based practice is based on research evidence. It is not based on medical director preferences, citations from the latest stroke certification visit summary, or the latest editorials in *The New England Journal of Medicine*.

166. **A) Urinary tract infection (UTI)**

UTI is the reason for many readmissions, and chronic UTIs can result in need for institutionalization. Depression and subluxation are common poststroke complications, but seldom require readmission or institutionalization. Osteoporosis is a very long-term consequence of immobility and unlikely to require hospitalization.

167. **B) Constipation**

Bowel motility is stimulated by ambulation and supported by hydration. Osteoporosis and pneumonia are benefited by ambulation, but not specifically by hydration. Spasticity can be impacted by hydration, but it must be sulfurous water in combination with other medical therapy, and the impact is not as significant as with constipation.

168. **A) Vessel dissection**

Vessel dissection has been associated with these maneuvers because of vascular torsion. The third cranial nerve arises from the brainstem and is not affected by hyperextension or manipulation maneuvers. Vessel spasm is generally the result of subarachnoid hemorrhage (SAH). Sudden sinus headache is not associated with neck and chiropractic manipulation maneuvers.

169. **A) Monitor level of consciousness (LOC) and prepare for intubation**

A large SAH increases intracerebral pressure (ICP), which diminishes consciousness quickly and puts the patient at risk of respiratory failure. ASRHs do not have neuro-specialized ICUs and do not admit a large volume of SAH patients. The nurse would be administering antihypertensive for BP much lower than 200 with SAH. In a patient with a large SAH, more action is required than just monitoring LOC and notifying provider if pulse ox falls below 100%.

170. **B) Prenotify the nearest certified stroke center and transport**

According to the algorithm, if the closest CSC or TSC is >30 minutes away, then take patient to nearest certified stroke center, regardless of level. Most state emergency medical services (EMS) protocols require that suspected strokes go to certified stroke centers, so patient choice is not applicable. Urgent care centers are not certified stroke centers.

Appendix: Neuroscience Glossary

Agnosia—Failure to recognize stimuli when the appropriate sensory systems are functioning adequately; commonly occurs in visual, tactile, and auditory forms

Antithrombotics—Medications that inhibit clot formation; two classes are anticoagulants and antiplatelet agents

Aphasia—Loss of ability to use language and to communicate thoughts verbally or in writing; receptive aphasia: inability to understand; expressive aphasia: inability to speak/write

Ataxia—Incoordination or clumsiness of movement that is not the result of muscular weakness; it is caused by vestibular, cerebellar, or sensory disorders

Aura—Subjective sensation preceding a paroxysmal attack; may precede migraines or seizures and can be psychic or sensory in nature

Clonic—Alternating contraction and relaxation of muscles

Collateral circulation—Circulation of blood established through enlargement of minor vessels and anastomosis of vessels with those of adjacent parts when a major vein or artery is functionally impaired (as by obstruction)

Comorbid conditions—Presence of one or more disorders in addition to the primary disorder, for example, a stroke patient with diabetes and hypertension—these are comorbid conditions

Contralateral—Originating in, or affecting, the opposite side of the body

Cortical—Referring to the outer layer of the cerebrum; predominantly gray matter

Decerebrate—Posture characterized by a rigid—possibly arched—spine, rigidly extended arms and legs, and plantar flexion; indicative of a brain-stem lesion

Decorticate—Posture characterized by a rigid spine, inwardly flexed arms, extended and internally rotated legs, and plantar flexion; indicative of a brainstem lesion

Delirium—Mental confusion and excitement characterized by disorientation for time and place, usually with illusions and hallucinations; possible causes are fever, shock, exhaustion, anxiety, or drug overdose

Dementia—An acquired, generalized, and often progressive impairment of cognitive function that affects the content, but not the level, of consciousness; may indicate pathology affecting the cerebral cortex, its subcortical connections, or both

Diplopia—Double vision; may indicate pathology involving the cranial nerves, eyeballs, cerebellum, cerebrum, or meninges

Dissection—Separation of the layers of an arterial or venous wall resulting in reduced lumen and possibly complete occlusion

Dysphagia—Difficulty swallowing or inability to swallow

Dysphasia—Impaired ability to communicate with verbal or written language; seldom used in clinical care, as aphasia has come to be used to represent not only the inability to communicate but also the impaired ability to communicate; dysphasia is often confused with dysphagia

Euthermia—Condition of having normal body temperature; synonym is normothermia

Fissure—Deep cleft or groove between segments of the cerebral cortex; larger than a sulcus

Gray matter—Largest portion of the brain; neuronal cell bodies and glial cells in the cortex and deep nuclei process information originating in the sensory organs or in other gray matter regions

Gyrus (plural is gyri)—Prominent convolutions on the surface of the cerebral hemispheres

Hemianopia—Loss of half of the visual field; homonymous hemianopia means that both right visual fields or both left visual fields are lost

Hemiparesis—Weakness affecting only one side of the body; may indicate an intracranial structural lesion

Hemiplegia—Paralysis affecting only one side of the body; may indicate pathology of upper motor neurons

Hemorrhagic transformation—Also called hemorrhagic conversion, that is, leakage of blood from vessels in the ischemic stroke bed; the presence of blood "transforms" an ischemic stroke into a hemorrhagic stroke on imaging, but improved imaging makes it possible to differentiate a primary hemorrhage from an ischemic stroke with hemorrhagic transformation

Hyperreflexia—Abnormally intense response to a stimulus; may indicate a lesion of the upper motor neurons and suggests lack of cortical control over the reflex

Ictal—Pertaining to or caused by a sudden attack such as acute epilepsy

Infarction—Irreversible damage or death of tissue

Intima—Innermost lining of an artery or vein

Intrathecal—Introduction of substance into the subarachnoid space of the brain or spinal cord; certain drugs are given this way to avoid the blood–brain barrier

Ipsilateral—Originating in or affecting the same side of the body

Ischemia—Insufficient blood flow to meet metabolic demand; if not corrected, leads to hypoxia and infarction

Myelin—White fatty material that encloses the axons of myelinated nerve fibers; acts as an insulator, increasing the speed of transmission of nerve signals

Myoclonic—Twitching or clonic spasm of a muscle or group of muscles

Nerve palsy—Neurological defect caused by dysfunction of the nerve that controls that part of the body; for example, third cranial nerve palsy is manifested by limited eye movements and ptosis

Normothermia—Normal body temperature; synonym is euthermia

Nystagmus—Involuntary, rhythmic, oscillating motions of the eyes

Parenchyma—Functional tissue of an organ, distinguished from connective and supporting tissue

Plateau—Point in recovery when progress slows or stops; often used as criterion for discontinuing therapy services

Postictal—Phase that follows an attack such as acute epilepsy; subjective sensation can be variable

Ptosis—Drooping eyelid

Recanalization—Restoration of blood flow to an arterial occlusion site

Spasticity—Unusual tightness, or stiffness, of muscle due to increased tone or hypertonia; occurs within days to weeks in 30% of stroke patients

Subcortical—Referring to the area below the cerebrum; predominantly white matter

Sulcus (plural is sulci)—Deep grooves on the surface of the cerebral hemisphere

Supratentorial—Refers to portions of the brain above the tentorium (see Tentorium)

Symmetry—Two sides having the same size and shape

Tentorium—Extension of the dura mater that separates the cerebellum from the inferior portion of the occipital lobes

Thrombolysis—Dissolution, or lysis, of a blood clot

Tonic—Pertaining to, or characterized by, tension or contraction, especially muscular tension

Ventricles—Four hollow spaces in the brain that are filled with cerebrospinal fluid

Vertigo—Sensation of moving around in space or having objects move around the person; indicates disturbance of the equilibratory apparatus

White matter—Bundles of myelinated axons that connect various gray matter areas of the brain and carry nerve impulses between neurons

Index